NOTES ON CANINE INTERNAL MEDICINE

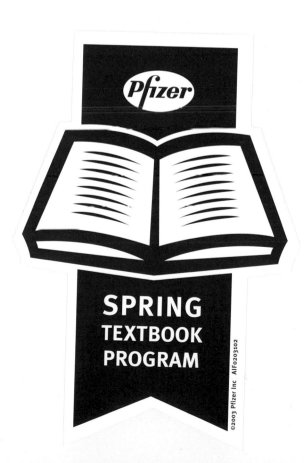

NOTES ON CANINE INTERNAL MEDICINE

Third Edition

E. J. Hall

K. F. Murphy

and

P. G. G. Darke

Blackwell
Science

© 2003 by Blackwell Science Ltd
a Blackwell Publishing company

Editorial offices:
Blackwell Science Ltd, 9600 Garsington Road,
Oxford OX4 2DQ, UK
    Tel: +44 (0) 1865 776868
Iowa State Press, a Blackwell Publishing
Company, 2121 State Avenue, Ames, Iowa
50014-8300, USA
    Tel: +1 515 292 0140
Blackwell Science Asia Pty Ltd, 550 Swanston
Street, Carlton, Victoria 3053, Australia
    Tel: +61 (0)3 8359 1011

First edition 1983 under the Wright Imprint
by IOP Publishing Limited, Techno House,
Radcliffe Way, Bristol, BS1 6NX
Second edition 1986 under the Wright Imprint
by IOP Publishing Limited, Techno House,
Radcliffe Way, Bristol, BS1 6NX
Third edition 2003

Library of Congress Cataloging-in-Publication
Data

Hall, E. J. (Edward J.)
Notes on canine internal medicine / E.J. Hall,
K.F. Murphy, P.G.G. Darke.-- 3rd ed.
        p. ; cm.
Rev. ed. of: Notes on canine internal medicine
/ P.G.G. Darke. 2nd ed. 1986.
Includes bibliographical references and index.
ISBN 0-632-05371-2 (pbk. : alk. paper)
1. Dogs--Diseases.
2. Veterinary internal medicine.
[DNLM: 1. Dog Diseases--Handbooks.]
I. Title: Notes on canine internal medicine.
II. Murphy, K. F. (Kathryn F.)
III. Darke, P. G. G.
IV. Darke, P. G. G. Notes on canine internal
medicine.
V. Title.

SF991.H17 2003
636.7'0896--dc21

                                    2003012133

ISBN 0-632-05371-2

A catalogue record for this title is available
from the British Library

Set in 9/11.5 pt Sabon
by Sparks Computer Solutions Ltd, Oxford
http://www.sparks.co.uk
Printed and bound in
India using acid-free paper
by Replika Press Pvt. Ltd. Kundli 131 028

For further information on Blackwell
Publishing, visit our website:
www.blackwellpublishing.com

Disclaimer
The authors and publishers cannot take
responsibility for information provided on
dosages and methods of treatment mentioned
in this book. Details of this kind must be veri-
fied by individual users from the appropriate
data sheets and literature.

CONTENTS

Section 2
Physical Abnormalities   85

Section 3
Laboratory Abnormalities   133

In 1983, the First Edition of this book provided a revolutionary new and simplified diagnostic approach to internal medicine problems. And it was not long before it was to be found in the pocket of every veterinary undergraduate in the UK, as well as being an important first source of information for the busy practitioner.

It is now over 15 years since the Second and last Edition and, in that time, our knowledge of canine internal medicine and our ability to investigate cases has grown almost exponentially. Indeed, the standard texts have swelled and often now fill two large volumes. Attempts have been made to condense them into pocket-size books for ready reference. Yet they continue to bulge from all but the most generous of pockets, and often fail to distinguish the possible from the most likely. We believe that actually knowing the three most likely differential diagnoses is of more use than knowing ten obscure and unlikely ones: to paraphrase an old saying, 'if you hear hoofbeats it's more likely horses than zebras'. Thus, in this book we list the 'Common causes' of medical problems. Nevertheless, we also list 'Uncommon causes', as zebras do exist!

The purists may criticise our attempt to make this a true handbook of Internal Medicine for its over-simplification and failure to explain the underlying pathophysiology that is essential to full understanding of disease. Whilst we readily accept the importance of pathophysiology, it must be found in more substantial texts than this, and we assume the reader already has a reasonable level of understanding. This handbook is an attempt, not to be comprehensive, but to highlight the more important diseases. We welcome corrections from readers about errors and omissions, but our experiences are personal and may differ, particularly as not every patient 'reads the textbook'.

The ultimate aims of this book remain the same as in previous editions: that is to provide fresh ideas:

- to stimulate clinicians to use thought rather than dogma
- to protect some dogs against excessively prolonged investigation or inappropriate therapy
- and to save a few lives, *perhaps*.

We also believe it is important to repeat the essential advice of the First Edition, 'that basic, careful history-taking and thorough and, if necessary, repeated clinical examination are fundamental procedures that may yield a diagnosis in a complicated or unresolved case'. We do not believe in a totally algorithmic approach as used in some texts, but using the results of history-taking, physical examination and basic laboratory tests should guide the clinician's investigation in the right direction.

This Edition discusses common specific diseases associated with specific organ systems as in earlier editions, although we have extended our remit to include systems lying outside the abdomen and thorax. However, sections listing differential diagnoses based on presenting complaints, physical findings and laboratory abnormalities precede this final section. For it is when common signs can be produced by more than one organ system that the unwary clinician can be misled and perform inappropriate investigations. For example, the understanding that hyperadrenocorticism is a more common cause of polydipsia than diabetes insipidus will prevent many dogs undergoing unnecessary – and potentially dangerous – water-deprivation tests. In addition, the use of laboratory testing has become routine, and we offer differential diagnoses lists based on important laboratory abnormalities.

Our personal experiences, and geographical location, inevitably bias our views on what are the most common diagnoses and what is the best diagnostic approach to any problem, and again the purists may criticise. But, as noted in the First Edition, the recognition that not everything in internal medicine is black-and-white is part of its challenge and stimulation. We hope that the reader – whether veterinary undergraduate or busy practitioner – finds something in this book to help them with their next puzzling case.

E.J.H., K.F.M. & P.G.G.D.
2003

ACKNOWLEDGEMENTS

The initial inspiration for this book remains Peter Darke's, and we are honoured to update it, and receive Peter's help in editing it. The book retains its original name to emphasise its aim to be an easily accessible *aide memoire* for the veterinary practitioner and student to assist their diagnostic investigations of medically ill dogs.

E.J.H., K.F.M.

We must inevitably acknowledge the patience and support of our respective families during the production of this volume. However, we wish to dedicate it to:

The late Dr Joan O'Brien, who inspired me and made me understand that there was always one more question to be asked, or one more investigation to be performed on that problem case, and yet to never be afraid to go back to the beginning and start again.

E.J. Hall

My colleagues and friends at the University of Bristol, past and present, who have encouraged my enthusiasm for internal medicine and taught me that there is always more to be learnt.

K. F. Murphy

Carole, my wife, for her endless patience over 38 years, and to Dr Christine Gibbs, Professor Donald Kelly, Mr Jim Pinsent and the late Professor Harold Pearson. The earlier editions were published whilst I was at Edinburgh, but they were my mentors when I took up the first Lectureship in Small Animal Medicine at Langford in 1973.

P.G.G. Darke

USING THIS BOOK

SECTION I – PRESENTING COMPLAINTS

In this section, the common presenting complaints are listed alphabetically according to a stylised format.

- Each problem is defined, and the expected clinical signs explained.
- Causes for the problem are divided into 'common' and 'uncommon' to guide the reader, but these are only the opinion of the authors, and clearly may vary in different geographical locations.
- For each problem a logical diagnostic approach is suggested.
- Clinical clues to look for in the history and physical examination are suggested in note form; but not every case will show every sign.
- Laboratory findings that aid the diagnosis are noted.
- Key results from imaging are noted.
- Special tests that may confirm the diagnosis are listed.

SECTION 2 – PHYSICAL ABNORMALITIES

In this section, significant findings from the physical examination are listed alphabetically.

- Each problem is defined.
- Common and uncommon causes are suggested for each problem.
- Related clinical signs are listed.
- For each problem a logical diagnostic approach is suggested.
- Key findings to look for in the history and physical examination are noted; not all will be present in every case.
- Laboratory findings that aid the diagnosis are noted.
- Key results of imaging are noted.
- Special tests that may confirm the diagnosis are listed.

SECTION 3 – LABORATORY ABNORMALITIES

In this section, laboratory abnormalities of haematology, serum biochemistry and urinalysis are listed alphabetically.

- The abnormality is defined.
- Causes are listed, and the likely degree of severity is suggested.
- The diagnostic interpretation for the abnormality is given.
- Adjunctive tests that may help confirm the diagnosis are given.

SECTION 4 – ORGAN SYSTEMS

The potentially relevant clinical presentations, physical abnormalities and laboratory abnormalities (identified in Sections 1, 2 and 3, respectively) are given for each major internal organ system. Then, the diagnostic approach and the methods of investigation of each organ system are briefly explained. Finally, the more common diseases of each system are covered alphabetically. For each, their aetiology, predisposition, historical clues, clinical signs, laboratory test results, treatment, sequelae and prognosis are given.

ABBREVIATIONS

ACE	angiotensin-converting enzyme (inhibitor)
ACT	activated clotting time
ACTH	adrenocorticotrophic hormone
ACh	acetylcholine
ADH	antidiuretic hormone, adrenal-dependent HAC
AF	atrial fibrillation
ALL	Acute lymphoblastic leukaemia
ALP/SAP	(serum) alkaline phosphatase
ALT	alanine aminotransferase
ANA	antinuclear antibody
ANP	atrial natriuretic peptide
aPTT	activated partial thromboplastin time
APUDoma	amine precursor uptake and decarboxylation -oma
ARD	antibiotic-responsive diarrhoea
ARF	acute renal failure
AS	aortic stenosis
ASD	atrial septal defect
AST	aspartate aminotransferase
AT III	Antithrombin III
AV	atrioventricular (valve) or arteriovenous (fistula)
BAER	brainstem auditory-evoked response
BAL	bronchoalveolar lavage
BID	twice daily (q. 12 h)
BMBT	buccal mucosal bleeding time
BPH	benign prostatic hypertrophy
bpm	beats per minute
CDI	central diabetes insipidus
CDRM	canine degenerative radiculomyelopathy
CDV	canine distemper virus
CHF	congestive heart failure
CHPG	chronic hypertrophic pylorogastropathy
CKCS	Cavalier King Charles spaniel
CLL	Chronic lymphocytic leukaemia
CNS	central nervous system
cPLI	canine pancreatic lipase immunoreactivity
CRF	chronic renal failure
CRT	capillary refill time
CSF	cerebrospinal fluid
CT	computed tomography
cTLI	canine pancreatic trypsin-like immunoreactivity
CVC	caudal vena cava
DCM	dilated cardiomyopathy
DDAVP	desmopressin
DDx	differential diagnosis
DIC	disseminated intravascular coagulation

DJD	degenerative joint disease
DKA	diabetic ketoacidosis
DM	diabetes mellitus
DMSO	dimethyl sulphoxide
DV	dorso-ventral (view)
ECG	electrocardiogram
EEG	electroencephalogram
EGE	eosinophilic gastroenteritis
EHBDO	extrahepatic bile duct obstruction
ELISA	enzyme linked immunosorbent assay
EMG	electromyogram
EOD	every other day (q. 48 h)
EPI	exocrine pancreatic insufficiency
EPO	erythropoietin
ETD	every third day (q. 72 h)
FB	foreign body
FCE	fibrocartilaginous embolism
FDP	fibrin degradation product
FNA	fine-needle aspiration
GA	general anaesthesia
G-CSF	granulocyte colony-stimulating factor
GDV	gastric dilatation-volvulus
GFR	glomerular filtration rate
GGT	gamma-glutamyl transferase
GH	growth hormone
GI	gastrointestinal
GME	granulomatous meningoencephalitis
GSD	German shepherd dog
HAC	hyperadrenocorticism
Hb	haemoglobin
HCT	haematocrit
HDDS	high-dose dexamethasone suppression test
HGE	haemorrhagic gastroenteritis
HHDDS	high-high dose dexamethasone suppression test
HPO	hypertrophic pulmonary osteopathy
HUC	histiocytic ulcerative colitis
IBD	inflammatory bowel disease
IBS	irritable bowel syndrome
ICH	infectious canine hepatitis
IDDM	insulin-dependent diabetes mellitus
i/m	intramuscular
IMHA	immune-mediated haemolytic anaemia
IMT (IMTP, ITP)	immune-mediated thrombocytopenia
IPSID	immunoproliferative small intestinal disease
ITP (IMT, IMTP)	immune-mediated thrombocytopenia
i/v	intravenous
IVU	intravenous urogram
LA	left atrial

LDDS	low-dose dexamethasone screening (suppression) test
LI	large intestine
LMN	lower motor neurone
LN	lymph node
LP	laryngeal paralysis
LPC	lymphocytic-plasmacytic colitis
LPE	lymphocytic-plasmacytic enteritis
LV	left ventricular
MCT	mast cell tumour
MCT	medium chain triglyceride
MDS	myelodysplastic syndrome
MG	myasthenia gravis
MO	megaoesophagus
MRI	magnetic resonance imaging
MV	mitral valve
MVD	mitral valve disease
NDI	nephrogenic diabetes insipidus
NIDDM	non-insulin-dependent diabetes mellitus
NPO	*nil per os*
nRBC	nucleated red blood cell
NSAIDs	non-steroidal anti-inflammatory drugs
OESD	Old English sheepdog
OHE	ovariohysterectomy
OSPT	one-stage prothrombin time
Pa	partial pressure
PCR	polymerase chain reaction
PCV	packed cell volume
PD	polydipsia
PDA	patent ductus arteriosus
PDH	pituitary-dependent HAC
PF_3	platelet factor 3
PIE	pulmonary infiltrate with eosinophils
PIVKA	proteins induced by vitamin K antagonism
PLE	protein-losing enteropathy
PLI	pancreatic lipase immunoreactivity
PLN	protein-losing nephropathy
PLR	papillary light response
PMI	point of maximal intensity
PO	*per os*
PPi	proton pump inhibitor
PPDH	peritoneo-pericardial diaphragmatic hernia
PR	peripheral resistance
PRAA	persistent right aortic arch
PS	pulmonic stenosis
PSS	portosystemic shunt
PT	prothrombin time
PTE	pulmonary thromboembolism
PTH	parathyroid hormone (parathormone)

PTHrP	PTH-related peptide
PTT	activated partial thromboplastin time
PU	polyuria
PU/PD	polyuria / polydipsia
QID	four times daily (q. 6 h)
RAAS	renin-angiotension-aldosterone system
RBC	red blood cell
RF	rheumatoid factor
SA	sinoatrial
SAM	S-adenosylmethionine
SAS	subaortic stenosis
s/c	subcutaneous
SG	specific gravity
SI	small intestine
SIBO	small intestinal bacterial overgrowth
SID	once daily (q. 24 h)
SLE	systemic lupus erythematosus
SMI	sphincter mechanism incompetence
SPE	serum protein electrophoresis
SRMA	steroid-responsive meningitis-arteritis
SV	stroke volume
SVT	supraventricular tachycardia
T4	thyroxine
TAP	trypsinogen activation peptide
TCT	thrombin clot time
TID	three times daily (q. 8 h)
TLI	trypsin-like immunoreactivity
TPMT	thiopurine methyl transferase
TP	total protein
TPR	temperature-pulse-respiration
TRH	thyroid-releasing hormone
TSH	thyroid stimulating hormone
TVT	transmissible venereal tumour
UDCA	ursodeoxycholic acid
UK	United Kingdom
UMN	upper motor neurone
URT	upper respiratory tract
UTI	urinary tract infection
VD	ventro-dorsal (view)
VPC	ventricular premature complex
VSD	ventricular septal defect
VWD	von Willebrand disease
vWf	von Willebrand factor
vWfAg	von Willebrand factor antigen
WBC	white blood cell
WHWT	West Highland White terrier
WNL	within normal limits

SECTION 1
PRESENTING COMPLAINTS

ABDOMINAL DISCOMFORT/PAIN

DEFINITION

The sensation of discomfort caused by stimulation of special nerve fibres in the abdomen, manifested either spontaneously or unmasked by abdominal palpation.
- Abdominal pain is caused by distension, chemical inflammation or infection of the abdominal viscera and/or peritoneal space.
- An 'acute abdomen' is the sudden onset of severe abdominal pain, that often requires surgical intervention.

CLINICAL SIGNS

- Abdominal distension
- Diarrhoea
- Grunting/groaning
- Occasional adoption of 'prayer position' if cranial abdominal pain
- Resents abdominal palpation
- Vomiting

COMMON CAUSES

- Any abdominal organ and/or peritoneum may be involved

Endocrine
- Hypoadrenocorticism (uncommon but important)

Gastrointestinal
- Foreign body
- Gastric dilatation-volvulus
- Gastric ulceration
- HGE
- IBD
- Intussusception
- Neoplasia
- Parvovirus

Peritoneal
- Acute pancreatitis

Splenic
- Ruptured splenic haematoma, haemangioma, haemangiosarcoma with bleeding
- Traumatic rupture

Urogenital
- Acute prostatitis
- Urethral obstruction

UNCOMMON CAUSES

Gastrointestinal
- Acute hepatitis
- Infarction
- Intestinal volvulus

Peritoneal
- Peritonitis
  - *Actinomyces* or *Nocardia* infection
  - Perforated gastric ulcer from NSAID administration
  - Ruptured biliary tract
  - Spontaneous rupture of GI tract
    - Intestinal neoplasia
    - Perforated gastric ulcer from mast cell tumour
    - Spontaneous ulcers in acute CNS disease
  - Traumatic perforation/rupture of GI tract
    - Avulsion of mesenteric vessels leading to ischaemic perforation
    - Migrating foreign body (e.g. cocktail stick, grass awn)
    - Surgical dehiscence
- Pansteatitis

Splenic
- Torsion of splenic pedicle

Toxicity
- Lead poisoning

Urogenital
- Acute renal failure (ARF)
- Acute pyelonephritis
- Ruptured kidney
- Ruptured pyometra
- Ruptured ureter/bladder
- Ureteral obstruction
- Testicular torsion

DIAGNOSTIC APPROACH

1   Distinguish benign causes that can be
    managed medically from conditions
    needing urgent surgery.
2   Exploratory surgery.

CLINICAL CLUES

- 'Prayer' position suggests cranial
  abdominal pain – gastric ulceration,
  pancreatitis.
- Painful lesions of the abdominal wall
  (e.g. bruising, cellulitis) may falsely
  give the appearance of intraperitoneal
  pain.
- Shock if acute haemorrhage or intestinal obstruction.
- Spinal pain may appear abdominal in
  origin, either because pain is referred
  or simply abdominal palpation causes
  painful spinal movement.

Predisposition
- GDV in large/giant, deep-chested dog
  breed (Great Dane, Wolfhound, Irish
  setter)
- Intestinal volvulus in Bloodhound and
  in GSD with EPI
- Splenic torsion in GSD and Great Dane
- Testicular torsion in cryptorchids

History
- Dietary indiscretion before pancreati-
  tis
- Intermittent GI signs in hypoadreno-
  corticism
- Large meal and exercise before GDV
- NSAID administration
- Pyometra in older unspayed bitches
  after oestrus
- Trauma: signs may be delayed by hours
  or days following known trauma

Physical examination
Observation
- Lethargic or collapsed
- Unproductive attempts to vomit in
  GDV

Inspection
- Distended abdomen
- Jaundice if bile peritonitis
- Pale mucous membranes
- Pyrexia
- Tachycardia

Palpation
- Absence of bladder if ruptured
- Caudal mass/pain in cryptorchid, if
  testicular torsion
- Hollow viscus on percussion in GDV
- Pain: cranial abdominal if gastric/
  pancreatic
  - Some dogs are quite stoical (e.g.
    Labradors) and may only manifest a
    small expiratory grunt on palpation
  - May vomit on palpation if severe
    peritonitis
- Splenic mass

LABORATORY FINDINGS

Haematology
- Anaemia if severe/recurrent bleeding
- Degenerative left shift if overwhelming
  sepsis (e.g. ruptured GI tract)

- Inappropriate number of nucleated RBCs (nRBCs) in lead poisoning
- Leukopenia (neutropenia) with no left shift in parvovirus
- Neutrophilia and left shift in inflammatory disease

Serum biochemistry
- Azotaemia if ruptured urinary tract, ARF
- Raised amylase and lipase may be seen in pancreatitis

Urinalysis
- Haematuria if trauma
- Pyuria in pyelonephritis, prostatitis

IMAGING

Plain radiographs
- Abdominal effusion

- Free intraperitoneal gas
- Gastric dilatation volvulus
- Obstructed bowel loops
- Intestinal volvulus
- Foreign body
- Splenic mass

Ultrasound examination
- Abdominal effusion
- Pancreatic disease
- Splenic mass or congestion if torsion present

SPECIAL TESTS

- Abdominocentesis
- Contrast GI study – use iodinated contrast if perforation suspected
- Excretory urogram
- Exploratory laparotomy
- Retrograde (vagino)-urethrogram

ALOPECIA

DEFINITION

Absence of hair from areas of skin that normally carry hairs, due either to a failure of production or to an increased loss of hair.

CLINICAL SIGNS

- Loss or absence of hair
- Self-trauma if pruritic skin disease

COMMON CAUSES

Primary follicular disease
- Bacterial folliculitis
- Dermatophytosis
- Demodectic mange
- *Malassezia*

Secondary follicular disease
- HAC
- Hypothyroidism
- Seasonal flank alopecia

Self-trauma if pruritic
- Atopy
- Fleas and flea allergic dermatitis
- Sarcoptic mange
- Secondary pyoderma

UNCOMMON CAUSES

Primary follicular disease
- Alopecia areata
- Autoimmune skin disease
  - Dermatomyositis
  - Sebaceous adenitis
- Black hair follicular dysplasia
- Colour mutant/dilution

- Congenital hypotrichosis
- Hairless breeds
- Injection reaction
- Pattern baldness

Secondary follicular disease
- Adrenal sex hormone imbalance/adrenal hyperplasia syndrome (alopecia X)
- Cicatricial (scar-related)
- Epitheliotrophic lymphosarcoma
- Hyposomatotropism (pituitary dwarf)
- Protein/calorie malnutrition
- SLE
- Telogen effluvium (e.g. post partum)
- Vitamin A deficiency

Self-trauma
- Acral lick/neurodermatitis
- *Cheyletiella*
- Food allergy
- Lice
- *Trombicula* (harvest mite)

DIAGNOSTIC APPROACH

1   Presence or absence of pruritus narrows the differential diagnosis.
    If pruritic:
    - Identification of infectious agents by sellotape strips, skin scrapes, hair plucks, and bacterial and fungal cultures.
    - After ruling out infectious causes, trial therapy for bacterial pyoderma, fleas and possibly also for *Sarcoptes*, is acceptable.
    - Intradermal skin testing is performed to identify atopic reactions.
    - If all negative, an exclusion food trial is indicated.
    If non-pruritic:
    - consider endocrinopathy or breed-related problem.
2   Skin biopsy is indicated if no cause is obvious.

CLINICAL CLUES

Predisposition
- Breed predisposition may suggest primary follicular diseases:
  - Canine hairless breeds: Chinese Crested, Mexican Hairless
  - Colour mutant alopecia in blue/fawn/red Dobermann, blue Great Dane, fawn Irish setter, blue Dachshund, blue Chow Chow, blue Whippet

History
- Colour mutant alopecia develops in young adults
- Congenital or hereditary hypotrichosis is usually evident from an early age
- Slow onset suggestive of endocrinopathy
- Other clinical signs (e.g. PU/PD, weight change) suggest a possible endocrinopathy

Physical examination
Observation
- Bilaterally symmetrical alopecia is considered the hallmark of an endocrinopathy, but pruritic skin disease can also appear symmetrical
- Evidence of pruritus:
  - positive scratch reflex
  - broken hairs, not hair loss
- Pattern of pruritus-induced self-trauma and hair loss can be informative

Distribution of self-trauma
- Dorso-lumbar with flea-allergic dermatitis
- Ear margins and elbows with sarcoptic mange
- Face, feet and ventrum with atopy
- Feet and ventrum with contact allergy
- Face, ears and feet with food allergy
- Face, ears, feet or multifocal with demodecosis
- Face, feet, mucocutaneous junctions with autoimmune skin disease

Localised distribution of hair loss
- Alopecia areata
- Cicatricial
- Demodecosis
- Dermatophytosis
- Injection reaction
- Pattern baldness
- Superficial pyoderma/bacterial folliculitis

Multifocal or diffuse but patchy distribution of hair loss
- Colour dilution
- Demodecosis
- Dermatomyositis
- Dermatophytosis
- Epitheliotropic lymphosarcoma
- Follicular dysplasia
- Superficial pyoderma/bacterial folliculitis

Symmetrical, generalised, diffuse distribution of hair loss
- Demodecosis
- Dermatophytosis
- Endocrinopathies
- Superficial pyoderma/bacterial folliculitis
- Telogen effluvium

Inspection
- Broken hairs if pruritic, otherwise hair absent
- Lesions secondary to self-trauma: erythema, excoriation, lichenification, hyperpigmentation

- Presence of fleas or flea dirt
- Pustules, erythema, scaling in pyoderma

Palpation
- Thickened skin in hypothyroidism
- Thinned skin in HAC

LABORATORY FINDINGS

Unremarkable unless underlying endocrinopathy:
- Bacterial and fungal cultures
- Hair plucks – *Demodex*, ringworm
- Hypercholesterolaemia and raised ALP in HAC
- Hypercholesterolaemia in hypothyroidism
- Skin scrapes – *Sarcoptes*, *Demodex*

IMAGING

- Usually unnecessary and unremarkable unless systemic signs (e.g. endocrinopathy)

SPECIAL TESTS

- Dynamic cortisol testing
- Exclusion diet trial
- Intradermal skin tests
- Sarcoptic mange antibody
- Skin biopsy
- Thyroid function tests

ALTERED CONSCIOUSNESS

DEFINITION

Consciousness is maintained by the ascending reticular activating system, located in the midbrain and projecting diffusely to the cerebral cortex.

- Normal consciousness reflects appropriate level of consciousness and level of arousal.
- Diffuse cerebral disease or midbrain disease can cause altered consciousness.

- Lesions of the medulla oblongata can cause altered consciousness if the cardiorespiratory centres are affected severely enough to produce hypoxia.
- Altered consciousness can be caused by:
  - cerebral oedema
  - increased intracranial pressure
  - herniation of brain tissue
  - metabolic disorders

CLINICAL SIGNS – GRADES OF DYSFUNCTION

Normal
- Alert
- Aware of surroundings
- Responds as expected to commands
- Responsive to external stimuli

Depressed
- Less responsive to its environment
- Lethargic
- Retains capability to respond in a normal manner

Disorientated/confused
- Can respond to environment but may do so in an abnormal manner

Stuporous
- Appears asleep when undisturbed, but can be aroused by strong stimulation, especially pain
- Seen with brainstem or bilateral cerebral injuries

Comatose
- Loss of consciousness and cannot be aroused
- Only reflex responses to stimuli, e.g. toe pinch may cause flexion reflex or increased extensor posturing, but will not lead to any behavioural response, e.g. crying or turning

- Seen with brainstem or bilateral cerebral injuries

Demented
- Aimless wandering
- Head pressing
- Inappropriate behaviour
- Loss of self-awareness
- Seen with cerebral or thalamic injury
  - Post-ictal (seizure)
  - Metabolic disease affecting the cerebrum
  - Structural cerebral disease

Vegetative
- Brainstem function is present
- Can be aroused
- Lack of awareness of the environment
- Loss of cortical function

Brain dead
- Apnoea
- Coma
- Electrocerebral silence – flat EEG and lack of response to evoked stimuli
- Lack of brainstem reflexes

COMMON CAUSES

Congenital/familial
- Hydrocephalus

Cranial trauma
- *Contre-coup* injury due to severe head-shaking
- Direct blow to head

Inflammatory
- Granulomatous meningoencephalitis

Metabolic disorders
- Acid–base imbalance
- Diabetes mellitus
- Heat stroke
- Hepatic encephalopathy
- Hypoglycaemia

- Hypothyroidism
- Hypoxia
- Uraemia

Neoplasia
- Primary CNS

Toxins/drugs
- Sedation and anaesthesia
  - Barbiturates, etc.

UNCOMMON CAUSES

Congenital/familial
- Lissencephaly
- Lysosomal storage disease

Cranial trauma
- Needle aspiration of CSF in animals with raised intracranial pressure

Inflammatory
- Distemper
- *Ehrlichia*
- Fungal/protozoal/bacterial infections
- Rabies
- Rocky Mountain Spotted fever

Metabolic disorders
- Hyperlipidaemia
- Osmolality imbalance

Neoplasia
- Metastasis to CNS

Toxins/drugs
- Ethylene glycol
- Cannabinoids and hallucinogens
- Lead

Vascular
- Bacterial emboli
- Coagulopathies
- Hypertension
- Ischaemia

Other
- Status epilepticus

DIAGNOSTIC APPROACH

1 Rule out metabolic causes by laboratory testing and perform neurological examination to localise primary CNS disease.
2 Cardiothoracic assessment for evidence of cardiorespiratory disease, which could have caused neurological signs secondary to hypoxia.
3 Then proceed to neurodiagnostics.

CLINICAL CLUES

History
- Pre-existing medical/neurological signs/disease?
- Trauma?
- Toxin/drug exposure?

Physical examination
Complete neurological examination
- Eye movements
- Level of consciousness
- Pupil size
- Respiratory pattern
- Skeletal motor responses
  - Development of extensor rigidity or opisthotonus = grave prognosis
  - Decerebrate rigidity = extensor rigidity of all four limbs, with stupor or coma, is due to severe midbrain or pontine injury to all the motor tracts

Pupillary light response
- Equal constricted pupils at rest, which constrict to light and dilate to darkness = metabolic disease
- Equal dilated pupils at rest, which constrict to light and dilate to darkness = sympathetic stimulation

- Equal dilated pupils at rest, no response to light and fixed and dilated in dark = midbrain, optic chiasm, optic nerve II, oculomotor nerve III, retina
- Anisocoria at rest, both constrict to light, both dilate to darkness = unilateral cerebral cortex lesion contralateral to larger pupil
- Equal constricted pupils at rest, fixed to light and no response to dark = pons, ophthalmic injury with iridospasm, bilateral sympathetic denervation (Horner's)
- Unequal, one fixed one dilated; in response to light dilated pupil is fixed, normal pupil constricts, in response to darkness dilated pupil is fixed, normal pupil dilates = unilateral oculomotor nerve III

Other associated signs
- Cerebral lesion
  - Cheyne-Stokes respiration
  - Decerebrate rigidity
  - Normal or constricted pupils that respond to light
  - Roving eye movements
  - Seizures
- Midbrain
  - Hyperventilation
  - Loss of oculocephalic response (requires intact vestibular nerves, brainstem, medial longitudinal fasciculus and cranial nerves for eye movements III, IV, VI): in a normal animal moving the head rapidly from side to side induces nystagmus with fast phase in the direction of motion; disappears when motion stops.
  - Negative caloric test – infusing warm or cold water into ear canal should induce nystagmus if intact oculocephalic response. Absence of nystagmus carries guarded/hopeless prognosis.
  - Pinpoint or dilated pupils that do not respond to light.
- Medulla
  - Cardiac arrhythmia (bradycardia)
  - Irregular respiration

LABORATORY FINDINGS

- Evaluate for metabolic cause of altered consciousness

IMAGING

- Skull radiographs to assess for evidence of trauma
- Thoracic and abdominal radiographs to assess for cardiorespiratory or metastatic disease, or systemic infection

SPECIAL TESTS/ INVESTIGATIONS

- CSF analysis – cytology, biochemistry, culture
- CT and/or MRI scans
- EEG or BAER (brainstem auditory evoked response)

ANOREXIA/INAPPETENCE

DEFINITION

- The decline of food intake through loss of appetite.
- Anorexia suggests a complete lack of food intake.
- Inappetence implies a decline in food intake through loss of appetite or a selective appetite.
- 'Pseudo-anorexia' is a condition where a dog wishes to eat but is unwilling or unable to do so because of neuromuscular dysfunction or pain.

CLINICAL SIGNS

- In pseudo-anorexia the dog may try to eat and stop quickly because of pain or difficulty swallowing.
- In true anorexia the dog will not attempt to eat, or may turn away as if nauseated.

COMMON CAUSES

True anorexia/inappetence
- Fever
- GI disease
- Hepatic disease
- Hypercalcaemia
- Hypoadrenocorticism
- Infectious/inflammatory disease
- Neoplasia
- Unpalatable diet
- Uraemia

Pseudo-anorexia
- Jaw fracture
- Oesophagitis
- Oral dysphagia/foreign body
- Retrobulbar abscess/periorbital cellulitis
- Temporal myositis

UNCOMMON CAUSES

True anorexia/inappetence
- Severe cardiac failure
- Intracranial disease
  - Anosmia
  - Hypothalamic disease
  - Psychological (food aversion)

Pseudo-anorexia
- Blindness
- Cranial nerve deficits

DIAGNOSTIC APPROACH

1 Determine from history and direct observation whether dog wants to eat, or not.
2 Pseudo-anorexia will be caused by a cranial nerve deficit or a lesion in the mouth, pharynx or oesophagus.
3 Complete examination is needed for true anorexia.

CLINICAL CLUES

Predisposition
- None

History
- Does dog attempt to eat and then drop or regurgitate food, or does it avoid food?
- PU/PD in liver and renal disease
- Trauma if jaw fracture
- Weight loss in excess of what is expected from not eating suggests increased energy usage, e.g. metabolic disease, neoplasia, etc.

Physical examination
Observation
- Depression, seizures if intracranial disease
- Drooling saliva, halitosis if oral disease
- Dyspnoea if cardiac failure
- Unilateral exophthalmos if retrobulbar abscess

Inspection
- Abnormal lung and heart sounds
- Temporal muscle atrophy

Palpation
- Abdominal masses
- Pain or resistance on opening mouth if myositis, foreign body or retrobulbar abscess

LABORATORY FINDINGS

- Variable, often WNL
  - Azotaemia
    - Plus isosthenuria in renal failure
    - Pre-renal in CHF
  - Hypercalcaemia most frequently associated with malignancy, especially lymphosarcoma
  - Hyponatraemia/hyperkalaemia in hypoadrenocorticism
  - Inflammatory leukogram with infection or inflammatory disease
  - Raised liver enzymes, bile acids ± bilirubin in liver disease

IMAGING

- Head and neck for causes of pseudo-anorexia
- Variable for other conditions

SPECIAL TESTS

- Multiple depending on suspected condition
- Neurological examination

ATAXIA

DEFINITION

A failure of muscular co-ordination or an irregularity of muscle action.
- It is not accompanied by spasticity, paresis or involuntary movement
- It is the result of disorders of:
  - the *vestibular* system, or
  - the *cerebellum*, or
  - conscious or unconscious *proprioceptive* systems

CLINICAL SIGNS

Cerebellar ataxia (motor)
- Ipsilateral ataxia with unilateral lesion
- Bilateral ataxia with bilateral lesion
- No proprioceptive deficits (conscious proprioceptive pathways to cerebrum are intact)
- No weakness (descending pathways, the upper motor neurones are intact)

- Spastic, non-coordinated gait
- Hypermetria
- Intention tremor

Proprioceptive ataxia (sensory)
- Wide-based stance
- Longer strides or stumbling
- Knuckling of the paws
- Weakness (involvement of descending pathways or upper motor neurones)
- Progression to paresis/paralysis
- Gait abnormalities most evident in spinal cord disease
- Postural reactions will best demonstrate central lesions with proprioceptive defects

Vestibular ataxia
- Head tilt – towards the side of the lesion (except with paradoxical vestibular disorder)
- Dog leans and falls to the side of the lesion
- Nystagmus may be present (fast phase away from lesion)

COMMON CAUSES

Proprioceptive
- Spinal cord disease, e.g. disc protrusion

Secondary to metabolic disease
- e.g. Hepatic disease, renal failure

Vestibular
- Peripheral vestibular disease, e.g. otitis media/interna
- Idiopathic vestibular syndrome

UNCOMMON CAUSES

Cerebellar
- Traumatic/vascular – damage to cerebellum and brainstem
- Neoplasia, e.g. choroid plexus papilloma
- Congenital hypoplasia
- Meningitis
- Cerebellar abiotrophy

Degenerative
- Storage disease
- Demyelinating diseases
- Neuronopathies

Multiple congenital
- Bilateral congenital vestibular disorders, e.g. in Doberman, Beagle and Akita

Toxic/drug-induced
- Aminoglycoside toxicity

Vestibular
- Central vestibular lesion, e.g. neoplasia, inflammatory disease
- Peripheral vestibular disease
  - Primary
  - Secondary to endocrinopathy or neuritis for example

DIAGNOSTIC APPROACH

1   Rule out metabolic disease by laboratory testing.
2   Confirm if ataxic or weak.
3   If truly ataxic, it is always neurological in origin and can be accompanied by other neurological signs, so perform full neurological examination to localise problem.
4   If dog's mental status is normal, the problem is likely to be spinal in origin.

CLINICAL CLUES

Predisposition
- Congenital disorders seen in young animals
- Degenerative disorders can take years to become apparent
- May be confused by metabolic disease
- Neoplastic disease more likely in older animals

History
- Use of ototoxic drugs

Physical examination

Observation
- Does the animal appear weak/fall to one particular side?
- Does it use structures to support itself on one side?
- Gait, e.g. hypermetria/dysmetria, knuckling, wide-based stance
- Head tilt (vestibular)
- Intention tremor (cerebellar)
- Is there swaying/swaggering gait ± hypermetria?

Inspection
- Full otic examination – pay particular attention to the external ear and tympanic membrane

- Neurological examination including thorough assessment of the cranial nerves and proprioceptive reflexes

Palpation
- Abdomen for organomegaly, e.g. liver, kidney (NB they may be decreased in size)
- Skull for any deformities, e.g. fractures

Auscultation
- Cardiovascular auscultation – serious arrhythmia can cause hypoxia secondary to poor cardiac output causing weakness which can be difficult to differentiate from ataxia

Ophthalmological examination
- Nystagmus if vestibular or cerebellar disease

LABORATORY FINDINGS

- Haematology, biochemistry (including glucose and electrolytes), and urinalysis will likely be unremarkable, but should be performed to rule out metabolic disease

IMAGING

Radiographs
- Skull
  - Open mouth rostro-caudal – ideal for viewing tympanic bullae
  - Ventro-dorsal – some information about tympanic bullae
- Spinal radiographs to assess for evidence of degenerative disc disease and narrowed disc spaces – myelogram to confirm spinal cord compression
- Thoracic/abdominal radiographs to assess for other disease
- Myelography if suspicious of spinal cause for ataxia ± decompressive surgery

MRI/CT scans
- More information on tympanic bullae
- Investigate suspected central cerebellar/vestibular lesions or spinal lesions

SPECIAL TESTS

- CSF analysis (cytology and protein)
- EEG

BLEEDING

DEFINITION

Losing blood: it is only of concern when it does not stop, or is recurrent.
- Local bleeding can result from traumatic injury, but may also arise spontaneously from ulcerated benign or neoplastic lesions.
- Spontaneous or prolonged bleeding is an abnormal condition resulting from a failure of the haemostatic mechanism, and can result from a deficiency in one or any of:
  - platelet numbers or function
  - the extrinsic or intrinsic coagulation pathways
  - vascular integrity

CLINICAL SIGNS

- Changes in urine/faecal colour
- Petechiation (not easy to recognise early)
- Prolonged bleeding after routine surgery or traumatic wounds
- Spontaneous bleeding from:
  - Gums
  - GI tract (melaena, haematochezia)

- Lungs (haemoptysis)
- Nose (epistaxis)
- Spontaneous intracavitary bleeding can be difficult to recognise except from associated clinical signs:
  - Abdominal distension
  - Dyspnoea (haemothorax)
  - Lameness or swelling if bleeding into joints or developing haematomas
  - Weakness/collapse

COMMON CAUSES

Anticoagulant ingestion
- Rodenticide toxicosis

Hereditary factor deficiency
- von Willebrand factor

Local injury
- Necrotic tumour
- Trauma
- Ulcerated tissue

Thrombocytopenia
- Primary immune-mediated
- Secondary immune-mediated, e.g. neoplasia, drugs

UNCOMMON CAUSES

- Disseminated intravascular coagulation (DIC)
- Hyperviscosity syndrome
- Primary hyperfibrinolysis
- Therapeutic anticoagulation

Hereditary factor deficiency
- Factor II, VII, VIII, IX, X, XI

Platelet dysfunction
- Drug-induced, e.g. phenylbutazone, plasma expanders
- Secondary to underlying disease, e.g. renal/hepatic failure, polycythaemia

- Thrombasthenia/thrombopathia

Thrombocytopenia
- Consumption, e.g. DIC, vasculitis
- Decreased/ineffective production or release from bone marrow
- Secondary immune-mediated to rickettsial disease

Vitamin K deficiency
- Fat malabsorption
- Liver disease

DIAGNOSTIC APPROACH

1 Determine whether bleeding is localised or generalised.
2 Differentiate platelet problems from coagulopathy by type of bleeding.
3 Assess platelet function and numbers and clotting times as appropriate.

CLINICAL CLUES

Predisposition
- Haemophilia in GSD, Scottish terrier
- Middle-aged animals more commonly acquire immune-mediated disease
- Older animals more likely to develop neoplastic disease
- Von Willebrand disease in Dobermann
- Young to middle-aged animals more prone to infectious causes
- Young pure-bred animals are more likely to have hereditary coagulopathies

History
Breed/family history of bleeding problems
- Hereditary coagulopathy is unlikely if there have been no problems after previous surgery, unless concurrent disease/drug administration exacerbates mild coagulopathy, e.g. von Willebrand disease and aspirin administration

PRESENTING COMPLAINTS

Current medication
- Acquired platelet destruction or dysfunction, e.g. aspirin, other NSAIDs
- Bone marrow suppression secondary to cytotoxic drugs, phenylbutazone, oestrogen
- Immune-mediated platelet destruction with sulphonamides
- Vaccination history, e.g. modified live vaccines can cause transient thrombocytopenia or platelet dysfunction

Environment
- Access to rodenticides
- Any other animals affected?

Nature and chronicity of problem
- Any previous problems?
- Profuse or seeping bleed, spontaneous or incited by minor trauma/severe trauma/surgery?
- Site of bleeding?
- Is the amount of bleeding proportional to the injury?
- Any signs consistent with pre-existing disease?

Trauma

Travel history
- Areas with rickettsial diseases

Physical examination
Observation
- Is bleeding localised – is there an adequate local cause?
- Petechiation/ecchymoses/mucosal bleeding (including melaena/epistaxis) – suggest platelet disorder
- Prolonged bleeding:
  - Epistaxis
  - Haematochezia/melaena
  - Haematuria
  - Haemoptysis
- Signs suggestive of coagulopathy:
  - Abdominal enlargement (intracavitary bleeding)

- Dyspnoea/tachypnoea (intracavitary bleeding)
- Haemarthrosis (joint bleeds)
- Haematomas
- Weakness or lameness

Inspection
- Examine skin and mucous membranes (oral, penile, vulval) for petechiae, ecchymoses
- Fundic examination – retinal lesions from infectious disease, e.g. rickettsial/fungal, or secondary to coagulopathies, hypertension or neoplasia
- Signs of trauma

Palpation
- Joint swelling
- Pain/deformity of face
- Abdomen for fluid thrill or hepatosplenomegaly
- Pulse for volume and rhythm

Auscultation
- Evidence of pleural/pericardial fluid with alterations in the lung sounds
  - Dullness on percussion and reduced sounds ventrally/over heart
  - Increased sounds dorsally

LABORATORY FINDINGS

Haematology
- Evidence of thrombocytopenia
- Is there evidence of regeneration if anaemic: polychromasia, anisocytosis, reticulocytosis?
- Platelet numbers and morphology should be assessed

Serum biochemistry
- Assess for other systemic disease which might cause coagulopathy, e.g. uraemia, hepatic disease
- Hyperglobulinaemia with ehrlichiosis, chronic inflammation and neoplasia

- Hypoproteinaemia with blood loss, severe liver disease

Urinalysis
- Haematuria may be a finding with co-agulopathies, but may be microscopic. Often found in association with thrombocytopenia
- Proteinuria with hyperglobulinaemias, immune-mediated disease

Haemostatic studies: see Section 4, Haemostatic system
- Activated clotting time (ACT)
- Antithrombin III (ATIII)
- Buccal mucosal bleeding time (BMBT)
- Coagulation profile to evaluate the intrinsic and extrinsic coagulation pathways
  - One-stage prothrombin time (OSPT) [extrinsic and common cascade]
  - Activated partial thromboplastin time (aPTT) [intrinsic and common cascade]
- D-dimer
- Fibrinogen and fibrin degradation products (FDPs)
- Platelet aggregation
- Specific factor assays
- Thrombin clot time
- Whole blood clotting time

Thoracic and abdominal radiographs
- Assess for intracavitary bleeding
- Assess for possible internal neoplasia

- Organomegaly, e.g. liver or spleen
- Radiographs of areas of localised bleeding (e.g. nose) or swelling (e.g. joints)

Ultrasonography
- Intra-abdominal masses or free fluid
- Liver/spleen for evidence of neoplasia

SPECIAL TESTS

- Antinuclear antibody (ANA)
- Anti-platelet antibody
- Bone marrow aspirate/core biopsy if cytopenia, abnormal circulating cells or paraproteinaemia
- Bronchoscopy if haemoptysis
- Clot retraction/platelet aggregation studies if considering thrombopathia; or further platelet studies or skin biopsy if considering vascular disorder
- Coagulation factor assays
- Coombs' test if also anaemic
- Knott's test and heartworm titre if travelled in endemic areas
- PIVKAs if suspect rodenticide intoxication or liver disease
- Plasmin activity, FDPs, antithrombin III, fibrinogen and D-dimer to assess for excessive fibrinolysis due to consumptive coagulopathy, e.g. DIC
- Reticulocyte count
- Rhinoscopy if epistaxis
- Serologic/PCR testing for infectious diseases, e.g. chrlichiosis
- SPE
- Ultrasound-guided aspirate/biopsy – risky with bleeding animal – to identify liver or splenic disease, or to confirm intracavitary bleeding

PRESENTING COMPLAINTS

CONSTIPATION

DEFINITION

Infrequent and difficult or absent defecation, with abnormal retention of faeces in the colon.

- Obstipation is prolonged, intractable constipation in which faeces have become so firm that defecation is no longer possible, and which ultimately leads to secondary degeneration of colonic musculature.

CLINICAL SIGNS

- Anorexia, lethargy and vomiting
- Dyschezia (pain or difficulty in defecation) – see p. 69
- Failure to pass faeces or small, hard, dry faeces
- Haematochezia if intraluminal cause
- Paradoxical diarrhoea (scant liquid faeces passed around the constipated mass)
- Tenesmus (straining to defecate) – see p. 69

COMMON CAUSES

Dietary
- Foreign material, e.g. bones, hair
- Insufficient fibre
- Inadequate water intake

Drug-induced
- Anticholinergics
- Kaolin-pectin
- Opioids

Environmental
- Dehydration
- Hospitalisation
- Inadequate exercise

Neuromuscular disease
- Lumbosacral disease

Obstruction
Extraluminal
- Healed pelvic fracture
- Prostatic enlargement – hypertrophy, abscess, neoplasia

Intraluminal
- Perineal hernia and rectal diverticulum
- Rectal tumour

Pain
Anorectal disease
- Anal sac impaction, abscess, cellulitis
- Perianal fistula

Orthopaedic disease (pain and failure to posture)
- Injury to pelvis, hip or pelvic limbs
- Spinal (lumbo-sacral disease)

Water-electrolyte abnormalities
- Dehydration
- Hypercalcaemia
- Hypokalaemia

UNCOMMON CAUSES

Obstruction
Extraluminal
- Pelvic collapse due to nutritional bone disease
- Prostatic or paraprostatic cyst
- Sublumbar lymphadenopathy

Intraluminal
- Benign stricture

Anorectal disease
- Anal or rectal stricture
- Anal sac adenocarcinoma

- Atresia ani
- Foreign body
- Pseudocoprostasis (faecal impaction due to matted hair)

Drug-induced
- Aluminium hydroxide
- Antihistamines
- Barium sulphate
- Diuretics
- Iron
- Phenothiazines
- Sucralfate

Neuromuscular disease
- Bilateral pelvic nerve damage
- Dysautonomia

Metabolic
- Hyperparathyroidism
- Hypothyroidism

DIAGNOSTIC APPROACH

1 Confirm constipation by abdominal and rectal palpation, and radiographs.
2 Identify underlying cause.

CLINICAL CLUES

Predisposition
- Benign prostatic hypertrophy in uncastrated older dogs
- Sedentary dogs on low-fibre diet

History
- Old pelvic trauma

Physical examination
Observation
- Dyschezia
- Hindleg weakness or pain with lumbosacral disease

- Haematochezia if intraluminal cause
- Tenesmus

Inspection
- Anal lesions

Palpation
- Faecal material in colon
- Paraprostatic cyst
- Pelvic deformity
- Prostatic enlargement

Rectal palpation
- Anal sac disease
- Dry, impacted faeces
- Paraprostatic cyst
- Pelvic canal narrowing
- Perineal hernia and rectal diverticulum
- Prostatic enlargement
- Rectal stricture

LABORATORY FINDINGS

- Hypokalaemia causing colonic muscle weakness
- Otherwise usually unremarkable

IMAGING

Radiographs
Plain
- Old pelvic fractures
- Prostatomegaly

Contrast
- Rectal stricture
- Colonic/rectal tumour

SPECIAL TESTS

- Thyroid function tests
- Proctoscopy

PRESENTING COMPLAINTS

COUGH

DEFINITION

A sudden expiratory effort resulting in a sudden, noisy expulsion of air from the lungs.
- It is an attempt to try and clear excess secretion or foreign material from the lungs, bronchi or trachea.

CLINICAL SIGNS

Associated signs
- Dyspnoea/tachypnoea – see p. 33
- Exercise intolerance/collapse
- Nasal/ocular discharge

Variable nature to the cough
- Acute coughing can often be assumed to be infectious in origin, until proved otherwise
- Non-productive moist or dry suggests upper airway
- Productive/non-productive moist or dry suggests pulmonary link
  - Animal may swallow excessively after coughing if productive
- Haemoptysis with coagulopathy, foreign body, neoplasia or trauma

COMMON CAUSES

Allergic/immune-mediated
- Reverse sneeze, sometimes mistaken for coughing

Cardiovascular
- Cardiomegaly with left atrial enlargement and bronchial compression

Inflammatory
- Acute or chronic inflammatory disease anywhere from pharynx to pulmonary tissue can stimulate coughing

- Acute secondary to infectious agents, e.g. infectious tracheobronchitis (kennel cough)
- Bronchopneumonia
- Chronic bronchitis
- Inhalation, secondary to oesophageal disease

Pleural effusion
- Very rarely causes coughing; dyspnoea is more important sign – see p. 33

Traumatic/physical
- Collapsing trachea
- Inhaled/ingested foreign body
- Laryngeal paralysis: coughing when drinking

UNCOMMON CAUSES

Allergic
- Asthma (much more common in cats than dogs)
- Eosinophilic inflammatory respiratory diseases (pulmonary infiltrate with eosinophils), e.g. eosinophilic bronchitis/bronchopneumonopathy/pneumonia

Cardiovascular
- Non-cardiogenic pulmonary oedema
- Pulmonary thromboemboli
- Left-sided failure causing pulmonary oedema (dyspnoea rather than coughing)

Inflammatory
- Abscess rarely
- Chronic pulmonary fibrosis, especially in WHWT
- Granulomatous disease
- Hilar lymph node enlargement

Neoplastic

- Mediastinal
- Metastatic (more commonly causes dyspnoea than cough)
- Primary
  - Tracheal
  - Laryngeal
  - Lymphosarcoma
  - Extrathoracic, e.g. rib/sternum/soft tissue

Parasitic

- *Dirofilaria immitis* (not currently in UK)
- *Angiostrongylus vasorum* – regional variation in prevalence in UK
- *Oslerus osleri* (lungworm)
- Others, e.g. *Crenosoma vulpis, Pneumocystis, Filaroides hirthii* are very uncommon
- Visceral larva migrans

Traumatic/physical

- Noxious gases
- Iatrogenic secondary to inhalation of liquids or solids, e.g. force-feeding, barium administration

DIAGNOSTIC APPROACH

1   Determine whether this is an upper or lower airway problem from signs and physical examination.
2   Rule out cardiac disease.
3   Rule out oesophageal disease.
4   Investigate airway disease by radiography, laboratory analysis and endoscopy.

CLINICAL CLUES

Predisposition

- Brachycephalics have obstructive upper-airway disease
- Idiopathic megaoesophagus in Great Dane, GSD, Irish setter

- Kennelled pets are at risk of infectious diseases
- Large/giant breed dogs
  - Dilated cardiomyopathy
  - Laryngeal paralysis
  - Megaoesophagus
  - Pneumonia
- *Oslerus* infection in young dogs
- Small dogs of mid-old age likely to have:
  - Chronic obstructive lung disease, e.g. chronic bronchitis
  - Collapsing trachea
  - Chronic mitral valve disease
  - Pulmonary interstitial fibrosis in WHWT

History

Associated dyspnoea
- Obstruction, and alveolar and pleural space disease

Duration of cough
- Acute (< 2 weeks' duration) = kennel cough
- Chronic (> 2 weeks' duration) cough

Environment: flare factors for cough
- Access to intermediate hosts of parasites
- Cough associated with walking on collar and lead: collapsing trachea
- Owners who are heavy smokers, causing passive smoking
- Potential exposure to other parasites if have been outside of UK
- Seasonality for allergic airway disease

Nature of cough
- Haemoptysis with coagulopathy, foreign body, neoplasia or trauma
- Regurgitation (and inhalation) in primary oesophageal disease
- Response to therapy
- Sound of the cough: 'wheezy' suggests small airways
- Terminal retch

- Terminal retch or vomiting can be confused with GI disease

Timing of the cough
- Any association with eating food/drinking fluids suggests larynx or oesophagus

Physical examination
Observation
- Abnormal respiratory sounds
- Airway noise
  - Inspiratory if upper airway
  - Expiratory if lower airway
- Dyspnoea
- Respiratory pattern, e.g. any abdominal effort
- Tachypnoea

Inspection
- Halitosis – often a feature with inhaled foreign bodies, megaoesophagus
- Ocular/nasal discharge

Palpation
- Cough elicited by tracheal pinch if upper airway
- Larynx, trachea and thorax for abnormalities

Auscultation
- Airway noise: localise origin
  - Trachea: abnormal respiratory sound
  - Thorax: adventitious respiratory sounds, e.g. crackles and wheezes
- Is there a murmur present? Consider cardiac cause of cough?

LABORATORY FINDINGS

- Eosinophilia may be associated with parasitic diseases and eosinophilic immune-mediated disorders
- Faecal examination may reveal the presence of parasitic larvae

- Increased serum globulins may be seen in certain inflammatory conditions, e.g. granulomatous disease
- Leukocytosis in pulmonary inflammatory disease
- Often unremarkable if upper-airway disease

IMAGING

Thoracic radiographs
- Assess heart size for cardiomegaly, especially the left atrium
- Assess tracheal diameter throughout its length: can carry out dynamic assessment under fluoroscopy for tracheal collapse
- Assess lung patterns as bronchial, interstitial, alveolar or mixed
- Assess for presence of mediastinal abnormalities
- Inflated radiographs under general anaesthesia may provide more information
- Right lateral and DV (lungs) or VD (heart) projections should be performed

SPECIAL TESTS

- Baermann faecal flotation for lungworm and *Angiostrongylus*
- Blood gas analysis (if available) – arterial to assess oxygenation
- Bronchoscopy
  - Bronchoalveolar lavage for cytological examination and culture
- Cardiovascular examination: ECG, echocardiography
- Fine-needle lung aspiration/biopsy
- Knott's test and/or serology for *Dirofilaria immitis*
- laryngoscopy under GA
- Nuclear scintigraphic studies of ventilation-perfusion
- Thoracocentesis
- Ultrasound of the larynx to assess for laryngeal paralysis

DIARRHOEA

DEFINITION

An increase in the water content of faeces with a consequent increase in their fluidity and/or volume and/or frequency.
- Diarrhoea can be:
  - Acute or chronic
  - Caused by primary GI pathology, or be secondary to disease elsewhere
  - Due to alterations in one or a combination of:
    - the osmotic content of the stool
    - intestinal secretion
    - intestinal mucosal permeability
    - motility
  - Self-limiting or life-threatening
  - The result of disorders of the small or large intestine, or both

CLINICAL SIGNS

- The consistency of diarrhoea can vary from soft with some retention of form, through 'cow-pat', to completely watery.

- Small intestinal (SI) diarrhoea is characteristically large volume, infrequent and watery, and may contain melaena (p. 49).
- Large intestinal (LI) diarrhoea is characteristically small volume, mucoid and may contain fresh blood (haematochezia, see p. 43). Dogs will show urgency, increased frequency of defecation, and will strain (tenesmus, see p. 69).

Associated signs
- Abdominal discomfort (p. 3), excessive borborygmi, flatus, and halitosis (p. 48) are non-specific signs
- Anorexia in the presence of diarrhoea is generally an indication of sinister disease
- Severe, chronic diarrhoea may be a protein-losing enteropathy with consequent hypoalbuminaemia and ascites/ oedema
- Vomiting can be associated with both SI and LI diseases

ACUTE DIARRHOEA

DEFINITION

Acute diarrhoea generally occurs abruptly in a previously healthy dog, and is typically of short duration. It will have been present continuously for less than 2 weeks, or intermittently for less than 4 weeks.
- It is frequently associated with vomiting, and often affects the whole GI tract.
- It is most often self-limiting, but can be life-threatening.

CLINICAL SIGNS

- Acute, often profuse, watery diarrhoea
- Associated vomiting
- Borborygmi
- Weight loss is not a feature

COMMON CAUSES

GI disease
Dietary
- Dietary indiscretion
- Food intolerance
- Overfeeding
- Sudden change in diet

Drug/toxin
- Antimicrobials
- NSAIDs

Idiopathic
- Haemorrhagic gastroenteritis (HGE)

Infection: bacterial
- *Campylobacter*
- *Clostridium*
- *E. coli*

Infection: parasitic
- *Ancylostoma* hookworms (not in UK)
- *Giardia*
- *Trichuris* whipworms (uncommon in UK)

Infection: viral
- Coronavirus (mild)
- Parvovirus

Obstructive (surgical)
- Foreign body
- Intussusception

Non-GI disease
- Hypoadrenocorticism: not common, but important

UNCOMMON CAUSES

GI disease
Dietary
- Food hypersensitivity

Drug/toxin
- ACE inhibitors
- Anthelmintics
- Anti-arrhythmics
- Anti-cancer agents
- Blue-green algae
- Digoxin
- Heavy metals
- Laxatives
- Organophosphates
- Phenylpropanolamine

Infection: bacterial
- *Bacillus piliformis*
- *Salmonella*
- *Yersinia*

Infection: parasitic
- Ascarids and cestodes (infection common, but rarely a cause of diarrhoea)
- *Cryptosporidium*
- *Isospora* (rarely primary pathogen, except in puppies)
- *Strongyloides*
- *Uncinaria* hookworms

Infection: rickettsial
- Salmon-poisoning disease, *Neorickettsia helminthica* and *elokominica* (geographically limited to Pacific NW USA)

Infection: viral
- Astrovirus (mild)
- Rotavirus (mild)

Obstructive (surgical)
- Incarcerated bowel loop (internal or external hernia)
- Intestinal volvulus
- Linear foreign body

Non-GI disease
- Acute hepatitis
  - Infectious canine hepatitis
  - Leptospirosis
- Acute pancreatitis
- Acute renal failure
- Canine distemper
- Pyometra

DIAGNOSTIC APPROACH

1   Differentiate between primary (GI) and secondary (non-GI) disease by history, physical examination and laboratory findings.

2 Dogs with distemper usually have concurrent respiratory signs, and dogs with leptospirosis also usually have hepatic and renal problems.

3 If primary GI disease is present, differentiate by history, physical examination and laboratory findings those that require only symptomatic support (e.g. anti-diarrhoeals, fluid therapy) from life-threatening causes that require either:

- aggressive medical therapy
  - Parvovirus
  - *Salmonella*
  - HGE

or

- surgical correction
  - Foreign body
  - Intussusception

CLINICAL CLUES

Predisposition
- Young, not fully immunocompetent
- Unsanitary environment
- Unvaccinated

History
- Access to toxins
- Acute onset of diarrhoea, etc.
- Contact with infected dogs
- Drug administration
- Other signs, e.g. vomiting
- Presence of blood in diarrhoea
- Scavenging
- Vaccination status

Physical examination
Observation
- Dull and depressed versus bright and alert indicates greater need for definitive diagnosis and aggressive treatment

Inspection
- Linear foreign body under tongue
- Oral ulcers from acute uraemia
- Pyrexia with infectious/inflammatory disease
- Signs of dehydration
  - Dry mucous membranes
  - Skin tenting
  - Slow capillary refill
  - Sunken eyes
  - Tachycardia

Palpation
- Abdominal pain: see p. 3
  - Cranial abdominal pain in pancreatitis
- Bunching of intestines with linear foreign body
- Fluid or gas-filled bowel loops
- Foreign body
- Mesenteric lymphadenopathy
- Sausage-shaped mass consistent with intussusception

Rectal examination
- Evidence of diarrhoea
- Evidence of melaena or haematochezia
- Abnormal faecal material
- Advanced ileo-colic intussusception

LABORATORY FINDINGS

Haematology
- Eosinophilia may be seen with parasitism
- Haemoconcentration indicative of dehydration (NB check total protein)
- Leukopenia in parvovirus infection (~60% of cases) or overwhelming sepsis
- Leukocytosis ± left shift with infectious/inflammatory disease
- Marked haemoconcentration with normal serum proteins suggests HGE
- Non-regenerative anaemia with peracute disease

Serum biochemistry
- Often unremarkable, but may be helpful in ruling out non-GI diseases
  - Hyperkalaemia and hyponatraemia suggestive of hypoadrenocorticism
  - Azotaemia in renal failure
  - Amylase and lipase may be elevated in pancreatitis
- Azotaemia may be pre-renal; check urine SG
- Decreased serum proteins may develop after rehydration in ulcerative/haemorrhagic diseases (parvovirus, HGE)
- Electrolyte abnormalities, especially hypokalaemia, gives information about the best choice of fluid therapy
- Hypoglycaemia sometimes seen in sepsis and in inadequate food uptake by puppies
- Increased liver enzymes secondary to intestinal inflammation, gut bacterial translocation
- Increased serum proteins in dehydration

Urinalysis
- Hypersthenuria in face of dehydration is appropriate
- Isosthenuria in face of dehydration is inappropriate, and indicates renal insufficiency
- Failure to concentrate urine fully is typical of hypoadrenocorticism

Faecal examination
- Bacterial culture may identify primary pathogen, and is indicated if there is haemorrhagic diarrhoea or pyrexia
- Faecal cytology is of limited value. *Campylobacter*-like organisms and sporulating *Clostridia* may be identified
- Flotation tests to identify endoparasites
  - Baermann: *Strongyloides* larvae
  - Sodium nitrate, or formalin-ether: nematode and cestode ova

- Sheather's sugar centrifugation: *Cryptosporidium*
- Three zinc sulphate flotations may be needed to identify *Giardia*

IMAGING

Radiographs
Plain
- Foreign body
- Free intraperitoneal gas indicates perforated viscus
- Intestinal distension with fluid or gas = ileus
  - Obstructive ileus with massively dilated, stacked bowel loops
  - Physiological ileus is less severe and reflects inflammation or metabolic abnormalities
  - Mesenteric torsion causes distension of all intestinal loops
  - Strangulation causes dilation of one segment of intestine
- Signs of obstruction
  - Fluid- or gas-filled, dilated bowel loop(s)
  - 'Gravel' sign
- Soft tissue density

Contrast
- Radiolucent foreign body
- Often no value over plain films

Ultrasound examination
- Foreign body/obstruction
- Intussusception – double concentric ring with hyperechoic centre
- Mesenteric lymphadenopathy
- Pancreatic pathology

SPECIAL TESTS

- ACTH stimulation test
- Assay for *Clostridium perfringens* and *Cl. difficile* toxins

- Endoscopic biopsy (rarely indicated in acute disease)
- Exploratory laparotomy
- Faecal ELISA for *Giardia* antigen

- Faecal ELISA for parvovirus
- Scanning electron microscopy of faeces for virus particles
- Serology – haemagglutination inhibition for parvovirus

CHRONIC DIARRHOEA

DEFINITION

Diarrhoea is defined as chronic if:
- It has been present continuously or intermittently for 2–4 weeks at least, and has not responded to symptomatic treatment;

or
- If there is a pattern of recurrent episodes.

CLINICAL SIGNS

- Diarrhoea
- Ascites (p. 94) occurs if a protein-losing enteropathy (PLE) causes significant hypoalbuminaemia (< 15 g/L)
- Frequent mucoid diarrhoea ± haematochezia with tenesmus suggests colitis
- Melaena may indicate upper GI haemorrhage, and in association with diarrhoea suggests SI bleeding
- Polyphagia in the presence of diarrhoea is suggestive of malabsorption
- Weight loss is characteristic of SI disease

NB Dogs with chronic LI disease may lose weight if the owner repeatedly withholds food

COMMON CAUSES

Chronic diarrhoea
GI disease
- Bacterial infection? (some potential pathogens may be commensals)
- Food intolerance

- Giardiasis
- Idiopathic inflammatory bowel disease
  - Lympho-plasmacytic enteritis (LPE) and/or colitis
  - Eosinophilic gastroenteritis (EGE)
- Irritable bowel syndrome (undiagnosed, functional diarrhoea)
- Small intestinal bacterial overgrowth (SIBO)

Non-GI disease
- Right-sided heart failure
- Chronic liver disease
- Exocrine pancreatic insufficiency (EPI)

UNCOMMON CAUSES

Chronic diarrhoea
GI disease
- Alimentary lymphosarcoma
- Chronic intussusception
- Food allergy
- Histoplasmosis (geographically limited to Ohio valley in USA)
- Idiopathic inflammatory bowel disease
  - Granulomatous enteritis
  - Histiocytic ulcerative colitis (Boxer and French bulldog only)
  - Immunoproliferative small intestinal disease (IPSID – Basenji only)
- Intestinal adenocarcinoma
- Lymphangiectasia
- Parasitic
- Hookworm (rare in UK)
- *Prototheca*
- *Strongyloides*

PRESENTING COMPLAINTS

PRESENTING COMPLAINTS

- Whipworm colitis (uncommon in UK)
- Pythiosis (geographically limited to southern USA)
- Short-bowel syndrome

Non-GI disease
- Chronic pancreatitis
- Gastrinoma (APUDoma)
- Hypoadrenocorticism
  - Classical, but previously masked by symptomatic therapy
  - Atypical, i.e. normal electrolytes as only hypocortisolaemia
- Hyperthyroidism
- Renal disease

DIAGNOSTIC APPROACH

1 Rule out non-GI causes by history, physical examination and laboratory testing.
2 Rule out simple causes, such as diet-induced and parasitism from history and faecal examination.
3 Perform TLI test to diagnose EPI *before* further investigations.
4 Anatomical localisation from history and faecal characteristics (see Table 1).
5 Suspect PLE from serum proteins – see Ascites p. 94.
6 Faecal culture often unhelpful.
7 Folate and cobalamin to screen for SIBO and infiltrative bowel disease – see p. 182.
8 Radiographs to screen for masses, partial obstruction.
9 Ultrasound examination to examine bowel wall thickness, and identify masses.
10 Endoscopic biopsy.
11 Exploratory laparotomy and biopsy if endoscopy unavailable or non-diagnostic, or focal disease found on imaging. Biopsy must always be performed, even if no gross abnormalities are found.

(See Table 1.)

CLINICAL CLUES

Predisposition
- Clostridial enterotoxicosis in stressed (e.g. hospitalised) dogs
- EPI – GSD, Collie, Chow chow, small terriers
- Inflammatory bowel disease
  - LPE – GSD, Shar pei
  - EGE – GSD
  - Immunoproliferative small intestinal disease (IPSID): Basenji
- Irritable bowel syndrome (IBS) – toy breeds, working dogs
- Lymphangiectasia – Yorkshire terrier, Rottweiler
- Neoplasia in older dogs

History
- Correlation with specific food
- Drug administration
- Full dietary history
- Mode of onset – abrupt versus gradual suggests an infectious aetiology
- Other signs – vomiting, weight loss
- Previous surgery, especially intestinal resection
- Response to previous treatment

Physical examination
Observation
- Demeanour
- Nature of faeces and style of defecation help localise to SI or LI
- Peripheral (ventral) oedema if severe hypoproteinaemia
- Weight loss

Inspection
- Pallor of mucous membranes due to blood-loss anaemia
- Poor quality hair coat secondary to malabsorption

Table 1 Classification of diarrhoea is made on a range of clinical signs and faecal characteristics

Sign	Small intestinal diarrhoea	Large intestinal diarrhoea
Faeces		
Volume	Markedly increased	Normal or decreased
Mucus	Rarely present	Common
Melaena	May be present	Absent
Haematochezia	Absent except in acute HGE	Fairly common
Steatorrhoea	Present with malabsorption	Absent
Undigested food	May be present	Absent
Colour	Colour variations occur	Colour variations rare; may be bloody
Defecation		
Urgency	Absent except if acute or very severe	Usually but not invariably present
Tenesmus	Absent	Frequent but not invariably present
Frequency	2–3 times normal for the patient	Usually greater than 3 times normal
Dyschezia (difficulty in defecation)	Absent	Present with distal colonic or rectal disease
Ancillary signs		
Weight loss	May occur in malabsorption	Rare except in severe colitis and diffuse tumours
Vomiting	May be present in inflammatory diseases, especially in cats	Probably occurs in ~30% of dogs with colitis
Flatulence and borborygmi	May occur	Absent
Halitosis in absence of oral disease	May be present with malabsorption	Absent unless perianal licking
Folate and cobalamin	May be abnormal	Normal

Palpation
- Abdominal masses
- Ascites in PLE
- Thickening of bowel loops suggests infiltration (IBD or lymphosarcoma)

Rectal examination
- Distal colonic mass or stricture
- Evidence of melaena or haematochezia
- Irregular mucosal texture due to inflammation or neoplasia

LABORATORY FINDINGS

Haematology
- Eosinophilia sometimes seen in eosinophilic enteritis, but many false positives and negatives). Consider parasitism or hypoadrenocorticism
- Haemoconcentration from intestinal fluid loss
- Leukocytosis (neutrophilia ± monocytosis) in severe inflammatory disease or perforation
- Lymphopenia with stress or lymphangiectasia
- Microcytic anaemia if chronic blood loss
- Non-regenerative anaemia with chronic disease/malnutrition

Serum biochemistry
- Commonly unremarkable in primary, chronic GI disease
- Hyperkalaemia and hyponatraemia seen in hypoadrenocorticism and sometimes in whipworm colitis
- Hypocalcaemia, reflecting hypoalbuminaemia
- Hypocholesterolaemia suggestive of malabsorption, especially lymphangiectasia
- Hypokalaemia of therapeutic importance
- Increased liver enzymes, secondary to intestinal inflammation
- Panhypoproteinaemia typical in PLE, although severe inflammatory disease may cause raised globulins, e.g. IPSID in Basenji

Urinalysis
- Rule out proteinuria as cause of hypoalbuminaemia

Faecal examination
- Faecal leukocytes on cytology indicate inflammation, but are not specific
- Presence of undigested food is non-specific and unhelpful
- Fungal culture and rectal cytology for histoplasmosis
- Occult blood test, but false-positives are common
- Faecal culture may give false-negatives and false-positives

IMAGING

Radiographs
Plain
- To identify mass or foreign body or partial obstruction

Contrast
- Barium follow-through studies generally unhelpful if just diarrhoea present and plain radiographs unremarkable
- Barium enema largely superseded by colonoscopy

Ultrasound examination
- Demonstrate free fluid or gas
- Identify masses, lymphadenopathy
- Measure bowel wall thickness

SPECIAL TESTS

- ACTH stimulation test
- Assay for *Clostridium perfringens* and *Cl. difficile* toxins
- Breath hydrogen for SIBO, but not readily available
- Endoscopic biopsy
- Exclusion diet trial
- Exploratory laparotomy and full-thickness biopsy
- Faecal alpha$_1$-protease inhibitor as a marker for a PLE
- Faecal ELISA for *Giardia* antigen
- Folate and cobalamin to screen for SIBO, and infiltrative bowel disease
- Serum thyroxine (but hyperthyroidism in dogs very rare)
- Trypsin-like immunoreactivity (TLI)
- Xylose absorption too insensitive to be useful

DROOLING

DEFINITION

Dribbling of saliva from the mouth.
- Pseudoptyalism is drooling due to failure to swallow normal amounts of saliva
- True ptyalism is increased production of saliva

CLINICAL SIGNS

- Drooling saliva from mouth
- Dysphagia
- Coughing, inappetence, etc. if non-pharyngeal disease

COMMON CAUSES

Pseudoptyalism
- As for causes of dysphagia (p. 31): oral ulcers, foreign body, masses and lip-fold deformities
- Oesophageal disease: oesophagitis, obstruction
- Pharyngeal foreign body

Ptyalism
- Local irritant (metronidazole, trimethoprim-sulpha)
- Nausea (see vomiting, p. 75)
- Physiological (anticipation of food)

UNCOMMON CAUSES

Pseudoptyalism
- Mandibular neuropraxia
- Myasthenia gravis
- Pharyngeal foreign body
- Tonsillar tumour

Ptyalism
- Gastric tumour
- Hypersialosis
- Ingestion of toxic/irritant substance and plants
  - *Amanita*, Dumb Cane (*Dieffenbachia*), *Philodendron*, *Poinsettia*, toads, etc.
  - Caustics
  - Ivermectin
  - Metaldehyde
  - Organophosphates
- Salivary gland infarction
- Sialoadenitis
- Rabies and pseudorabies

DIAGNOSTIC APPROACH

1 Distinguish oropharyngeal, oesophageal and gastric disease. See dysphagia, regurgitation and vomiting (pp. 31, 61, 75).

DYSPHAGIA

DEFINITION

Difficulty or inability to prehend, chew or swallow food. Due to:
- Physical failure to open and close jaw and move food into oesophagus
- Pain

CLINICAL SIGNS

- Coughing and/or nasal discharge if secondary inhalation
- Drooling (hypersalivation or failure to swallow saliva)
- Dropping food from mouth
- Extension or lowering of head and neck
- Failure to prehend food

- Halitosis if food retained
- Pain on opening mouth

COMMON CAUSES

Structural or functional diseases of the mouth and/or temporo-mandibular joint and/or pharynx

- Dental and/or periodontal disease
- Foreign body, including linear foreign body
- Mandibular fracture/luxation
- Neoplasia (see Oral mass, p. 115)
- Oral ulceration
- Pharyngitis/tonsillitis
- Retropharyngeal abscess or lymphadenopathy
- Temporal myositis

Oesophageal disorders

- See Regurgitation, p. 61

UNCOMMON CAUSES

- Craniomandibular osteopathy
- Cricopharyngeal achalasia
- Hypersialosis
- Hypothyroidism
- Mandibular neuropraxia ('trigeminal paralysis')
- Myasthenia gravis
- Nutritional secondary hyperparathyroidism ('rubber jaw')
- Rabies and Aujeszky's disease (pseudo-rabies)
- Salivary gland infarction
- Sialoadenitis
- Temporo-mandibular dysplasia/jaw locking
- Trigeminal sensory neuropathy
- Uraemic ulceration

DIAGNOSTIC APPROACH

1 Distinguish from regurgitation and vomiting.
2 Confirm difficulty in swallowing.
3 Distinguish morphological causes from functional causes by inspection.
NB Rabies should always be considered as a potential diagnosis in endemic areas.

CLINICAL CLUES

Predisposition

- Craniomandibular osteopathy in WHWT
- Trauma in younger dogs
- Uraemia, neoplasia in older dogs

History

- Concurrent signs of renal failure (anorexia, PU/PD), if uraemic ulcers
- Mandibular neuropraxia may follow excessive chewing of bones, etc., and leads to failure to close jaw
- Potential exposure to rabies is important outside UK
- Swollen painful muscles precede atrophy in temporal myositis
- Trauma (road traffic accident, or fall from height) can cause oral fractures/luxations

Physical examination
Observation
- Observe patient eating to confirm dysphagia and assess jaw motion

Inspection
- Check extent of jaw tone, width of opening and presence of pain on opening mouth
- Check neurological function (jaw and tongue movements, gag reflex) if no structural disease obvious *before* sedation/GA

- Thorough oral examination checking under tongue for linear foreign body; complete examination may require sedation/GA

Palpation
- Mandibular, retropharyngeal and cervical LNs if oral mass present
- Salivary glands for pain or swelling
- Temporal muscles for swelling or atrophy
- Tonsils may be hard if infiltrated with tumour

Auscultation
- Chest for secondary inhalation pneumonia
- Throat for upper airway obstruction

LABORATORY FINDINGS

Haematology and serum biochemistry
- Creatine kinase elevated in myositis
- Look for inflammatory and systemic diseases

Oral and pharyngeal cultures
- Rarely helpful

IMAGING

Radiographs
Plain
- Chest radiographs essential if oral mass present
- Head and neck radiographs only helpful for structural abnormalities

Contrast
- To assess swallowing function

SPECIAL TESTS

- Acetylcholine receptor antibody titre for myasthenia gravis
- Barium swallow, preferably with fluoroscopy, for functional dysphagia
- Biopsy or fine-needle aspirate of oropharyngeal masses and LNs
- CSF tap
- EMG and muscle biopsy
- Thyroid function

DYSPNOEA

DEFINITION

Respiratory distress associated with inappropriate degree of breathing effort reflected by changes in respiratory rate, rhythm and character.
- Exertional, paroxysmal or continuous.
- Orthopnoea indicates breathing difficulty whilst in a recumbent position.
- Tachypnoea refers to an increased rate of breathing but does not necessarily indicate dyspnoea.

CLINICAL SIGNS

- Coughing may indicate airway or pulmonary disease
- Cyanosis
- Increased expiratory effort (lower-airway obstruction)
- Increased inspiratory effort (upper-airway obstruction)
- Pallor suggests haemorrhage

COMMON CAUSES

Haematological disorders
- Anaemia

Lower-airway disorders
- Bronchial disease, e.g. chronic bronchitis
- Left atrial enlargement causing bronchial compression
- Tracheal collapse

Mediastinal disorders
- Neoplasia

Peritoneal cavity disorders
- Ascites (severe)
- GDV
- Pregnancy

Pleural/body wall disorders
- Diaphragmatic rupture
- Pleural effusion
- Thoracic wall trauma/pneumothorax

Pulmonary parenchymal disorders
- Allergic/immune-mediated disease, e.g. eosinophilic pneumonopathy (PIE)
- Metastatic neoplasia
- Pneumonia – inhalational, infectious, parasitic
- Pulmonary oedema
  - CNS trauma
  - Heart failure
  - Shock
  - Toxic
- Pulmonary thromboembolism (increasingly common, but probably still under-recognised), e.g. DIC, heartworm, HAC, neoplasia
- Trauma/bleeding disorder

Upper-airway disorders
Brachycephalic airway disease
(common in brachycephalic breeds)
- Stenotic nares
- Everted laryngeal saccules
- Laryngeal collapse
- Over-long soft palate
- Tracheal hypoplasia

Cervical tracheal disease
- Collapse
- Tracheal foreign body

Laryngeal disease
- Laryngeal oedema
- Laryngeal paralysis

UNCOMMON CAUSES

Haematological disorders
- Methaemoglobinaemia

Lower-airway disorders
Tracheal diseases affecting thoracic trachea
- As for cervical trachea below

Extraluminal intrathoracic tracheal and/or bronchial compression
- Heart base mass
- Lymphadenopathy

Mediastinal disorders
- Mediastinal mass
- Mediastinitis
- Pneumomediastinum

Nasal cavity obstruction
- Neoplasia
- Rhinitis – see nasal discharge, p. 51
NB Nasal cavity obstruction may cause open-mouth breathing.

Peritoneal cavity disorders
- Organomegaly/morbid obesity

Pleural/body wall disorders
- Congenital body wall disorder
- Peritoneo-pericardial diaphragmatic hernia (PPDH)
- Thoracic wall trauma/neoplasia/paralysis

Pulmonary parenchymal disorders
- Lung lobe torsion
- Non-cardiogenic pulmonary oedema, see p. 123
- Paraquat poisoning
- Primary pulmonary neoplasia

Upper-airway disorders
Cervical tracheal disease
- Tracheal hypoplasia (common in brachycephalics)
- Tracheal neoplasia very rarely
- Tracheal parasites (*Oslerus*)

Laryngeal disease
- Laryngeal neoplasia

Miscellaneous
- CNS disorder
- Fear/pain
- Metabolic acidosis
- Peripheral nerve, neuromuscular, muscular disorder

DIAGNOSTIC APPROACH

1   The over-riding concern is not to make the dyspnoea worse by investigations.
2   Check for upper-airway obstruction, and treat.
3   Characterise intrathoracic disease by imaging.

CLINICAL CLUES

Predisposition
- Brachycephalic dogs – stenotic airway syndrome
- Congenital disorders usually less than 1 year old
- Laryngeal paralysis – old, large breed dogs, especially retrievers, setters

- Metastatic pulmonary neoplasia usually older animals (haemangiosarcoma, mammary, prostatic)
- Tracheal collapse in small breed middle- to old-aged dogs

History
- Environment/geographical location, e.g. access to potentially infectious/toxic agents
- History of trauma, recent or old (undiagnosed diaphragmatic rupture)

Physical examination
Observation
- Abnormal discharges, deformities or lesions
- Airway noise suggests obstruction
- Change in voice if disease of larynx or affecting recurrent laryngeal nerve
- Orthopnoea suggests effusion or heart failure
- Pattern of dyspnoea, e.g. inspiratory versus expiratory
- Rate and rhythm of respiration
- Restrictive versus obstructive

Inspection
- Cyanosis
- Evidence of trauma
- Oculo-nasal discharges

Palpation
- Abdomen: feels 'empty' with ruptured diaphragm
- Compressibility of the cranial mediastinum (in small dogs) – loss of 'spring' can suggest a mass lesion
- Larynx/trachea
- Ribs for evidence of trauma, fractures, masses
- Thoracic wall percussion for alteration in resonance, e.g. increased with pneumothorax, decreased with thoracic fluid or consolidated tissue

Auscultation
- 'Fluid line' with effusions: increased breath sounds dorsally and muffled ventrally
- Cardiac auscultation for murmurs, tachycardia, arrhythmias
- Crackles suggest small airway disease
- Heart sounds may be muffled with pleural fluid
- Normal or abnormal breath sounds localise airway obstruction
- Wheezes suggest large-airway disease

Percussion
- Dull with pleural or pericardial effusion
- 'Fluid line' with effusions
- Hyper-resonant with pneumothorax
- Lung consolidation

LABORATORY FINDINGS

- Bacterial bronchopneumonia – may be leukocytosis, left shift and degenerate neutrophils
- Coagulation panel helpful if bleeding disorder, DIC
- Dark, brown blood with Heinz body anaemia suggests methaemoglobinaemia
- Eosinophilia may suggest parasitic disease or eosinophilic disorder
- Often within normal limits

IMAGING

- Airway disease – radiography as in Cough (see p. 20)
- Fluoroscopy to investigate dynamic airway collapse
- Nasal lesions – see nasal discharge/sneezing
- Ultrasonography to identify pulmonary/mediastinal mass lesions ± ultrasound-guided aspirate/biopsy

SPECIAL TESTS

- Angiography/nuclear perfusion studies to investigate pulmonary vascular disease
- Blood gas analysis for pulmonary thromboembolism (plus tests of coagulation function), metabolic disorders, and parenchymal diseases
- Examination of laryngeal/pharyngeal region under anaesthesia
- Exploratory thoracotomy and lung biopsy
- Radiography/bronchoscopy/bronchoalveolar lavage as for coughing if suspect airway ± pulmonary parenchymal disease
- Specific tests for parasites
- Thoracocentesis and fluid analysis (cytology ± culture)

DYSURIA

DEFINITIONS

Painful or difficult urination.
- Bladder atony frequently arises from neurological disease, but can be caused by detrusor muscle dysfunction.
- Urinary tract obstruction can be mechanical or functional (neuromuscular).
- Usually caused by inflammatory or obstructive lower-urinary tract disease.

CLINICAL SIGNS

- Dysuria may be manifested as one or a combination of:
  - haematuria: presence of blood in urine
  - pollakiuria: frequent urination (even in the absence of polyuria)
  - stranguria: slow or painful urination with increased straining

- urinary tenesmus – straining to urinate
- Oliguria is the reduced production of urine, and may be associated with dysuria
- Urinary retention: the failure of the bladder to empty completely
- Urinary incontinence may be seen if the bladder is atonic and there is urine overflow (see p. 73)

COMMON CAUSES

- Infection/inflammation
  - Cystitis/urethritis
  - Juvenile vaginitis
  - Prostatitis/prostatic abscess
- Neurological disorders causing bladder atony
  - Lower motor neurone disease
  - Upper motor neurone disease
- Obstruction
  - Benign prostatic hypertrophy
  - Neoplasia
  - Prostatic carcinoma
  - Transitional cell tumour of bladder or urethra
  - Urolithiasis
    - Cystic and/or urethral

UNCOMMON CAUSES

- Infection
  - Secondary to congenital anomaly, e.g. ectopic ureter, urachal defects
- Neurological
  - Reflex dyssynergia
- Obstruction
  - Neoplasia
    - Transmissible venereal tumour
    - Vaginal leiomyoma or leiomyosarcoma
  - Retroflexion of bladder into perineal hernia
  - Urethral stricture

- Sterile inflammation
  - Cyclophosphamide-induced cystitis
- Trauma
  - Ruptured bladder/urethra
  - Urethral stricture

DIAGNOSTIC APPROACH

1 Dysuria must be distinguished from urinary incontinence.
2 Distinguish inflammatory from obstructive disease by noting the dog's ability to pass urine and whether the bladder tends to be full or empty.
3 Urinalysis to detect inflammatory and neoplastic disease.
4 Radiographs and ultrasonography to image the lower-urinary tract, and detect urolithiasis, neoplasia and structural abnormalities.

CLINICAL CLUES

History
- Presence or absence of urination, tenesmus and haematuria

Physical examination
Observation
- Check whether dog strains to urinate, and whether it actually passes urine

Inspection
- Urine staining of perineum is more suggestive of incontinence than dysuria

Palpation
- A full bladder despite attempts to urinate indicates either an obstruction or a hypotonic bladder
- If not obstructed, the bladder can be expressed or catheterised
- Check prostate for size, symmetry, pain, and fluctuance by rectal examination

LABORATORY FINDINGS

Haematology and serum biochemistry
- Azotaemia if urinary obstruction or polyuric renal failure
- Generally unremarkable

Urinalysis
- Inflammatory sediment
- Bacteria
- Blood
- Neopastic cells
- Low urine SG suggests underlying PU/PD

IMAGING

- Pneumocystogram
- Positive contrast retrograde (vagino)-urethrogram
- Ultrasound examination of bladder and prostate

SPECIAL TESTS

- Myelogram
- Neurological examination
- Passage of urinary catheter
- Urodynamic pressure profile

EXERCISE INTOLERANCE

DEFINITION

A reduced ability to exercise.
- Decreased stamina
- Reluctance to exercise

CLINICAL SIGNS

- Muscle weakness/wasting
- Musculoskeletal pain
- Panting/tachypnoea
- Prolonged recovery from exercise
- Pyrexia
- Reduced stamina at exercise
- Reluctance to exercise

COMMON CAUSES

Cardiac disease (see Syncope p. 78)

Endocrine disease
- HAC
- Hypoadrenocorticism
- Hypothyroidism

Generalised weakness
- Anaemia
- Chronic inflammation or infection or wasting
- Drugs, e.g. anticonvulsants, antihistamines, diuretics, vasodilators, anti-arrhythmics
- Neoplasia
- Nutritional deficiency
- Obesity
- Parasitism
- Pyrexia

Metabolic disease
- Hypercalcaemia
- Hypo/hyperkalaemia
- Hypo/hyperglycaemia
- Hyponatraemia

Muscular disease
- Myopathies, e.g. Labrador retriever myopathy

Neurological/spinal disease
- Cervical spondylopathy
- Intervertebral disc protrusion
- Vestibular disease

Neuromuscular disease
• Myasthenia gravis

Respiratory disease (see Syncope p. 78)

Skeletal disease
• Cruciate ligament disease/rupture
• Degenerative joint disease

UNCOMMON CAUSES

Endocrine disease
• Diabetic ketoacidosis
• Insulinoma
• Phaeochromocytoma

Metabolic disease
• Acidosis
• Hepatic encephalopathy
• Hyperthermia (exercise-induced)
• Malignant hyperthermia

Muscular disease
• Muscular dystrophy
• Polymyositis
• Scottie cramp

Neurological/spinal disease
• Cerebellar disease
• Discospondylitis
• Fibrocartilaginous embolism
• Narcolepsy/cataplexy
• Neoplasia
• Peripheral polyneuropathies
• Spinal trauma

Skeletal disease
• Hypertrophic osteodystrophy
• Panosteitis
• Polyarthritis

DIAGNOSTIC APPROACH

1 Thorough history to discern any other clinical signs apart from exercise intolerance which itself is non-specific.
2 Complete physical examination covering all body systems.
3 Exercise test once cardiorespiratory diseases and lameness have been ruled out.

CLINICAL CLUES

• See Stiffness and joint swelling, p. 68
• See Weakness and syncope, p. 78

LABORATORY FINDINGS

• Elevated CPK/AST in muscle disease, e.g. polymyositis
• See Weakness and syncope, p. 78

IMAGING

• See Weakness and syncope, p. 78

SPECIAL TESTS

• Malignant hyperthermia – exercise test will induce hyperlactacidaemia, hyperthermia, haemoconcentration, mild respiratory alkalosis included by short period exercise (c.f. normal animals after long, strenuous exercise)
• Scottie cramp – administer serotonin antagonist to induce episode in affected dogs – give 0.3 mg/kg orally of methysergide and exercise 2 hours later
• See Section 4, Myasthenia gravis, p. 290
• See Syncope, p. 78

PRESENTING COMPLAINTS

FAECAL INCONTINENCE

DEFINITION

The involuntary passage of faecal material, due to an inability to retain faeces. The cause can be:
- Anatomical, as the result of reduced capacity or compliance of the rectum.
- Neurological sphincter mechanism incontinence.

CLINICAL SIGNS

- Dyschezia
- Haematochezia
- Involuntary passage of faeces
- Perineal staining
- Tenesmus
- Other signs of neurological deficits

COMMON CAUSES

Anal disease
- Incontinence associated with constipation
  - Perineal hernia
  - Anal sac disease
- Perianal fistulae
- Previous local surgery

Neurogenic sphincter mechanism incontinence
- Lumbosacral disease
  - Degenerative myelopathy (CDRM)
  - Disc herniation

UNCOMMON CAUSES

Neurogenic sphincter incontinence
- Congenital malformation

- Fibrocartilaginous embolism (FCE)
- Lumbosacral disease
- Polyneuropathy
- Sacrocaudal dysgenesis (brachycephalic breeds)
- Spina bifida
- Spinal trauma

Neoplasia
- Perineal, rectal or colonic

Myopathy
- Polymyopathy

DIAGNOSTIC APPROACH

1 Distinguish inappropriate defecation (e.g. improper house training) from true incontinence by observing defecation.
2 Rule out rectal/anal disease by presence of straining and physical findings.
3 Evaluate local and general neurological function if no obvious anatomical cause.

CLINICAL CLUES

Predisposition
- Lumbosacral disease and CDRM in GSD
- Perineal hernia in intact male dogs

History
- Chronic progressive with most neurological disease except FCE and trauma
- Tenesmus, dyschezia and haematochezia with local rectal/anal disease

Physical examination
Observation
- Other neurological deficits – tail carriage, proprioception, etc.

Inspection
- Perineal masses, bulges

Palpation
- Rectal examination to determine anal tone and local disease

LABORATORY FINDINGS

- Usually unremarkable

IMAGING

Radiographs
Plain
- Vertebral abnormality

Contrast
- Myelography often inadequate to image lumbosacral disease
- Epidurography and MRI scan preferred for lumbosacral disease

SPECIAL TESTS

- Electromyography
- Lumbar CSF collection
- Biopsy of masses

HAEMATEMESIS

DEFINITION

Vomiting blood. See Vomiting, p. 75. The blood is either:
- due to a generalised bleeding problem
- swallowed

or
- comes from gastric and/or upper GI ulceration.

CLINICAL SIGNS

- Epistaxis, bleeding oral lesion or coughing if swallowed blood
- Vomiting of fresh or changed blood
  - Large volumes and very fresh blood will appear bright red
  - After a few minutes in gastric acid, blood is changed and the dog will vomit brown granular material ('coffee grounds')

COMMON CAUSES

Endocrine
- Hypoadrenocorticism (not common but important)

Gastric ulceration
- NSAIDs
- Acute and chronic gastritis
- Abrasive gastric foreign body
- Gastric carcinoma
- Uraemic gastritis
- Portal hypertension in end-stage liver disease

Generalised bleeding problem – see Bleeding, p. 14

GI disease
- Acute pancreatitis
- HGE
- Parvovirus infection

PRESENTING COMPLAINTS

Swallowed blood
- Epistaxis – see Nasal discharge, pp. 51
- Oral bleeding

UNCOMMON CAUSES

Gastric ulceration
- Gastric lymphosarcoma
- Gastric leiomyoma/sarcoma
- Mast cell tumour
- Gastrinoma

Swallowed blood
- Following haemoptysis

DIAGNOSTIC APPROACH

1   Distinguish vomiting of gastric blood from swallowed blood or a generalised bleeding problem.
2   Treat symptomatically but investigate by endoscopy, etc. if severe or not improving.

CLINICAL CLUES

Predisposition
- Gastric carcinoma more common in 7- to 10-year-old Collies, Labradors, Belgian shepherd and Bull terrier

History
- Anorexia and weight loss if severe gastric ulceration, and especially if gastric carcinoma
- Diarrhoea and weight loss with gastrinoma
- Known administration of NSAIDs or exposure to infection or toxins

Physical examination
Observation
- Bleeding at other sites if generalised
- Epistaxis or oral bleeding
- 'Prayer position' if cranial abdominal pain due to ulceration

Inspection
- Skin masses (possible mast cell tumour)

Palpation
- Cranial abdominal pain in acute pancreatitis, severe gastric ulceration
- Upper GI mass

LABORATORY FINDINGS

- Anaemia and hypoproteinaemia if severe bleeding
- Microcytic anaemia if chronic bleeding and iron deficiency
- Leukocytosis if pancreatitis or peritonitis associated with incipient ulcer perforation
- Amylase/lipase unreliably elevated in acute pancreatitis

IMAGING

- As for Vomiting, p. 75

SPECIAL TESTS

- Buccal mucosal bleeding time, clotting profile
- As for Vomiting, p. 77

HAEMATOCHEZIA

DEFINITION

Presence of fresh blood in faeces.
- Usually an indicator of LI or perianal disease.
- Rarely seen with SI haemorrhage, and only if this is massive and/or rate of intestinal transit is increased.

CLINICAL SIGNS

- Abnormal stool shape/size if rectal mass
- Concurrent diarrhoea, often with mucus if colitis
- Normal stool consistency with blood on surface if rectal polyp
- Passage of bright red fresh blood

COMMON CAUSES

Anal disease
- Anal sac infection
- Perianal adenoma

Generalised bleeding disorder – see Bleeding, p. 14

Generalised GI disease
- HGE

Large intestinal disease
- Colitis
- Colonic or rectal neoplasia
- Ileo-colic intussusception
- Rectal polyps
- Rectal prolapse
- *Trichuris* whipworms

UNCOMMON CAUSES

- Anal sac adenocarcinoma
- *Ancylostoma* hookworms (rare in UK)
- Blood vessel malformation (e.g. AV fistula)
- Caecal inversion
- Foreign body
- Perianal carcinoma

DIAGNOSTIC APPROACH

1 Rule out generalised bleeding.
2 Localise problem to external anus or distal intestine.

CLINICAL CLUES

Predisposition
- Rectal prolapse most common in young dogs with colitis

History
- Absence of diarrhoea helps rule out colitis
- Spotting of blood between bowel movements indicates anal disease or lesion close to anus

Physical examination
Observation
- Dyschezia if anal sac inflammation
- Tenesmus if inflammatory or neoplastic rectal disease

Inspection
- Anal masses
- Bleeding at other sites if generalised
- Protrusion of severe ileo-colic intussusception
- Rectal prolapse

PRESENTING COMPLAINTS

Palpation
• Colonic mass

Rectal palpation
• Anal sac disease
• Rectal polyp or neoplasia

LABORATORY FINDINGS

• Haematology and serum biochemistry usually unremarkable

Faecal examination
• Culture rarely helpful

• Parasitology for whipworms and hookworms

IMAGING

• Sublumbar lymphadenopathy if metastasis from rectal tumour

SPECIAL TESTS

• Barium enema (rarely performed nowadays)
• Proctoscopy/colonoscopy

HAEMATURIA AND DISCOLOURED URINE

DEFINITION

Discoloured urine indicates a change in colour from the normal yellow-amber to red, brown or a combination of these colours.

Haematuria is the presence of blood in urine. It may be microscopic and only detected by urinalysis or cause gross discoloration.

CLINICAL SIGNS

• May be associated with dysuria (p. 36)
• Passage of abnormally coloured urine
• Signs of underlying disease
  • Dyspnoea if anaemic
  • Icterus
  • Weakness

COMMON CAUSES

Red discoloration
RBC – haematuria
• Generalised bleeding disorder
• Lower-urinary tract infection
• Neoplasia of bladder or prostate

• Oestrus
• Trauma
• Urolithiasis

Haemoglobin
• Early haemolytic anaemia

Brown/red-brown discoloration
• Haemoglobin – as above
• RBC – as above

Yellow/brown/orange discoloration
• Any cause of icterus including haemolytic anaemia, hepatic disease and posthepatic causes (see Jaundice, p. 108)
• Bilirubinuria

UNCOMMON CAUSES

Red discoloration
RBC – haematuria
• Pyelonephritis
• Renal calculi
• Renal neoplasia
• Renal infarction
• Renal cysts?

- Idiopathic renal haemorrhage
- Renal telangiectasia
- Cyclophosphamide-induced cystitis
- Vaginal or penile lesions
  - Trauma
  - Transmissible venereal tumour (TVT)
- Parasites (*Capillaria*) – not in UK

Myoglobin
- Severe muscle trauma
- Exertional rhabdomyolysis

Exogenous substances
- Food dyes
- Drugs

Brown/red-brown discoloration
Myoglobin

Methaemoglobin
- Paracetamol (acetaminophen) toxicosis

Urate crystalluria (may precipitate)
- Chronic liver disease
- Portosystemic shunt

DIAGNOSTIC APPROACH

1 Confirm presence of RBC/haemoglobin/myoglobin by urine dipstick. Check a fresh urine sample sediment for RBCs; cells may be lysed if sample is too old.
2 If haematuria is present, check for generalised bleeding, and examine external genitalia, vagina or prostate. Renal haemorrhage is more likely to cause sufficient blood loss to result in significant anaemia.
3 Haemoglobinuria suggests massive haemolysis, and a haemolytic anaemia will be present.
4 Muscle pain and weakness will be present if there is myoglobinuria. Myoglobin can be detected chemi-

cally, but elevated muscle enzymes (CK, AST) help localise the problem.
5 Significant bilirubinuria indicates icterus is present; this can be detected by clinical and serum biochemical examination. See p. 108 for diagnostic approach.

CLINICAL CLUES

History
- Consider lower-urinary tract disease if discoloured urine is accompanied by dysuria
- Exposure to drugs including cyclophosphamide or paracetamol
- Weakness, laboured breathing if anaemic

Physical examination
Inspection
- Look for pale mucous membranes, icterus

Palpation
- Hepatosplenomegaly if haemolytic jaundice
- Prostatic mass on rectal examination
- Renal mass

Auscultation
- Flow murmur if anaemic

LABORATORY FINDINGS

Haematology and serum biochemistry
- Anaemia if haemolysis, or idiopathic renal haemorrhage
- Hyperbilirubinaemia if icteric
- Inflammatory leukogram if prostatic abscess or pyelonephritis
- Raised CK and AST if myoglobinuria
- Usually unremarkable if lower-urinary tract disease

Urinalysis
- Bizarre cells – neoplasia
- RBC – haematuria
- WBC – infection, calculi

IMAGING

Radiographs
Plain
- To look for calculi, masses

Contrast
- Intravenous excretory urography
- Positive contrast retrograde (vagino)-urethrogram

Ultrasound examination
- Kidneys, bladder and prostate

SPECIAL TESTS

- Coagulation profile: see pp. 255–7
- Coombs' test
- Exploratory laparotomy and cannulation of ureters to identify renal haemorrhage
- Ultrasound-guided or transurethral catheter biopsy of prostate
- Urine culture and antibiotic sensitivity
- Vaginal cytology to confirm oestrus

HAEMOPTYSIS

DEFINITION

Coughing up blood or blood-tinged sputum.

CLINICAL SIGNS

- Coughing with blood
- Associated signs
  - Dyspnoea/tachypnoea
  - Exercise intolerance/collapse
  - Melaena if significant volume of swallowed blood

COMMON CAUSES

- Acute pulmonary oedema: frothy, bloody fluid
- Coagulopathies
- Pulmonary neoplasia
- Tracheal/bronchial foreign bodies
- Trauma/pulmonary contusions

UNCOMMON CAUSES

- Abscess
- Bacterial bronchopneumonia rarely

Parasites
- *Dirofilaria* (not yet in UK)
- Other parasites, e.g. *Angiostrongylus*, *Oslerus*

Pulmonary thromboembolism
- Increasingly common but probably still under-recognised, e.g. heartworm, HAC, DIC, neoplasia

DIAGNOSTIC APPROACH

1 Differentiate from haematemesis, gingival bleeding and nasopharyngeal bleeding.
2 Determine whether this is an upper- or lower-airway problem from signs and physical examination.
3 Investigate by radiography, laboratory analysis and endoscopy.

CLINICAL CLUES

History
- Current medication
- Heartworm status
- Known trauma
- Previous exercise intolerance to suggest cardiorespiratory disease?
- Toxin exposure
- Travel history

Physical examination
Thorough examination of:
- Cardiac and respiratory system
- Oral cavity

LABORATORY FINDINGS

Haematology
- Eosinophilia ± basophilia if parasitism
- Regenerative anaemia if chronic bleeding
- Thrombocytopenia if ITP

Serum biochemistry profile
- Usually unremarkable

Haemostatic studies
- To check for generalised bleeding problem, see pp. 255–7

IMAGING

Thoracic radiographs
- Can be normal despite severe pulmonary disease, e.g. acute trauma and PTE
- Cardiomegaly
- Cavitating lesions may appear as soft tissue entities, unless they contain any gas
- Foreign bodies
- Pleural effusion: coagulopathy or extension of pulmonary disease
- Pruning of pulmonary arteries, e.g. PTE, *Dirofilaria*
- Pulmonary contusions
- Pulmonary oedema
- Rib fractures

SPECIAL TESTS

- Blood gas analysis
- Bronchoscopy and BAL
- Cardiac investigation
- Evaluate coagulation and haemostasis
- Exploratory thoracotomy
- Faecal parasitology
- Heartworm tests
- Lung biopsy

HALITOSIS

DEFINITION

Offensive, foul-smelling breath.

COMMON CAUSES

High-protein meals
- Can produce halitosis naturally

Oral diseases/conditions
- Can predispose to bacterial proliferation in necrotic tissue or retained food particles

- Dental tartar or periodontal disease
- Food retention in lip folds, etc.
- Oral foreign body
- Oral neoplasia – beware the non-healing gingival lesion after tooth loss
- Stomatitis/pharyngitis

Oral contact with contaminated site
- Licking of impacted anal sacs, infected skin wounds, etc.

UNCOMMON CAUSES

Remote causes producing exhalation of malodorous breath
- GI disease: malabsorption, liver disease, gastritis
- Oesophageal disease: megaoesophagus with food retention
- Pulmonary disease: inhalation pneumonia, inhaled foreign body

CLINICAL SIGNS

- Offensive breath
- Retained food associated with masses, ulcers
- Oral pain may indicate periodontal disease, inflammation or neoplasia
- Coughing if inhalation pneumonia
- Vomiting and/or diarrhoea if GI disease

DIAGNOSTIC APPROACH

- As for Dysphagia, see p. 31

HEAD POSTURE ABNORMALITIES

DEFINITION

Continuous or intermittent carriage of the head in an abnormal position. If continuous there is resistance to straightening of the head on examination.
- Head turn is an abnormal head posture where the ears are on the same horizontal plane.
- Head tilt is an abnormal head posture where the ears are not on the same horizontal plane.

CLINICAL SIGNS

Head tilt
- Unilateral vestibular disease
  - Ataxia and broad-based stance
  - Nystagmus
    - horizontal or rotatory in lesions of the receptors or the vestibular nerve – does not change with head position
    - any direction, which changes with head position in lesion of vestibular nuclei and associated structures

Head turn
- Cervical pain
- Neurological deficits, e.g. circling, hemi-neglect

COMMON CAUSES

Intermittent
- Ear mites
- Oral pain
- Otitis externa/media

Continuous
Head turn
- Spasm of cervical muscles secondary to spinal cord or nerve root disease

Head tilt
- Central – brainstem or cerebellum
- Peripheral – inner ear or cranial nerve VIII

UNCOMMON CAUSES

Intermittent
- Ear laceration
- Facial injuries

DIAGNOSTIC APPROACH

1   Aim to identify underlying ear dis-
    ease which might explain the head
    tilt.
2   Usually unilateral except in congeni-
    tal anomalies and occasionally in
    inflammatory diseases.

CLINICAL CLUES

Physical examination
• Assess for facial injury or oral pain
• Complete neurological examination
  (see Section 4, Neurological System,
  Vestibular disease, for further informa-
  tion)
• Head tilt (to the side of the lesion):
  • accentuated if remove visual or tac-
    tile proprioceptive compensation

LABORATORY FINDINGS

• Likely to be unremarkable

IMAGING

Radiographs
• Lateral, AP and open-mouth views for
  the tympanic bullae to assess crudely
  for middle ear disease
• Spinal radiographs ± myelogram to assess for spinal cord compression

FURTHER INVESTIGATIONS

• CSF tap
• MRI scan
• Myringotomy

MELAENA

DEFINITION

Black tarry faeces due to the presence of
partially digested blood, either from upper
GI haemorrhage or swallowed blood.

CLINICAL SIGNS

• Dark, tarry faeces
• Haematemesis
• Signs of hypovolaemia and/or anaemia
  if severe bleeding

COMMON CAUSES

Endocrine
• Hypoadrenocorticism (not common
  but important)

Generalised bleeding problem – see Bleeding, p. 14

Gastric ulceration
• Abrasive gastric foreign body
• Acute and chronic gastritis
• Gastric carcinoma
• NSAIDs
• Portal hypertension in end stage liver
  disease
• Uraemic gastritis

Intestinal disease
• Inflammatory bowel disease

Intestinal neoplasia
• Adenocarcinoma
• Leiomyoma/sarcoma
• Lymphosarcoma

Swallowed blood
- Epistaxis
- Oral bleeding

UNCOMMON CAUSES

Gastric ulceration
- Gastric leiomyoma/sarcoma
- Gastrinoma
- Mast cell tumour

Intestinal disease
- Chronic intussusception
- GI ischaemia
  - Infarction
  - Mesenteric avulsion
  - Shock
  - Vascular malformation
  - Volvulus
- Polyps
- Severe hookworm infestation (not in UK)

Pancreatic disease
- Severe acute pancreatitis

Swallowed blood
- Haemoptysis

Severe oesophageal disease
- Neoplasia
- Oesophagitis

DIAGNOSTIC APPROACH

1 Any cause of haematemesis is likely to produce melaena, and the diagnostic approach is similar – see Haematemesis, p. 41
2 The presence of diarrhoea in association with melaena suggests intestinal disease.

NB Some medications (iron, metronidazole, tylosin, bismuth) can give faeces a dark colour. The outside of an old faecal sample will become oxidised and become darker in appearance

CLINICAL CLUES

Predisposition
- As for Haematemesis, see p. 41

History
- Diarrhoea and weight loss with intestinal disease, gastrinoma
- Epistaxis, bleeding oral lesion or coughing if swallowed blood
- Haematemesis if gastric lesion

Physical examination
- As for Haematemesis, see p. 41

Palpation
- Abdominal mass

LABORATORY FINDINGS

- Haematology and serum biochemistry as for Haematemesis, see p. 41

IMAGING

- As for Haematemesis, see p. 41

SPECIAL TESTS

Occult blood test
- Indicates presence of haemoglobin in faeces
- It cross reacts with all dietary blood, and so the dog must be on a meat-free diet for at least 72 hours before the test can be interpreted
- It is also unnecessary if there is overt melaena

NASAL DISCHARGE

DEFINITION

An increase in the volume of nasal secretion produced, so that it drains from the external nares. The nature of the discharge can be:
- Haemorrhagic (epistaxis)
- Mucoid
- Purulent
- Serous

or a combination of these types.

CLINICAL SIGNS

- Epistaxis – bleeding from the nose
- Nasal/facial bone distortion or pain
- Nasal planum erosion/depigmentation
- Discharge often not appreciated as animal licks it away
- Reduced air flow – check each nostril for unilateral or bilateral disease
- Sneezing
- Stertor (snoring) – noise arising from turbulent airflow in nose or nasopharynx
- Unilateral/bilateral nasal discharge

Associated signs
- Atrophy temporal/masseter muscles
- Coughing/gagging or retching
- Difficulty prehending/masticating food
- Facial irritation/pawing at face
- Ocular discharge

COMMON CAUSES

Unilateral
- Foreign body
- Neoplasia
- Inflammatory (rhinitis)
- Oronasal fistula

Bilateral/unilateral
- Bleeding disorder/coagulopathy, especially:
  - Anticoagulant poisoning
  - Thrombocytopenia
- Infectious/inflammatory disease (viral, secondary bacterial infection)
- Allergic/hyperplastic rhinitis
- Mycotic (Aspergillosis)
- Trauma

UNCOMMON CAUSES

- Bleeding disorder/coagulopathy, especially:
  - DIC
  - Ehrlichiosis
  - Hyperviscosity syndrome
  - von Willebrand disease
- Cleft palate
- Dental disease
- Intranasal parasites
- Oesophageal disease
  - Megaoesophagus and aspiration pneumonia
  - Oesophageal stricture
- Pneumonia

DIAGNOSTIC APPROACH

1 Identify nature of nasal discharge.
2 Localise to one or both nasal chambers.
3 Rule out dental and oesophageal disease or generalised bleeding problem.
4 Radiograph nose under GA.
5 Anterograde nasal endoscopy and retrograde nasopharyngoscopy.
6 Nasal flushings for cytology and/or nasal biopsy.

NB Culture from nasal cavity rarely identifies a primary cause.

PRESENTING COMPLAINTS

PRESENTING COMPLAINTS

CLINICAL CLUES

Predisposition
- Brachycephalic dogs have increased risk of upper-respiratory tract disease
- Congenital lesions in young animals
- Hyperplastic rhinitis associated with Irish Wolfhound
- Neoplasia and dental disease in older dogs

History
- Environment
- Onset, duration and type nasal discharge
- Previous skull trauma/surgery?
- Response to therapy
- Sneezing/reverse sneezing – onset and duration
- Unilateral/bilateral

Physical examination
Observation
- Facial distortion
- Nature of nasal discharge – mucoid, mucopurulent, haemorrhagic
- Ocular discharge
- Unilateral/bilateral

Inspection
- Facial pain
- Nasal planum for discharge/depigmentation/erosion
- Reduced air flow
  - Look for condensation on cool glass slide or listen/feel for air flow from each nostril with the other occluded; observe movement of cotton wool
- Thorough oro-nasal examination particularly hard palate (for defects, e.g. cleft palate), soft palate and periodontal area and the oral mucosa

Palpation
- Nasal/sinus regions/oral cavity for distortion/swelling/pain

Auscultation
- Thoracic airway auscultation for signs of lower-airway disease

LABORATORY FINDINGS

- May help to identify systemic diseases causing nasal discharge
- Rarely any specific abnormalities

IMAGING

Plain radiographic views
- Open-mouth DV
  - Good nasal turbinate detail, view maxillary sinuses and identify disease side
- Intra-oral (non-screen film) gives good detail of turbinates and maxillary sinuses. Aids in localising disease to a side of the nasal chamber
- Rostro-caudal (sky-line) radiograph – localises disease affecting the frontal sinuses, e.g. filling or bony defects
- Oblique views are helpful to view teeth roots

Radiographic changes
Increased density
- Infection
- Neoplasia
- Granuloma
- Foreign body
- Blood

Decreased density
- Turbinate destruction
  - *Aspergillus*/fungal rhinitis
  - Chronic dental disease
  - Tooth root lysis

CT or MRI scans
- To identify the mass
- To assess the extent of invasion

SPECIAL TESTS

- *Aspergillus* serology (and other fungal diseases)
- Coagulation profile if epistaxis with no specific nasal explanation
- Nasal bacterial and fungal cultures – difficult to interpret because of commensal organisms
- Nasal cytology – useful for some neoplasia (e.g. lymphosarcoma) and some fungal diseases
- Nasal flushing, catching fluid in the pharynx
- Nasal biopsy: to biopsy, use small pinch biopsy forceps or catheter biopsy (suction through side holes of polyethylene catheter). NEVER go past the level of the medial canthus
- Rhinoscopy – anterior and posterior
- Rhinotomy – last resort

PAIN

DEFINITION

The sensation of discomfort caused by stimulation of special nerve fibres. General stimuli for pain are heat, ischaemia, inflammation, chemicals, trauma and mechanical forces. Pain may be generalised or localised.

CLINICAL SIGNS

- Aggression
- Decreased activity
- Inappetence
- Lame or stiff and hunched up
- Tachycardia
- Tachypnoea
- Whining
- Yelping when moving or being moved
- Other clinical signs are related to the cause and site of pain
- Associated signs
  - Pyrexia with infectious/inflammatory disease

COMMON CAUSES

Generalised
- Meningitis
- Polyarthritis

Localised
Abdominal pain (See p. 3)

Anorectal pain
- Anal or rectal stricture
- Anal sac impaction, abscess
- Constipation/obstipation – see p. 18
- Perianal fistula

Cutaneous/subcutaneous pain
- Cellulitis
- Foreign body
- Trauma

Head/oral pain
See also Dysphagia p. 31
- Neoplasia
- Otitis (especially aural foreign body)
- Temporal myositis
- Trauma

Limb pain
- Hip dysplasia
- Osteoarthritis
- Osteochondrosis
- Trauma

Spinal pain
- Discospondylitis
- Intervertebral disc disease
- Lumbosacral instability

PRESENTING COMPLAINTS

UNCOMMON CAUSES

Generalised
- Pansteatitis
- Polymyositis
- Polyneuritis

Localised
Cutaneous/subcutaneous pain
- Immune-mediated erosive/ulcerative diseases
- Panniculitis

Head pain
- CNS disease

Limb pain
- Hypertrophic osteopathy
- Metaphyseal osteopathy
- Multiple myeloma
- Myositis
- Nerve compression
- Osteomyelitis
- Osteosarcoma
- Panosteitis
- Thrombosis

Muscular pain
- Exertional myopathy in greyhounds

Spinal pain
- Atlanto-axial instability
- Cervical vertebral instability
- Meningitis
- Neoplasia

Thoracic pain
- Oesophagitis
- Pericarditis
- Pleural effusion
- Pulmonary thromboembolism
- Tracheobronchitis

DIAGNOSTIC APPROACH

1   Localise pain.
2   Investigate local disease by appropriate combination of physical examination, laboratory tests, imaging, biopsy, etc. depending on site and cause of pain.

CLINICAL CLUES

Predisposition
- Metaphyseal osteopathy in growing dogs
- Hip dysplasia in large breed dogs
- Legg-Perthe's disease in toy breed dogs
- Panosteitis in large breed dogs during adolescence

History
- Known trauma

Physical examination
Localisation of pain
- Heat
- Swelling
- Decreased joint mobility

LABORATORY FINDINGS

- Inflammatory leukogram if generalised inflammatory disease

IMAGING

- Joint swelling
- Specific bone and soft tissue changes

SPECIAL TESTS

- CSF tap
- EMG
- Nerve/muscle biopsy

POLYPHAGIA

DEFINITION

Eating in excess of normal caloric needs, either in response to a physiological or pathological increase in energy expenditure, or to a failure to absorb sufficient energy despite increased intake.

CLINICAL SIGNS

- Coprophagia (ingestion of faeces) and pica (bizarre intake) can be considered forms of polyphagia
- Increased appetite and even scavenging

COMMON CAUSES

Drugs
- Anticonvulsants
- Glucocorticoids

Endocrine disease
- Diabetes mellitus
- HAC

Gluttony
- Boredom
- Competition

Malabsorption
- Exocrine pancreatic insufficiency
- Intestinal malabsorption

Physiological
- Cold environment
- Increased exercise
- Lactation
- Poor-quality food
- Pregnancy

UNCOMMON CAUSES

Metabolic
- Acromegaly
- Hyperthyroidism (very rarely functional tumour; more commonly iatrogenic)
- Insulinoma (mild increase in appetite)

Drugs
- Amitraz
- Benzodiazepines
- Progestagens

Psychogenic
- Destruction of satiety centre in hypothalamus (neoplasia, trauma)

DIAGNOSTIC APPROACH

1   If there is weight loss, first consider malabsorption, especially if diarrhoea is present.
2   If there is weight gain ± PU/PD, consider endocrinopathy.

CLINICAL CLUES

Predisposition
- EPI and SIBO in GSD

History
- Coprophagia is seen most frequently in EPI and SIBO
- Increased appetite and thirst in diabetes mellitus and HAC
- Ravenous appetite typical of EPI and benign causes of malabsorption

Associated signs
- Diarrhoea and weight loss
  - EPI and malabsorption

PRESENTING COMPLAINTS

- Physiological stress (exercise, lactation), poor diet
- PU/PD
  - HAC, diabetes mellitus
- PU/PD, vomiting and diarrhoea, weight loss, tachycardia
  - Hyperthyroidism
- Weakness, lethargy and seizures
  - Insulinoma
- Weight gain
  - Overeating
  - Hypothyroidism
  - HAC
  - Insulinoma
- Weight loss
  - EPI
  - Malabsorption
  - Hyperthyroidism

Physical examination
- Normal if behavioural or physiological
- Weight gain or weight loss

Observation
- Emaciation if EPI or severe/prolonged malabsorption
- Pot belly and hair loss in hyperadrenocorticism

Inspection
- Thin skin, secondary pyoderma and comedones in HAC

Palpation
- Abnormal body condition
- Thyroid mass if hyperthyroid

LABORATORY FINDINGS

- Hypercholesterolaemia and high ALP in HAC
- Hyperglycaemia and glycosuria in diabetes mellitus
- Hypoglycaemia in insulinoma

IMAGING

- Hepatomegaly in endocrinopathy

SPECIAL TESTS

- Dynamic cortisol testing
- Folate/cobalamin for malabsorption
- Intestinal biopsies
- Serum insulin
- Serum T4
- TLI test for EPI

POLYURIA/POLYDIPSIA (PU/PD)

DEFINITION

- Polydipsia (PD) is a daily fluid intake of greater than 100 ml/kg/day.
- Polyuria (PU) is a daily urine output of greater than 50 ml/kg/day.
- Most common is primary polyuria and secondary polydipsia.

CLINICAL SIGNS

- Excessive fluid intake or urine output
- Nocturia is inappropriate urination at night that usually reflects PU/PD
- Differentiate from urinary incontinence/increased frequency of urination (pollakiuria)
- PU/PD may be the only clinical sign
- Other signs depend on cause of PU/PD

COMMON CAUSES

Primary polydipsia
- Fever
- Hepatic encephalopathy

Primary polyuria
Osmotic diuresis
- Diabetes mellitus
- Diuretic administration
- Fluid administration

Renal insensitivity to ADH = nephrogenic diabetes insipidus (NDI)
- Secondary NDI
  - Glucocorticoid administration
  - Hepatic disease (hepatoencephalopathy)
  - HAC
  - Hypercalcaemia
  - Hypoadrenocorticism
  - Pyometra
  - Renal insufficiency/failure

UNCOMMON CAUSES

Primary polydipsia
- Acromegaly
- Exocrine pancreatic insufficiency/malabsorption (polydipsia noted occasionally)
- Neurological – lesion in the thirst centre of the hypothalamus
- Pain
- Psychogenic

Primary polyuria
ADH deficiency = central diabetes insipidus (CDI)
- Idiopathic
  - Congenital
  - Neoplastic
  - Trauma-induced

Renal insensitivity to ADH
- Primary NDI

- Secondary NDI
  - Drugs
  - Hyperviscosity syndrome
  - Hypokalaemia
  - Pyelonephritis
  - Renal medullary solute washout (?)

Osmotic diuresis
- Primary renal glucosuria
- Fanconi's syndrome
- Post-obstructive diuresis

DIAGNOSTIC APPROACH

1 Confirm PU/PD by measuring water intake and urine SG.
2 Rule out pyometra by history, physical examination, laboratory results and imaging.
3 Serum biochemistry to rule out renal disease, hypercalcaemia and diabetes mellitus.
4 Dynamic cortisol testing for HAC.
5 Water deprivation test (see p. 232) only when safe, i.e. *after* ruling out the above.

CLINICAL CLUES

Predisposition
- CDI generally reported in middle-aged animals
- HAC most common in middle-aged dogs
- Hypercalcaemia is commonly reported as part of paraneoplastic syndrome, e.g. lymphosarcoma
- Primary NDI is a congenital disease with animals presenting at a young age
- Primary renal glycosuria reported in 1- to 6-year-old Basenji, Norwegian elkhound, Shetland sheepdog and Schnauzers
- Pyometra reported in bitches at 1–3 months post oestrus

History

- Differentiate polyuria from urinary incontinence or pollakiuria
- Females – oestrus activity – when was the last season?
- Is it appropriate polydipsia?
  - Environmental changes in temperature
  - Change in diet from moist to dry will increase water intake
- Owner should quantify the polydipsia – difficult in multi-animal households, this must be done in normal environment without external stresses
- Other clinical signs noticed by the owner suggesting any organ involvement
- Polyphagia in HAC and EPI

Physical examination

Observation
- Behavioural abnormalities, e.g. hepatic encephalopathy, pituitary neoplasms
- Body condition
- Dermatological changes, e.g. alopecia with HAC
- Panting – HAC

Inspection
- Eyes
  - Cataracts – diabetes mellitus
  - Jaundice – hepatic disease
  - Corneal lipidosis – HAC
  - Papilloedema – pituitary neoplasm
  - Retinal vessel tortuosity – hyperviscosity syndrome
- External genitalia for discharge, e.g. pyometra
- Mucous membranes
- Oral cavity – ulceration/stomatitis secondary to uraemia
- Skin/hair coat for thin skin, comedones, hair loss in HAC

Palpation
- Lymph nodes for enlargement, e.g. lymphosarcoma
- Anal sac, mammary glands, thyroid gland area (parathyroid tumour) for masses – hypercalcaemia can be associated [paraneoplastic syndrome]
- Hepatomegaly – diabetes mellitus, hyperadrenocorticism, some liver diseases
- Kidneys – not usually easy to palpate in the dog – if enlarged, consider neoplasia, pyelonephritis, portosystemic shunt (PSS)
- Uterine enlargement – pyometra

Auscultation
- Tachycardia with toxaemia, dehydration
- Bradycardia with hyperkalaemia secondary to renal failure or hypoadrenocorticism

LABORATORY FINDINGS

Haematology

- Neutrophilia with left shift – pyometra ± pyelonephritis
- Neutrophilia, eosinopenia, lymphopenia – stress leukogram in HAC
- Neutropenia, eosinophilia, lymphocytosis in hypoadrenocorticism
- Non-regenerative anaemia – chronic renal failure, hypoadrenocorticism, hepatic disease
- Polycythaemia – hyperviscosity syndrome (distinguish from dehydration elevating PCV)
- In association with hypercalcaemia, look for any signs of lymphoma, e.g. circulating lymphoblasts

Serum biochemistry

- Albumin
  - Decreased with liver disease, nephrotic syndrome
  - Increased with dehydration
- Globulin
  - Increased with hyperviscosity syndrome, liver disease

- Creatinine and urea
  - Increased with chronic renal failure, severe dehydration, hypoadrenocorticism, hypercalcaemia
- Urea
  - Decreased with liver disease
- Phosphate
  - Decreased with primary hyperparathyroidism, malignancy associated hypercalcaemia
  - Increased with chronic renal disease, vitamin D toxicosis, severe dehydration, hypoadrenocorticism
- Calcium
  - Decreased with chronic renal failure, hypoalbuminaemia
  - Increased with malignancy, hypoadrenocorticism, primary hyperparathyroidism, vitamin D toxicosis, chronic renal failure (especially juvenile nephropathy)
- Alkaline phosphatase
  - Increased with HAC, liver disease
- Alanine aminotransferase
  - Increased with liver disease, toxaemia, e.g. pyometra
- Total bilirubin
  - Increased with liver disease
- Cholesterol
  - Increased with HAC, DM, liver disease, nephrotic syndrome
- Glucose
  - Increased with DM, acromegaly, HAC
- Potassium
  - Decreased with post-obstructional diuresis, diuretic administration, diabetes mellitus
  - Increased with chronic renal failure, hypoadrenocorticism, severe diabetic ketoacidosis
- Sodium and chloride
  - Decreased with hypoadrenocorticism, ketoacidotic diabetic, (psychogenic polydipsia)

- Increased with primary nephrogenic diabetes insipidus, central diabetes insipidus, dehydration

Urinalysis
- Urine SG:
  - If SG > 1.030, the dog is not likely to have a concentrating defect; the polydipsia is to replace non-renal losses
  - If SG is 1.008 to 1.012 (isosthenuria, i.e. same osmolality as plasma) and the dog is dehydrated, suggests severe impairment of renal concentrating ability
  - If SG < 1.007 (hyposthenuria) implies tubular function is present as urine is being actively diluted
- Urine chemistry analysis, e.g. glucose, ketones, excessive bilirubin, protein
- Sediment analysis
- Urine culture
- Urine protein:creatinine ratio to quantify proteinuria

IMAGING

Radiographs
Abdominal radiographs
- Abnormal soft tissue masses, e.g. enlarged adrenal glands, spleen, mesenteric/sublumbar lymph nodes
- Liver size
  - Decreased with chronic liver diseases, PSS (± renomegaly) – see p. 114
  - Increased with diabetes mellitus, HAC or infiltrative disease – see p. 103
- Renal size
  - Decreased with chronic interstitial nephritis, juvenile nephropathy
  - Increased with pyelonephritis, congenital PSS, neoplasia, amyloidosis
- Uterine enlargement suggests pyometra

PRESENTING COMPLAINTS

Thoracic radiographs
- Mediastinal lymph node involvement if hypercalcaemic

Ultrasonography
- Assess renal, hepatic, adrenal tissues, etc.

SPECIAL TESTS

- Amino acid quantification in urine for identification of tubular disease, e.g. Fanconi's.
- Bone marrow aspirate in hypercalcaemic cases with no identifying cause.
- Measurement of plasma ADH – not readily available.

- Modified water deprivation test – never perform in azotaemic animals. It is advisable to completely rule out HAC before performing this test (see p. 232).
- Parathyroid hormone assay (PTH) if hypercalcaemic.
- Rule out hyperadrenocorticism: urine cortisol:creatinine ratio, ACTH stimulation test. If suggestive of hyperadrenocorticism further tests: low-dose dexamethasone suppression test, high-dose dexamethasone suppression test, endogenous ACTH.
- Tissue biopsy, e.g. liver, kidney, lymph node.
- Urine and plasma osmolality: osmolality is not affected by particle size, unlike the SG.

PRURITUS

DEFINITION

Itching: the sensation that elicits the desire to scratch.

CLINICAL SIGNS

- Visible signs are the end-result of persistent scratching
  - Alopecia
  - Erythema
  - Excoriation
  - Lichenification

COMMON CAUSES

- Acral lick
- Atopy (inhaled allergens)
- Demodectic mange
- Dermatophytosis
- Fleas and flea allergic dermatitis
- *Malassezia* infection

- Pyoderma
- Sarcoptic mange

UNCOMMON CAUSES

- *Cheyletiella*
- Contact dermatitis
- Drug eruptions
- Endoparasitic migration (*Uncinaria*)
- Food allergy
- Harvest mites
- Lice
- Psychogenic

DIAGNOSTIC APPROACH

1 Identification of infectious agents by sellotape strips, skin scrapes, hair plucks, and bacterial and fungal cultures.
2 After ruling out infectious causes, and trial therapy for bacterial pyo-

derma, fleas and possibly also for *Sarcoptes*, is acceptable.

3 Intradermal skin testing is performed to identify atopic reactions.

4 If negative, an exclusion food trial is indicated.

CLINICAL CLUES

Predisposition
- Infectious disease in young dogs
- Atopy in WHWT
- Demodecosis in short-haired breeds, especially Sharpei, Bull terrier

History
- Contact with infected animals
- Quality of flea control
- Owner with pruritus is suggestive of fleas, *Sarcoptes*, *Cheyletiella*, dermatophytosis

Physical examination
Observation
- Pruritic animals will scratch spontaneously, or the scratch reflex may be stimulated. The pinnae are often particularly sensitive in *Sarcoptes* infection

Inspection
- Excoriations, erythema, alopecia and lichenification
- Presence of fleas or flea dirt
- Lesions secondary to self-trauma – erythema, excoriation, lichenification, hyperpigmentation

Palpation
- Thickened skin in areas of repeated self-trauma

Distribution of lesions
- Symmetric lesions involving:
  - Lumbosacral areas and thighs suggests fleas
  - Ear margins and elbows with sarcoptic mange
  - Face, feet and ventrum with atopy
  - Feet and ventrum with contact allergy
  - Face, ears and feet with food allergy
  - Face, ears, feet or multifocal with demodecosis
  - Face, feet, mucocutaneous junctions with autoimmune skin disease

LABORATORY FINDINGS

- Blood tests usually unremarkable
  - Eosinophilia may be present in allergic skin disease
- Sellotape strips – *Cheyletiella* and *Malassezia*
- Skin scrapes – *Sarcoptes*, *Demodex*
- Hair plucks – *Demodex*, ringworm
- Bacterial and fungal cultures

SPECIAL TESTS

- Exclusion diet trial
- Intradermal skin tests
- In-vitro allergy testing
- Skin biopsy

REGURGITATION

DEFINITION

Passive expulsion of saliva/ingesta from the oesophagus. It is exclusively a sign of oesophageal disease.

CLINICAL SIGNS

- It is essential to distinguish regurgitation from dysphagia and vomiting
- Food prehension, chewing and swallowing are normal

- Food is returned passively with no abdominal heave
- Food may be tubular in shape and should not be acidic or contain bile unless there is preceding gastro-oesophageal reflux
- Cachexia may develop in chronically malnourished cases
- Dog is usually keen to re-eat food unless there is pain on swallowing (e.g. oesophagitis)
- Pseudoptyalism occurs through inability to swallow saliva
- Secondary signs may develop from inhalation of inadequately swallowed food
  - Coughing (inhalation)
  - Halitosis
  - Nasal discharge

COMMON CAUSES

Intraluminal obstruction
- Foreign body

Megaoesophagus
- Focal myasthenia gravis
- Idiopathic

Oesophagitis
Gastric reflux
- Acute and persistent vomiting
- During anaesthesia
- Spontaneous reflux oesophagitis

Ingestion
- Foreign bodies

UNCOMMON CAUSES

Extraluminal obstruction
- Anterior mediastinal mass
- Persistent right aortic arch

Intraluminal obstruction
- Stricture

Oesophagitis
Ingestion
- Caustics
- Hot liquids and food
- Irritants

Gastric reflux
- Hiatal hernia

Mural disease
- Diverticulum
- Gastro-oesophageal intussusception
- Hiatal hernia
- Primary neoplasia
- *Spirocerca lupi* granuloma

Secondary causes of megaoesophagus
Myopathies
- Dermatomyositis
- Dystrophin deficiency
- Polymyositis
- Systemic lupus erythematosus (SLE)
- Toxoplasmosis

Neuropathies/junctionopathies
- Bilateral vagal damage
- Brainstem disease
  - Hydrocephalus
  - Meningoencephalitis
- Botulism
- Dysautonomia (rare in dogs)
- Giant axonal neuropathy
- Polyradiculoneuritis
- Tick paralysis

Toxins
- Anticholinesterase
- Acrylamide
- Lead
- Thallium

Miscellaneous
- Distemper

- Glycogen storage disease Type II
- Hypoadrenocorticism
- Hypothyroidism?
- Thymoma
- Toxoplasmosis

DIAGNOSTIC APPROACH

1   Distinguish regurgitation from vomiting
2   Investigate first by:
    - plain radiographs and/or
    - endoscopy
3   Fluoroscopic assessment of swallowing motion

CLINICAL CLUES

Predisposition
- Gastro-oesophageal intussusception in Shar pei breed
- Idiopathic megaoesophagus is most common in GSD, Great Dane and Irish setter
- Persistent right aortic arch is most common in GSD, Great Dane and Irish setter and signs appear at weaning

History
- A recent history of ingestion of caustics or a GA (with presumed reflux) may precede oesophagitis or stricture.
- Regurgitation may occur immediately after eating or hours later depending on whether the oesophagus is inflamed or dilated.

Physical examination
Observation
- Depressed and dyspnoeic if inhalation pneumonia is present
- Halitosis if retention of food in megaoesophagus or inhalation pneumonia
- May regurgitate and re-eat food

Inspection
- Nasal discharge and coughing if inhalation present
- A dilated oesophagus may occasionally be seen ballooning in the left cervical area

Palpation
- Gag reflex may be absent if pharynx also affected

Auscultation
- May hear food/liquid slopping in dilated oesophagus
- Moist lung sounds if inhalation pneumonia
- Normal heart sounds with PRAA

LABORATORY FINDINGS

Haematology
- Usually mild inflammatory leukogram with inhalation pneumonia

Serum biochemistry
- Usually unremarkable

IMAGING

Radiographs
Plain
Plain radiographs of conscious dog to show:
- Radio-dense foreign body
- Dilated, gas-filled oesophagus in megaoesophagus
NB Beware of over-interpretation of passive dilatation under GA.

Contrast – Barium swallow
After plain films, to show:
- Radiolucent foreign body
- Stricture

PRESENTING COMPLAINTS

SPECIAL TESTS

- Acetylcholine receptor antibody titre for focal myasthenia gravis

- Anti-nuclear antibody for SLE
- Creatine kinase for polymyositis
- Manometry
- Oesophagoscopy
- Thyroid function tests

SEIZURES

DEFINITION

Clinical manifestation of an excessive, paroxysmal discharge of hyperexcitable cerebrocortical neurones.
- Epilepsy is any non-progressive intracranial disorder that induces recurrent seizure activity
- Generalised seizures
  - Widespread onset within both cerebral hemispheres
  - Loss of consciousness, recumbency and general motor signs
- Partial seizures
  - Focal onset in one cerebral hemisphere and limited spread to the rest of the brain
  - Simple, partial seizures do not have alteration in consciousness

CLINICAL SIGNS

Generalised tonic-clonic seizures
1 May be able to identify a prodromal phase
   - Can last from minutes to days before ictus (fit)
   - May have change in behaviour, vocalisation, restlessness, etc.
2 Loss of consciousness
   - Pupils are fixed and dilated, jaws can be open or closed
3 Tonic phase with increased muscle tone – dog will fall to its side
   - Symmetrical orofacial movements may precede the tonic phase

4 Clonic phase with intense muscle jerking
   - During clonic phase there may be violent jaw movements, excessive salivation, involuntary urination or defecation
   - Following clonic phase, walking or running movements can be seen
5 Postictal phase
   - Dog remains lying down or in a deep sleep for a period of time
   - Dog usually stands after a few minutes, but is disorientated and unresponsive
   - Bewilderment and may appear blind and/or deaf
   - Normalises, but often extremely hungry or thirsty

Partial seizures
- Simple partial seizures – motor signs predominate with twitching of individual muscle groups, tonus or clonus of an individual limb or turning of the head.
- Complex partial seizures accompanied by loss of consciousness, pupils may dilate, often facial muscle twitching and behavioural alteration.

Other seizures
- For absence seizures, myoclonic, clonic or tonic seizures, consult more specific texts

COMMON CAUSES

Intracranial
- Idiopathic epilepsy (diagnosis by exclusion of other causes)
- Inflammatory, e.g. encephalitis, meningitis
- Neoplasia
- Trauma

Extracranial
- Hypoglycaemia
  - Exogenous insulin overdose
- Liver disease (hepatic encephalopathy)

UNCOMMON CAUSES

Intracranial
- Congenital malformations, e.g. hydrocephalus
- Degenerative conditions, e.g. storage diseases
- Cerebral infarction
- Nutritional disorders
- Toxicoses, e.g. lead, organophosphate poisoning

Extracranial
- Hypocalcaemia
- Hypoglycaemia
  - Hepatoma
  - Insulinoma
  - Leiomyoma/myosarcoma, secreting insulin-like substance
- Renal disease (uraemic encephalopathy)
- Hyperlipoproteinaemia
- Hyperthermia

DIAGNOSTIC APPROACH

1 Distinguish intracranial and extracranial causes of seizures by laboratory testing.
2 Full neurological examination.
3 Neurological examination will be normal in inter-ictal phase with idiopathic epilepsy.

CLINICAL CLUES

Predisposition
- Epilepsy inheritance proven in Beagle
- Hypoglycaemia – cause of seizures in juvenile toy breeds or hunting dogs
- Hydrocephalus prevalent in toy/brachycephalic breeds
- Idiopathic epileptics should have the first seizure between 6 months and 5 years
- Increased incidence of idiopathic epilepsy in the following breeds – Golden retriever, Irish setter, Saint Bernard, German Shepherd, American cocker spaniel, Wirehaired fox terrier, Alaskan malamute, Siberian Husky and Miniature poodles
- No apparent sex predilection for idiopathic epilepsy
  - Except higher incidence of epilepsy seen in male GSD in the UK
  - Increased severity of seizures seen in females during oestrus or pregnancy
- Suggestion of genetic predisposition in other breeds, e.g. Belgian Shepherd dog, GSD, Keeshond, Collie dogs

History
- Seizure history
  - Age at onset: idiopathic epilepsy usually 6 to 36 months of age
  - Seizure character – good description from the owner is essential
  - Initial seizure frequency
- Vaccination history: possibility of prior CDV infection
- Previous illness/injuries/trauma
- If very young puppy – were there problems with the birth?
- Current frequency of seizures, duration, etc.

- Dog's behaviour between seizures: normal in idiopathic epilepsy
- Is there a relationship between feeding and seizure activity?
- Any toxic access, e.g. lead paint, metaldehyde, ethylene glycol?
- Family history of seizures?

Physical examination
Observation
- Gait
- Mentation

Inspection
- All body systems for evidence of disease
- Neurological examination
  - Idiopathic epilepsy: dogs are neurologically normal between seizures (leave a few days between last seizure and examination)
  - Dogs with CNS disease (inflammation, neoplasia) and metabolic causes of seizures may not have other neurological abnormalities
- Ophthalmological examination including retinal examination
  - Lesions consistent with chorioretinitis, e.g. viral, fungal, protozoal CNS infection
  - Papilloedema from increased intracranial pressure with congenital or acquired hydrocephalus, neoplasia or CNS inflammation
  - Differentiate pseudopapilloedema seen normally in some breeds (e.g. Collies) from true papilloedema

Palpation
- Skull for deformities associated with trauma, tumours, congenital defects, e.g. open fontanelle (hydrocephalus)

Auscultation
- Thorough cardiac auscultation should be performed. It is sometimes not possible based on the owner's description of episodes to conclusively identify seizure versus syncope. Serious arrhythmias could cause severe hypoxia and seizure activity might result.
- With primary neurological disease no abnormalities would be expected.

LABORATORY FINDINGS

Haematology
- Probably normal with intracranial disease
- Specific changes related to specific extracranial causes

Serum biochemistry to assess extracranial, metabolic or systemic causes
- Azotaemia
- Blood electrolytes
- Cholesterol/triglycerides
- Dynamic bile acid assay
- Hypocalcaemia
- Hypoglycaemia
- Liver enzymes (ALT, ALP)

Faecal examination
- In puppies – heavy intestinal parasite burdens have been associated with seizures

IMAGING

Plain radiographs
- Abdominal radiograph to assess organ disease or for the presence of lead-containing objects
- Skull radiographs if suspect cranial trauma. (NB Seizures can start years after the traumatic episode)
- Thoracic radiographs to assess for cardiac or respiratory disease and metastases i.e. metastases from primary CNS tumour or metastasis to both CNS and lungs

Abdominal ultrasound
- If hepatic/renal or metabolic causes of the seizures are suspected

SPECIAL TESTS

- Blood lead quantification
- CSF analysis – cytology, protein quantification, bacterial (mycotic) culture
- CT or MRI scans for specific anatomical information

- EEG (not routinely available)
- Infectious disease titres, e.g. canine distemper, *Cryptococcus* on CSF
- Portovenography/rectal scintigraphy to confirm the presence of portal vascular anomalies
- Serum titres for toxoplasmosis, neosporosis
- Stereotactic-guided brain biopsy (not currently available in the UK)

SNEEZING

DEFINITION

Sneezing is an involuntary airway protective reflex (like coughing), propelling air at high velocity through the nasal chambers. It is initiated via stimulation of subepithelial receptors.

Reverse sneezing is associated with violent, paroxysmal inspiratory efforts attempting to move secretions/debris from nasopharynx into oropharynx to allow swallowing.

CLINICAL SIGNS

- Sneezing
  - Intermittent
  - Paroxysmal
  - Continuous
- See Nasal discharge, p. 51

COMMON CAUSES

Expiratory – sinus/intranasal disease
- Infectious/inflammatory – see Nasal discharge, p. 51
- Neoplasia

Inspiratory – reverse sneeze
- Normal
- Nasopharyngeal disease, e.g. foreign body

UNCOMMON CAUSES

Expiratory – sinus/intranasal disease
- Dental disease
- Parasites

Inspiratory – reverse sneeze
Nasopharyngeal disease
- Parasites (not currently in the UK)
- Airborne irritant

Sinus disease

DIAGNOSTIC APPROACH

- As for Nasal discharge, see p. 51

STIFFNESS AND JOINT SWELLING

DEFINITION

An abnormality of the gait which manifests as restricted movement or a reluctance to rise after rest/lying down. Joint swelling/heat/pain may not be obvious.

CLINICAL SIGNS

- Pain – see p. 53.
- Degenerative joint disease (DJD) – should be limited to orthopaedic signs.
- Erosive polyarthritis particularly affects the distal weight-bearing joints, e.g. carpus, tarsus. Can be migratory/shifting. Pain on rising and walking, localised hot painful swellings over joints/periarticular tissue. Accompanied by pain, pyrexia, malaise, lymphadenopathy and muscle wasting.
- Immune-mediated polyarthritis generally accompanied by systemic signs, e.g. pyrexia, malaise, leukocytosis, and may be associated with other systemic immunologically mediated disease.
- Non-erosive polyarthritis – pyrexia, malaise, stiff/stilted gait, anorexia, lameness/weakness. May be associated with SLE, so look for concurrent disease, e.g. anaemia, glomerulonephritis, mucocutaneous lesions.

COMMON CAUSES

- Osteoarthritis
  - Immune-mediated (non-septic) joint disease
    - Non-erosive (idiopathic, drug-induced)
  - Non-inflammatory DJD
- Joint disease
- Spinal disease

UNCOMMON CAUSES

- Osteoarthritis
  - Infectious (septic) joint disease
  - Immune-mediated (non-septic) joint disease
    - Erosive
- Myasthenia gravis (usually weakness, but confusion from abnormal gait)
- Polymyositis

DIAGNOSTIC APPROACH

1   Determine if any pain is articular or muscular in origin.
2   Localised or generalised arthritis.
3   Investigate arthritis by:
- Imaging
- Joint tap

CLINICAL CLUES

Predisposition

- Doberman receiving potentiated sulphonamides are at risk of developing drug-induced immune mediated disease, particularly polyarthritis.
- Erosive polyarthritis most commonly seen in small breed dogs aged between 2 and 6 years.
- Non-erosive polyarthritis (idiopathic) seen in dogs aged 6 years old, with no sex predisposition. Breed predisposition suggested for GSD, Dobermann, Collies, Spaniels, Retrievers and Poodles.

History

- Any concurrent systemic illness, e.g. anorexia
- Any shifting nature to the signs
- Recent drug administration/vaccination history

- Travel history – possible exposure to exotic infectious agents

Physical examination
Observation
- Gait
  - 'Any particular limb affected
  - DJD generally worse after rest following exercise
  - Type of gait abnormality

Inspection
- Concurrent disease

Palpation
- Joints and bones for heat, pain, swelling, decreased range of movement

Auscultation
- Should be within normal limits

LABORATORY FINDINGS

- Haematology, serum biochemistry, urinalysis in all cases of non-erosive polyarthritis for evidence of other primary disease, e.g. in SLE – anaemia, thrombocytopenia, proteinuria.
- Hyperglobulinaemia and mild to marked neutrophilia are also common in cases with polyarthritis.
- Increased CPK and AST with muscle disease.
- Unremarkable with DJD.

IMAGING

Radiographs
- Affected areas, e.g. joints, to differentiate erosive from non-erosive polyarthritis and DJD

Echocardiography
- Suspected immune-mediated disease for evidence of bacterial endocarditis

SPECIAL TESTS

- Acetylcholine receptor antibody titre/edrophonium response test if suspect myasthenia gravis
- Antinuclear antibody in suspected immune mediated polyarthritis
- Arthroscopy/arthrotomy ± biopsy
- Blood cultures
- EMG, etc. to investigate muscle disease
- Joint tap for cytology, protein and culture
- Rheumatoid factor in suspected immune-mediated polyarthritis
- Serological testing to differentiate idiopathic polyarthritis from chronic infectious/inflammatory, e.g. *Borrelia burgdorferi*, *Dirofilaria immitis*, rickettsial diseases, systemic mycotic disease
- Urine culture

TENESMUS AND DYSCHEZIA

DEFINITION

- Tenesmus is straining to defecate or urinate.
- Dyschezia denotes pain or difficulty in defecation.

- A combination of dyschezia and tenesmus suggests distal LI and/or perianal disease.

CLINICAL SIGNS

Primary signs
Straining to pass faeces
- Straining after defecation if there is colono-rectal inflammation or mass
- Straining before passing stool and may ultimately pass small volume material if constipated

Straining to pass urine
- Production of a few drops of urine

Associated signs
Faecal tenesmus
- Anorexia and vomiting if severely constipated
- Blood and mucus mixed in faeces if colitis
- Blood on surface of faeces if focal bleeding lesion, e.g. polyp
- Distorted faecal shape if mass/stricture is present
- May stop straining abruptly and/or cry out if dyschezia is present

Urinary tenesmus
- Bladder empty if inflammatory disease
- Bladder full if obstructed

COMMON CAUSES

Faecal tenesmus and dyschezia
- All causes of Constipation (see p. 18)
- Anal sac
  - Impaction
  - Abscess/perineal cellulitis
- Colorectal disease
  - With diarrhoea
    - Acute colitis
    - Chronic colitis
- Pelvic fracture
- Perineal disease
  - Perianal fistula/anal furunculosis
  - Perineal hernia and rectal diverticulum

- Prostatic enlargement
- Spinal cord injury

Urinary tenesmus
- Prostatic enlargement (see p. 121)
- Urethral disease
  - Obstruction (tenesmus only)
  - Urethritis

UNCOMMON CAUSES

Faecal tenesmus and dyschezia
- Anorectal stricture
- Anal sac adenocarcinoma
- Colorectal disease
  - With blood and/or faecal deformation (indented or ribbon-shape)
    - Rectal polyp
    - Rectal tumour
- Idiopathic megacolon
- Paraprostatic cyst
- Rectal foreign body

Urinary tenesmus
- Paraprostatic cyst

DIAGNOSTIC APPROACH

1 Distinguish between urinary and faecal tenesmus by history and observation.
2 Examine perineum and perform rectal examination if faecal.
3 Look for underlying cause of constipation.
4 Examine urine or try to catheterise if anuric.

CLINICAL CLUES

Predisposition
- Anal sac adenocarcinomata in middle-aged female dogs
- Perineal hernia in male dogs

History
- Confirm whether dyschezia or dysuria is cause of tenesmus by observation and physical examination

Physical examination
Observation
- Distinguish attempted urination from defecation
- May strain and cry out, stop, walk around and try again

Inspection
- Distended abdomen
- Perianal fistula
- Perineal swelling

Palpation
- Distended colon if constipated
- Full bladder if obstructed
- Small bladder if cystitis/urethritis

Rectal examination
- Anal sac disease
- Constipation
- Pain
- Perineal hernia
- Prostatomegaly
- Rectal mass
- Retroflexed bladder within perineal hernia

LABORATORY FINDINGS

- Haematology and serum biochemistry usually unremarkable

IMAGING

Plain radiographs
- Extent of colonic impaction
- Bladder distension and identifies urethral calculi
- Identifies:
  - Pelvic and some spinal lesions
  - Abnormal faecal material (e.g. bones)
  - Prostatic enlargement
  - Sublumbar lymphadenopathy

Ultrasound examination
- Investigation of prostatic enlargement

SPECIAL TESTS

- Barium enema
- Colonoscopy
- Myelogram
- Retrograde (vagino)urethrogram

TREMORS

DEFINITION

Tremors are involuntary, repetitive, rhythmic, muscular oscillations. The contraction of muscles with opposing functions gives tremor its biphasic nature, which differentiates it from other movement abnormalities.

- Resting, intention or action tremors can be identified and classified as:
  - localised – limited to single limb or area of the body
  - generalised – involve the entire body
- Shivering is involuntary, physiological high frequency muscle contraction and relaxation.

CLINICAL SIGNS

- Tremors occurring at rest, with intention or action
- Other neurological signs
  - Cerebellar signs – dysmetria, ataxia, nystagmus, absent menace response

COMMON CAUSES

Cerebellar disease
- Abiotrophy
- Degenerative
- Hypoplastic
- Infectious
- Inflammatory, e.g. granulomatous meningoencephalitis (GME)
- Neoplastic

Idiopathic
- Senile limb tremor

Infectious disease
- Canine distemper

Metabolic causes of brain dysfunction
- Hepatic encephalopathy
- Hypoadrenocorticism
- Hypocalcaemia
- Hypoglycaemia

Muscle weakness
Secondary to:
- Spinal cord or peripheral nerve compression/entrapment
- Systemic illness
- Multiple drug therapy

Neuropathies

Toxin-/drug-induced
- Lead
- Organophosphates
- Metaldehyde

UNCOMMON CAUSES

CNS disease
- Head tremor/bob
  - Coarse tremor recognised particularly in the Doberman, disappears at rest. Usually appears at <1 year
- Little White Shakers (idiopathic cerebellitis)
  - Acute onset in adult, small breed white dogs, tremors worsen with exercise
- Lafora's disease in Wire-haired Dachshund
- Lysosomal storage diseases (accompanied by other cerebellar signs)

Myelination disorders (hypomyelinating or dysmyelinating)
- Action tremors are worse with excitement or at the start of movement and improve with rest
- Clinical signs with hypomyelination are usually evident in first few weeks of life

Physiological (normal)
- Low-amplitude tremulous movement secondary to cardiac activity – occurs even at rest, but difficult to see. Accentuated by drugs/stress that increase cardiac activity
- Higher amplitude tremor of unknown aetiology

Toxin-/drug-induced
- Mycotoxicoses
- Strychnine can cause tremors before seizures

DIAGNOSTIC APPROACH

1 Rule out toxic and metabolic causes.
2 Neurological examination.

CLINICAL CLUES

Predisposition

- Cerebellar abiotrophy in Kerry Blue terriers
- Hypomyelinating disorders usually show clinical signs within a few weeks of birth
- Little White Shakers – white, toy breed dogs, e.g. Maltese terrier, WHWT, Poodle
- Myelination disorders identified in many breeds, e.g. Springer spaniel, Chow chow, Weimaraner, Samoyed, Lurcher, Bernese mountain dog, Dalmatian
- Lafora's disease in Wire-haired Dachshund

History

- Association of tremor with food/water
- Do the tremors increase in the presence of food or drink (intention tremors)? This localises the lesion to the cerebellum.
- Do tremors improve with rest?
- Litter mates – are any others affected? Often, more than one pup in a litter may be affected with hypomyelination
- Recent drug administration/toxic access?
- Vaccination history – distemper infection can cause demyelination

Physical examination

Observation
- Gait
- Does tremor improve with rest?

Inspection
- Make a thorough neurological/ophthalmological examination

Palpation
- Spine – is there pain?

Auscultation
- No abnormalities would be expected

LABORATORY FINDINGS

- Often unremarkable
- Look for metabolic diseases

IMAGING

Radiographs

- Plain spinal ± contrast myelography where indicated to identify spinal cord compression

SPECIAL TESTS

- CSF analysis for cytology, protein analysis, serology for infectious diseases, e.g. distemper.
- MRI/CT scanning for further structural assessment.
- Nerve biopsy.
- Skin fibroblast cultures for diagnosis of lysosomal storage disease.

URINARY INCONTINENCE

DEFINITION

Urinary incontinence is the loss of voluntary control of urination, i.e. an inability to store and void urine.

Enuresis is the involuntary passage of urine during sleep.

NB Nocturia is excessive urination at night, usually due to polyuria, and is not necessarily due to incontinence.

CLINICAL SIGNS

- Constant or intermittent, unconscious dribbling
- Repeated attempts to urinate whilst only voiding small volumes despite retention of a large volume in the bladder
- Spontaneous involuntary urination
- Urine staining of perineum

COMMON CAUSES

Incontinence with no bladder distension
- Stranguria due to cystitis (not true incontinence)
- Urethral sphincter mechanism incompetence (SMI)

Incontinence with bladder distension
- Detrusor atony, e.g. following prolonged obstruction
- Neurogenic (urinary retention and overflow)
  - Sacral cord and peripheral nerve damage

UNCOMMON CAUSES

Incontinence with no bladder distension
- Bladder hypercontractility ('unstable' bladder)
- Reduced bladder storage due to chronic cystitis or neoplasia
- Ectopic ureters
- Persistent patent urachus
- Urethrovaginal fistula

Incontinence with bladder distension
- Neurogenic
  - Brainstem and spinal cord
  - Dysautonomia

- Reflex dyssynergia
- Partial physical obstruction
  - Urolithiasis

DIAGNOSTIC APPROACH

1 Rule out PU/PD and inflammatory urinary tract disease by urinalysis and culture, and minimum database.
2 Assess whether bladder remains distended after urination.
3 Assess neurological function.
4 Examine urinary tract by contrast radiography and urethral pressure profile.

CLINICAL CLUES

Predisposition
- Ectopic ureters in Golden retriever, OESD

History
- Ectopic ureters usually cause signs from early age
- SMI seen in ageing spayed bitches

Physical examination
Observation
- Dysuria is suggestive of inflammatory or neoplastic disease
- Spontaneous urination with incomplete bladder emptying is suggestive of a neurogenic cause

Inspection
- Proprioceptive and/or cranial nerve deficits
- Staining of perineum

Palpation
- Bladder empty or full?
- Can bladder be expressed easily?

LABORATORY FINDINGS

- Haematology and serum biochemistry unremarkable unless there is underlying PU/PD
- Urinalysis will indicate if inflammatory disease is present

IMAGING

- Intravenous urogram to detect ectopic ureters

- Retrograde vaginourethrogram
  - Congenital anatomical abnormalities
  - Bladder neck position in SMI
  - Thickening or neoplasia of lower urinary tract

SPECIAL TESTS

- Neurological examination
- Urethral pressure profile

VOMITING

DEFINITION

Vomiting is a reflex act characterised by forceful expulsion of gastric ± small intestinal contents from the stomach, and co-ordinated by the vomiting centre in the medulla.

The multiple afferents to the vomiting centre mean vomiting can be caused by primary GI disease or disease elsewhere in the dog.

CLINICAL SIGNS

- Usually preceded by nausea: hypersalivation, frequent swallowing, restlessness/anxiety
- Repeated contractions of diaphragm and abdominal wall
- Expulsion of gastric contents
  - Digested or undigested food
  - Bile and mucus
  - Blood (see Haematemesis, p. 41)

COMMON CAUSES

Acute vomiting
Primary GI disease
- Dietary indiscretion (change in diet, overindulgence)
- Gastric foreign body
- Haemorrhagic gastroenteritis (HGE)
- Intestinal obstruction: foreign body, intussusception
- Parvovirus infection
- Gastric dilatation-volvulus – ineffective attempts to vomit

Secondary vomiting
- Acute pancreatitis
- Acute renal failure and post-renal obstruction
- Diabetic ketoacidosis
- Hypoadrenocorticism (perhaps not common, but too important to be overlooked!)
- Pyometra
- Toxins/drugs, e.g. organophosphates, digoxin, morphine
- Vestibular disease, motion sickness

Chronic vomiting
Primary GI disease
- Chronic gastritis of unknown aetiology (*Helicobacter*?)
- Chronic hypertrophic pylorogastropathy (CHPG)
- Gastric neoplasia
- Gastric ulceration
  - NSAIDs
- Inflammatory bowel disease

Secondary vomiting
Chronic liver disease
- Chronic pancreatitis
- Head trauma
- Hypercalcaemia

Uraemia

UNCOMMON CAUSES

Acute vomiting
Primary GI disease
- Intestinal volvulus
- Peritonitis
- Psychogenic

Secondary vomiting
- Acute hepatitis
- Diaphragmatic rupture
- Distemper

Chronic vomiting
Primary GI disease
- Gastric ulceration
  - Gastrinoma
  - Mast cell tumour
- Obstipation
- *Physaloptera* (not in UK)
- Pyloric stenosis

Secondary vomiting
- Hypocalcaemia
- Raised intracranial pressure (hydrocephalus, tumour)

- Salmon-poisoning (not in UK)
- Septicaemia

DIAGNOSTIC APPROACH

1 Distinguish vomiting versus regurgitation by clinical clues below.
2 Rule out secondary causes of vomiting.
3 Treat acute vomiting symptomatically unless surgical disease is suspected.
4 Investigate chronic vomiting by laboratory tests and endoscopy.

CLINICAL CLUES

Predisposition
- Gastric carcinoma is more common in 7- to 10-year-old Collies, Belgian shepherd and Bull terrier
- Intussusception is more common in immature dogs
- Parvovirus infection is more likely in young, unvaccinated dogs
- Pyloric stenosis seen most often in brachycephalic dogs and soon after weaning
- Pyometra and diabetes mellitus more common in middle-aged to older unspayed females
- Scavenging is more common in Labradors

History
- Access to garbage, or history of roaming
- Lethargy and weight loss in hypoadrenocorticism
- Metoestrous phase for pyometra
- Systemic illness if secondary vomiting, e.g. PU/PD in diabetes mellitus
- Timing of vomition – the more frequent and sooner after feeding, the more acute and nearer to the stomach the cause

Clinical examination
Observation
- Content of vomit – bile, partially digested food, worms, blood
- Distinguish vomiting from regurgitation by presence of prodromal nausea and abdominal heaving
- 'Prayer position' with cranial abdominal pain – see p. 3

Inspection
- Assess degree of dehydration
- Bradycardia if hypoadrenocorticism
- Jaundice if hepatopathy
- Pale mucous membranes and tachycardia if bleeding gastric ulceration

Palpation
- Abdominal masses
- Foreign body
- Pain if pancreatitis, peritonitis or gastric ulceration

Auscultation
- Absence of gut sounds indicates ileus and possible peritonitis

LABORATORY FINDINGS

Haematology
- Inflammatory leukogram if pyometra, pancreatitis, peritonitis or gastric ulceration
- Neutropenia if parvovirus infection or acute peritonitis (bowel perforation)
- Degenerative left shift in peritonitis, bowel perforation
- PCV dramatically elevated in HGE
- PCV increased in dehydration

Serum biochemistry
- Amylase and lipase may be elevated in pancreatitis
- Azotaemia and isosthenuria in uraemia
- Electrolyte disturbances if prolonged vomiting
- Hyperglycaemia and glycosuria if diabetes mellitus
- Hyponatraemia/hyperkalaemia in hypoadrenocorticism

IMAGING

Radiographs
Plain
- Abdominal fluid (peritonitis)
- Abdominal mass
- Free abdominal gas (GI perforation)
- Obstructive GI gas pattern
- Pyometra
- Radiopaque foreign bodies

Contrast
- Low yield
- Only indicated if unremarkable plain films and laboratory studies are non-diagnostic

Ultrasound examination
- Abdominal masses
- Foreign body
- Gastric tumour
- Intussusception

SPECIAL TESTS
- ACTH stimulation test
- Gastroscopy only indicated in chronic vomiting after ruling out systemic disease, and for foreign body removal
- Exploratory laparotomy

WEAKNESS-LETHARGY-COLLAPSE/SYNCOPE

DEFINITION

Weakness can be due to:
- lassitude/fatigue (lack of energy)
- generalised muscle weakness (asthenia – true reduction in muscle tone)

Lethargy is a state of drowsiness, with delayed response to external stimuli, but no loss of consciousness.

Syncope is weakness due to a sudden transient loss of consciousness caused by deprivation of energy substrates, either oxygen or glucose, which briefly impairs cerebral metabolism. It usually results from impaired cerebral blood flow.

CLINICAL SIGNS

Weakness/lethargy
- Cachexia
- Generalised muscle weakness

Syncope
- Flaccid collapse with short period of loss of consciousness
- Most dogs will remain motionless with relaxed skeletal muscles
- Progressive ataxia
- Rapid recovery (± short period of confusion)
- Some cases may progress to tonic spasms and incontinence
- Vocalisation may occur

COMMON CAUSES

The causes of weakness and lethargy are too numerous to list. Causes of syncope are listed.

Cardiac disease
Outflow obstruction
- Valvular stenosis (aortic, etc.)

Arrhythmia
- Bradyarrhythmia
  - AV block
  - Sick-sinus syndrome
- Tachyarrhythmia
  - Supraventricular tachycardia
  - Ventricular tachycardia

Myocardial disease
- Dilated cardiomyopathy

Pericardial disease
- Pericardial effusion
- Constrictive pericarditis

Endocrine/metabolic
- Hypoadrenocorticism
- Hypoglycaemia

Haematological
- Acute blood loss anaemia (e.g. ruptured splenic mass)
- Polycythaemia – as a result of increased blood viscosity

Peripheral vascular dysfunction
- Vasovagal syncope

Respiratory tract disease
- Hypoxia
  - Secondary to brachycephalic airway syndrome or severe respiratory tract/ pleural cavity disease

UNCOMMON CAUSES

Cardiac disease
Severe AV valve incompetence
- Secondary to degenerative valvular changes or congenital AV valve disease

Endocrine/metabolic
- Hyperkalaemia
- Hypokalaemia

- Hypocalcaemia
- Phaeochromocytoma

Iatrogenic
- Drug administration, e.g. phenothiazines or drugs which affect systemic blood pressure

Neurological
- Myasthenia gravis causes weakness
- Narcolepsy/cataplexy

Peripheral vascular dysfunction
- Carotid sinus hypersensitivity, e.g. brachycephalic dogs, carotid sinus inflammation/neoplasia
- Hyperventilation
- Iliac thrombosis

Respiratory tract disease
- Pulmonary hypertension
- Cough syncope
- Cerebral neoplasia, thromboembolism

DIAGNOSTIC APPROACH

1 History
   - Does dog go flaccid?
   - Is it normal between episodes?
   - Is it otherwise unwell?
2 Confirm whether dog loses consciousness.
3 Absence of historical evidence of seizures.
4 Confirm presence or absence of respiratory signs.
5 Rule out metabolic disease by laboratory testing.
6 Investigate suspected cardiac disease.

CLINICAL CLUES

Predisposition
- Aortic stenosis in Boxer, Golden retriever

- Brachycephalic dogs: hypoxia from upper airway obstruction, vasovagal syncope
- DCM in large and giant breed dogs

History
- Characterise type of collapse
  - Presence or absence of consciousness during collapse
    - Remains conscious if locomotor disorder
  - Association with
    - feeding or starvation – endocrine, metabolic
    - exercise or excitement – cardiorespiratory
    - rest or waking – neurological
  - Duration of event
  - Altered behaviour before or after episode
  - Mucous membrane colour during episode
    - Cyanosis – respiratory or seizure (see p. 100)
    - Pallor – circulatory, anaemia
  - Frequency of episodes
    - episodic collapse – circulatory
    - continuous weakness – metabolic, systemic
  - Pattern of episodes
- Differentiate from seizures, this is important and sometimes difficult
- Drug/chemical/parasite exposure
- Familial history of congenital heart disease, seizures
- Other clinical signs, e.g. polydipsia, altered appetite, dysphagia, vomiting, polyuria, incontinence, altered defecation, respiratory disease, weight loss or gain suggestive of concurrent disease

Physical examination
Observation
- Gait abnormalities
- Weight loss

Inspection
- Mucous membrane colour and capillary refill time
- Neurological system including reflexes, etc.
- Inspect skin for any evidence of endocrinopathies

Palpation
- Femoral arteries for pulse
- Peripheral pulse volume and rhythm
- Lymph nodes
- Musculoskeletal system

Auscultation
- Cardiac evaluation for murmurs, etc.
- Assess for any pulse deficit/arrhythmia
- Abnormal respiratory noise/effort
- Abnormal percussion suggesting fluid/consolidation in thoracic cavity

LABORATORY FINDINGS

Haematology
- To assess for anaemia or polycythaemia. NB In acute blood loss, the PCV may remain normal for 12–24 hours.
- Check total proteins in conjunction.

Serum biochemistry
- To assess in particular:
  - Glucose
  - Electrolytes (sodium, potassium, calcium, magnesium)
  - Muscle enzymes (CPK, AST) elevated by muscle disease and prolonged seizure
  - Blood urea
  - Liver enzymes (ALT, ALP)

IMAGING

Radiography
- Inspiratory films to assess cardiac size and lung fields
- Expiratory films or fluoroscopy to assess dynamic airway collapse
- Skeletal radiographs may be indicated by the results of physical examination
- Contrast radiography, e.g. angiography, myelography may be indicated in specific cases

Ultrasound examination
- Abdominal ultrasound
- Adrenal ultrasound in suspected adrenal disorders, e.g. phaeochromocytoma
- Echocardiography in suspected cardiac disease

SPECIAL TESTS

- Acetylcholine receptor antibody titres or edrophonium response test if MG is suspected
- Adrenal function tests, e.g. ACTH stimulation test to investigate hypoadrenocorticism
- Blood gas analysis, resting, pre- and post-exercise
- CSF analysis for suspected neurological causes of syncope or true seizures
- ECG – routine or using telemetry or Holter monitors or event recorders
- Electromyography (EMG), nerve conduction velocities and muscle and nerve biopsies in investigation of neuromuscular disease
- Exercise testing
- Hypoglycaemia: high normal or increased insulin in face of hypoglycaemia is diagnostic for insulinoma
- Liver function tests, e.g. bile acids
- Respiratory tract investigation, e.g. bronchoscopy and BAL
- Thyroid function tests to investigate hypothyroidism (more a cause of exercise intolerance)

WEIGHT GAIN/OBESITY

DEFINITION

Weight gain occurs through the accumulation of fat, muscle mass or fluid, or by the growth of large masses.
- Weight gain occurs when caloric intake is increased and/or if energy use is decreased
- Obesity is usually defined as an increase in body fat such that body weight is at least 15% greater than ideal

CLINICAL SIGNS

- Increased body mass
  - Ascites
  - Increased fat deposition
  - Large mass
- Associated lethargy/exercise intolerance

COMMON CAUSES

- Decreased exercise (osteoarthritis)
- Hepatosplenomegaly
- HAC
- Hypogonadism, especially in bitches after ovariohysterectomy
- Hypothyroidism
- Overeating/overfeeding
- Peripheral oedema/ascites
- Pregnancy

UNCOMMON CAUSES

- Acromegaly
- Insulinoma
- Large mass (e.g. lipoma, haemangiopericytoma, granulosa cell tumour)
- Pyometra

DIAGNOSTIC APPROACH

1 If an increase in body weight is noted which cannot be reduced by decreasing dietary intake, or if there are concurrent clinical signs, then a pathological cause should be sought.
2 If over-feeding can be ruled out, and there is no obvious mass, an endocrinopathy is most likely.

CLINICAL CLUES

Predisposition
- Acromegaly in dogs treated with progesterone or in metoestrus
- HAC in middle-aged to older dogs
- Hypogonadism after neutering
- Insulinoma in middle-aged to older bitches
- Osteoarthritis in older dogs

History
- Administration of progesterone or recent oestrus in acromegaly
- Increased appetite in HAC, diabetes mellitus, insulinoma
- Lethargy in hypothyroidism
- PU/PD in diabetes mellitus
- Recent mating in pregnancy
- Recent oestrus in pyometra

Physical examination
Observation
- Alopecia in hypothyroidism and HAC
- Obesity

Inspection
- Increased subcutaneous fat and associated clinical signs, etc. seen in hypothyroidism
- Increased appetite in HAC, diabetes mellitus, insulinoma

- Intra-abdominal fat accumulation and a pot-belly characteristic of HAC
- Subcutaneous oedema
- Thin skin in HAC
- Thickened skin in hypothyroidism
- Weakness and/or seizures in hypoglycaemia caused by insulinoma

Palpation
- Abdominal mass if neoplasia
- Ascites
- Enlarged uterus or foetuses in pregnancy
- Tubular structure if pyometra

LABORATORY FINDINGS

Haematology
- Inflammatory leukogram sometimes in pyometra
- Stress leukogram in HAC

Serum biochemistry
- Hyperglycaemia and glycosuria in diabetes mellitus
- Hypoalbuminaemia if ascites/oedema
- Raised ALP in HAC

IMAGING

- Adrenal mass(es)
- Hepatosplenomegaly
- Occult thoracic and abdominal masses
- Pregnancy and pyometra

SPECIAL TESTS

- Dynamic cortisol testing
- Raised serum insulin in face of hypoglycaemia
- Thyroid function tests

WEIGHT LOSS

DEFINITION

A dog will lose weight when its energy use or loss exceeds its energy intake, and can therefore occur with:
- Increased energy use/loss
- Decreased energy intake/absorption
- Or both.

CLINICAL SIGNS

- A weight loss of more than 10% of body weight is considered significant
- Emaciation is more severe and equates to approximately 20% loss of body weight when bony prominences are noticeable
- Cachexia denotes extreme weight loss with associated weakness and depression

- Other signs may be associated with the primary cause, e.g. diarrhoea in malabsorption, dyspnoea in cardiac failure, pyrexia, etc.

COMMON CAUSES

Normal to increased food intake
Physiological
- Exercise
- Lactation
- Pregnancy (weight gain later)

Pathological
- Chronic blood loss
- Dysphagia and regurgitation (dog tries to eat but cannot swallow)
- Malabsorption
  - EPI
  - SIBO

- Mild IBD
- Non-ketotic diabetes mellitus

Normal to decreased food intake
- Fever
- Heart failure (cardiac cachexia)
- Hypoadrenocorticism
- Ketoacidotic diabetes mellitus
- Malabsorption
  - Severe IBD
- Liver disease
- Neoplasia (cancer cachexia)

UNCOMMON CAUSES

Normal to increased food intake
- Cold environment
- Deliberate or inadvertent underfeeding
- Hyperthyroidism (rare functional tumour; iatrogenic occasionally)
- Malabsorption
  - Lymphangiectasia
- Poor-quality food
- Protein-losing nephropathy

Normal to decreased food intake
- Malabsorption
  - Alimentary lymphosarcoma
- Oral disease
  - Oral neoplasia
  - Severe dental disease
  - Temporal muscle myositis
  - Temporomandibular joint dysplasia
- Severe intestinal parasitism
- Severe pyoderma

DIAGNOSTIC APPROACH

1   The differential diagnoses can be divided up on the basis of whether the dog wants to eat or is anorexic.

2   Weight loss due to lack of food intake causes an expected weight loss of 2% body weight per week.

3   Weight loss in excess of 2% body weight per week indicates increased energy loss or usage.

4   Other signs may help localise the organ system involved.

CLINICAL CLUES

Predisposition
- CHF in small breeds (especially CKCS) with valvular endocardiosis, and large breeds with DCM
- EPI in GSD
- Internal malignancies most commonly seen in Boxer, Flat coat retriever, Bernese Mountain dog
- Malabsorption through IBD in GSD, Retriever
- Malabsorption through lymphangiectasia in Lundehund, Rottweiler, Yorkshire terrier
- PLE ± PLN in Soft-coated wheaten terrier

History
- Abnormal faeces in malabsorption and EPI
- Cough/dyspnoea/ascites in CHF
- Inadequate intake identified in history
- Increased appetite in malabsorption and EPI

Physical examination
Inspection
- Bony prominences obvious when emaciated
- Jaundice if liver disease

Palpation
- Abdominal mass if neoplasia

PRESENTING COMPLAINTS

LABORATORY FINDINGS

Haematology
- Anaemia may suggest chronic blood loss
- Eosinophilia suggests presence of parasites
- Leukocytosis suggests inflammation or infection

Serum biochemistry
- Azotaemia if renal disease
- Faecal examination for parasites
- Glycosuria if diabetes mellitus
- Hyperglycaemia if diabetes mellitus
- Hypoproteinaemia suggests PLE, PLN or liver disease
- Increased liver enzymes ± hyperbilirubinaemia if liver disease
- Proteinuria if PLN

IMAGING
- CHF
- Occult thoracic and abdominal masses
- To identify effusions

SPECIAL TESTS
- Bile acids for non-icteric liver disease
- Folate and cobalamin for malabsorption
- Intestinal biopsy for malabsorption
- Serum T4 for hyperthyroidism
- Serum TLI for EPI

SECTION 2
PHYSICAL ABNORMALITIES

ABDOMINAL ENLARGEMENT

DEFINITION

Distension of the abdomen by fat, fluid, gas, or organ enlargement, and/or by weakness of the abdominal musculature.

- Ascites is the accumulation of free fluid within the peritoneum that may be a transudate, modified transudate or exudate, and which may contain blood, bile, chyle, pus or urine. These conditions are covered in Ascites (p. 94).
- Any fluid accumulation may be intraluminal or free, intraperitoneal fluid.
- The causes can be remembered by the mnemonic of the 6 Fs:
  - Faeces
  - Fat
  - Flatus
  - 'Flotsam' (i.e. masses)
  - Fluid
  - Foetus

CLINICAL SIGNS

- Acute enlargement with gas accumulation, e.g. in GDV and ruptured organ/viscus
- Chronic progressive enlargement in most cases

COMMON CAUSES

Fat accumulation
- Diabetes mellitus
- HAC
- Obesity

Fluid
Ascites
- Exudate
- Modified transudate
- Transudate

Haemoperitoneum
- Coagulopathy
- Haemangiosarcoma
- Traumatic rupture of liver/spleen

Intraluminal
- Pyometra

Uroperitoneum
- Traumatic rupture of bladder

Gas
- Gastric dilatation/volvulus

Muscle weakness
- HAC
- Malnutrition

Organomegaly
Hepatomegaly
- Congestion (right-heart failure)
- Diabetes mellitus
- HAC
- IMHA
- Neoplasia

Splenomegaly
- Barbiturate anaesthesia
- Haematoma
- Neoplasia – haemangioma, haemangiosarcoma, lymphosarcoma
- Reactive – IMHA, ITP

Uterine enlargement
- Pregnancy
- Pyometra

Intestinal enlargement
- Constipation/obstipation

Urinary tract
- Renomegaly
  - Neoplasia
  - Portosystemic shunt
- Distended bladder
  - Urethral obstruction

PHYSICAL ABNORMALITIES

UNCOMMON CAUSES

Fluid
Bile peritonitis
- Rupture of gallbladder or bile duct(s)

Chylous effusion
- Congestion – right-heart failure
- Lymphangiectasia (± concurrent chylo-thorax)
- Neoplasia (phaeochromocytoma)

Septic peritonitis
- *Nocardia/Actinomyces*

Uroperitoneum
- Traumatic rupture of kidney or ureter

Gas
Pneumoperitoneum
- Penetrating wound
- Post-operative
- Ruptured viscus

Muscle weakness
- Primary myopathy

Organomegaly
Gonadal
- Ovarian carcinoma
- Tumour of retained testicle

Intestinal enlargement
- Mesenteric lymphadenopathy – lymphosarcoma
- Neoplasia – lymphosarcoma, adenocarcinoma, leiomyoma/sarcoma
- Obstruction
- Pancreatic mass – carcinoma, chronic fibrosing pancreatitis

Splenomegaly
- *Babesia*
- *Leishmania*
- Myeloproliferative disease
- Splenic torsion

Urinary
- Hydronephrosis
- Prostatic and paraprostatic cyst

Uterine enlargement
- Leiomyoma/sarcoma
- Mummification

DIAGNOSTIC APPROACH

1   Identify free fluid and organomegaly/mass by abdominal palpation and ballottement.
2   Confirm by radiographs, ultrasound and abdominocentesis.

CLINICAL CLUES

Predisposition
- GDV in large/giant, deep-chested dogs
- Haemangiosarcoma in GSD

History
- Anorexia, vomiting if uroperitoneum
- Collapse/shock(recurrent/intermittent) if ruptured haemangiosarcoma
- Lack of urination if uroperitoneum or urethral obstruction
- Possibility of mating if pregnant
- PU/PD if pyometra
- Pyometra in older unspayed bitches after oestrus
- Unproductive retching in GDV

Physical examination
Observation
- Distended abdomen
- Feminisation if Sertoli cell tumour in retained testicle
- Movement of free fluid
- Tachypnoea/dyspnoea if right heart failure

Inspection
- Icterus if pancreatic mass obstructing common bile duct or bile peritonitis
- Jugular pulses if right-heart failure or cardiac tamponade
- Muffled heart sounds if cardiac tamponade
- Pyrexia if peritonitis or large mass with necrotic centre

Palpation
- Ballottement of free fluid or masses
- Presence of enlarged organ or mass
- Rectal palpation may reveal paraprostatic cyst
- Tympany

NB – Beware fat redistribution with abdominal muscle weakness in HAC which can feel like free fluid.

LABORATORY FINDINGS

Haematology
- Inflammatory leukogram if septic peritonitis or large necrotic mass
- Regenerative anaemia if bleeding mass

Serum biochemistry
- Azotaemia if uroperitoneum or urinary obstruction
- Raised liver enzymes with primary hepatopathy or secondary to inflammatory disease elsewhere in abdomen

IMAGING

Plain radiographs
- Abdominal mass
- Chest radiographs should be taken if ascites present to look for metastatic and cardiac disease
- Foetal skeletons after day 45 of pregnancy
- Loss of detail if free intraperitoneal fluid, and therefore not very helpful in ascites
- Uterine enlargement in pyometra and pregnancy

Ultrasound examination
- Abdominal masses
- Free fluid
- Organ enlargement/infiltration
- Pyometra or pregnancy
- Torsion of splenic pedicle

SPECIAL TESTS

- Abdominocentesis
- Coagulation profile
- Exploratory laparotomy
- FNA of abdominal mass

ANAEMIA

DEFINITION

Anaemia is the absolute lack of circulating RBCs. Anaemia results from:
- Depressed RBC production
- RBC loss
- RBC destruction

CLINICAL SIGNS

Acute anaemia
- Acute collapse
- Dyspnoea
- Pallor of mucous membranes
- Sudden weakness/exercise intolerance
- Tachypnoea

PHYSICAL ABNORMALITIES

PHYSICAL ABNORMALITIES

Chronic anaemia
- Anorexia
- Depression
- Dyspnoea
- Lethargy
- Pale mucous membranes
- Vague illness
- Weakness

CLASSIFICATION

RBC survival time is 100–120 days in the dog.

Regenerative/responsive anaemia
With RBC loss or excessive destruction
- Anisocytosis
- Polychromasia
- Reticulocytosis

Note:
- It takes 72 hours after the onset of anaemia until an increase in reticulocytes is seen.
- It takes 5–7 days for peak reticulocytosis to occur.
- Haemolysis often results in greater degree of reticulocytosis than haemorrhage because the iron is available for reuse.
- Nucleated RBCs in the absence of reticulocytosis do NOT indicate regeneration.

Non-regenerative/non-responsive anaemia
- Acute or chronic
- Lack of reticulocytosis
- RBC size can be microcytic, normocytic or macrocytic
- RBC may be hypochromic or normochromic

Degree of anaemia
- Mild   PCV 30–37%
- Moderate   PCV 20–29%
- Severe   PCV 13–19%
- Very severe   PCV <13%

COMMON CAUSES

Regenerative anaemia: blood loss/haemorrhage
Coagulation disorders
- Anticoagulant intoxication (e.g. warfarin – vitamin K antagonist)
- Thrombocytopenia

Gastrointestinal blood loss
- Gastric/duodenal ulcers
- Ulcerated neoplasia

Neoplasia
- Intracavitary bleeding (haemangiosarcoma)

Trauma
- External blood loss
- Internal blood loss

Regenerative anaemia: haemolysis
Immune-mediated disease
- Primary (idiopathic) IMHA
- Secondary to another disease process, e.g. lymphoma

Mechanical fragmentation
- Haemangiosarcoma

Non-regenerative anaemia
Hypoplastic anaemia – selective depression of RBC production, i.e. secondary to
- Anaemia of chronic disease (infection, inflammation, neoplasia)
- Chronic liver disease
- Chronic renal disease
- Hypoadrenocorticism
- Hypothyroidism

Immune-mediated disease
- Immune-mediated disease against RBC precursor

Nutritional deficiencies
- Iron
  - Chronic blood loss (initially regenerative, i.e. reticulocytosis, but later microcytosis)

Pancytopenia
- Chemical agents
  - Oestrogen
- Myelophthisis (myelodysplasia, myelofibrosis, neoplasia)

Pure red cell aplasia
- Idiopathic disease/immune-mediated

UNCOMMON CAUSES

Regenerative anaemia: blood loss/haemorrhage
Coagulation disorders
- DIC
- Factor deficiency

Gastrointestinal blood loss
- Hookworms (not in UK)
- Inflammatory bowel disease
- Secondary to other disease, e.g. pancreatitis

Neoplasia
- External bleeding

Urinary tract bleeding
- Haemorrhagic cystitis
- Idiopathic renal haematuria
- Neoplasia

Regenerative anaemia: haemolysis
Blood parasites/infectious diseases (not in UK)
- Babesiosis
- Ehrlichiosis
- *Dirofilaria immitis*

- *Haemobartonella canis* (only if splenectomised?)
- Leptospirosis

Chemical or toxic injury
- Heinz body anaemia
  - Kale
  - Onion intoxication
  - Urinary antiseptics containing methylene blue
  - Vitamin K$_1$
- Hypophosphataemia
- Ketoacidosis
- Lead poisoning
- Snake venom toxicity
- Zinc toxicity

Immune-mediated disease
- Isoimmune haemolytic disease of neonates
- Secondary to another disease process, e.g. lymphocytic leukaemia, bacterial/fungal/viral infections, granulomatous disease, SLE
- Secondary to drug administration, e.g. cephalosporins, potentiated sulphonamides, modified live virus vaccines, possibly to any drug
- Transfusion reaction

Intracorpuscular problem
- Hereditary non-spherocytic anaemia of beagles and poodles
- Hereditary stomatocytosis of Alaskan malamute
- Phosphofructokinase deficiency, e.g. English Springer and American Cocker spaniel
- Predisposition to oxidant injury, e.g. high potassium levels and low glutathione levels in RBCs, e.g. Akita
- Pyruvate kinase deficiency, e.g. Basenji, WHWT

Mechanical fragmentation
- Dirofilariasis
- Splenic disease, e.g. torsion

Non-regenerative anaemia
Nutritional deficiencies
- Folic acid
- Iron
  - Nutritional deficiency
- Vitamin B$_{12}$ deficiency, e.g. Giant Schnauzer, Border collie

Pancytopenia
- Bone marrow neoplasia
- Chemical agents
  - Alkylating agents
  - Chloramphenicol
  - Griseofulvin
  - Phenylbutazone
  - Trimethoprim-sulpha
- Ehrlichiosis
- Idiopathic
- Ionising radiation
- Myelophthisis (myelodysplasia, myelofibrosis, neoplasia)
- Parvovirus

Pure red cell aplasia
- Congenital
- Drug-induced

DIAGNOSTIC APPROACH

- Classify anaemia as mild, moderate, severe or very severe.
- Identify underlying causes of mild anaemia.
- Classify moderate-severe anaemia as regenerative or non-regenerative.
- If regenerative:
  - identify internal or external blood loss
  - identify haemolytic disease
- If non-regenerative:
  - look for underlying disease
  - examine bone marrow

CLINICAL CLUES

Predisposition
- See breed-related intracorpuscular diseases p. 91

History
- Any localising signs of disease
- Any possible trauma
- Any potential toxin exposure
- Duration – acute versus chronic
- Previous drug administration/vaccination
- Travel history

Clinical examination
Observation
- Body condition
- Faeces for melaena (or severe haematochezia) suggesting significant intestinal blood loss
- Physical strength/weakness

Inspection
- Mucous membranes
  - Capillary refill time – prolonged with poor cardiac output and hypovolaemia
  - Colour (pallor in an alert animal is more suggestive of chronic disease)
  - Evidence of icterus suggesting a haemolytic process
  - Evidence of petechiae/ecchymoses suggesting thrombocytopenia
- Retinal examination for haemorrhage (non-specific finding)
- Skin for evidence of petechiae/ecchymoses

Palpation
- Pulse for strength, rate, assess for pulse deficits or arrhythmias
- Spleen and liver for enlargement, e.g. immune-mediated haemolytic anaemias, secondary to neoplastic infiltration, etc.

Auscultation
- Heart murmur either due to pre-existing disease or as a result of decreased blood viscosity and increased turbulence due to the anaemia
- Increased heart and respiratory rates

LABORATORY FINDINGS

Haematology
- RBC count and indices, platelet count, WBC count and differential, smear evaluation

Packed cell volume (PCV)/Haematocrit (HCT)
Degree of anaemia see p. 90
- HCT is calculated by cell counter from RBC numbers and MCV
- PCV is calculated as % cells after microcentrifugation
- ↓ PCV and total protein (TP) indicates blood loss
  - GI or intracavitary blood loss: bigger ↓ in PCV as proteins are reabsorbed

Mean cell volume (MCV)
- An indication of the overall RBC size
- Increased MCV in regenerative anaemia = macrocytosis
- Decreased MCV = microcytosis
  - Low MCV is normal in Japanese Akita and Shiba Inu
  - Microcytosis is seen in young animals with congenital portosystemic shunts in the absence of anaemia

Mean corpuscular haemoglobin concentration (MCHC)
- Indicates the concentration of haemoglobin (Hb) per unit volume of RBCs
  - MCHC ↓ and MCV ↓ – iron deficiency
  - MCHC ↓ and MCV ↑ – with other signs suggests regeneration

- ↑ MCHC suggests haemolysis or laboratory error

Reticulocyte count
- Indicates the degree of regeneration, interpreted in view of the individual's PCV
- Stain with supravital stain, e.g. new methylene blue
- It takes 72 hours for reticulocytosis to occur after acute RBC loss
- Peak reticulocytosis within 5–7 days
NB – Regenerative anaemias can appear non-regenerative during this lag phase
- Reticulocyte responses (%)
  - Normal   1
  - Slight   1–4
  - Moderate   5–20
  - Marked   21–50

Reticulocyte indices
- Correlate reticulocyte response to the degree of anaemia
- Corrected reticulocyte percentage (CRP) = % reticulocytes × patient's PCV/normal PCV
- Reticulocyte index (RI) = CRP/life span of reticulocytes (1 day @ PCV =45; 1.5 day @ 35%; 2 days @ 25%, etc.)
  - RI > 1 indicates regeneration
  - RI > 3 indicates marked regeneration

Absolute reticulocyte count
- This is a more consistent indicator of bone marrow response
  - Normal 60×10^9/L
  - Slight 150×10^9/L
  - Moderate 300×10^9/L
  - Marked $>500 \times 10^9$/L

Agglutination
- Differentiate from rouleaux formation – mix one part EDTA blood with one part 0.9% NaCl and observe with microscope for agglutination (clumping) versus rouleaux (stacking)
- Agglutination in an anaemic animal indicates an immune-mediated process

Smear evaluation
- Basophilic stippling and nucleated RBCs: lead poisoning
- Blood parasites may be seen
- Heinz bodies
- Neutrophilia and thrombocytosis are often seen with regenerative anaemia: non-specific bone marrow stimulation
- Nucleated RBCs in the absence of reticulocytosis indicate bone marrow or splenic disease
- Nucleated RBCs with other signs of regeneration suggest regenerative anaemia
- Number of nucleated RBCs inappropriate for degree of anaemia suggests heavy metal (lead) poisoning
- Platelet assessment for numbers, clumps, etc.
- Polychromatic cells suggest regeneration
- RBC agglutination
- Schistocytes – may indicate DIC or other microangiopathic anaemias
- Spherocytes – IMHA

Serum biochemistry
- ALT/ALP/bile acids for underlying hepatic disease
- Cholesterol for suggestion of endocrinopathy, e.g. hypothyroidism
- Serum bilirubin if suspect haemolytic disease
- Serum electrolytes, e.g. for hypoadrenocorticism
- Urea/creatinine for underlying renal disease

IMAGING

Plain radiographs
- Thoracic and abdominal radiographs to identify any internal abnormalities not detected on physical examination

Ultrasound
- Assess hepatosplenomegaly

SPECIAL TESTS

- ACTH stimulation test
- Antinuclear antibody (ANA) test
- Bone marrow aspirate/core biopsy
- Clotting assessment if considering toxic access to anticoagulants or DIC
- Coombs' test for investigation of IMHA
- Exploratory laparotomy for assessment/biopsy of spleen
- Faecal examination for occult blood loss (limited use)
- Infectious disease identification, e.g. serology for *Ehrlichia*, *Babesia*, fungal diseases, etc.
- Hepatic/renal biopsy if suggested as cause of anaemia
- Thyroid hormone assessment for hypothyroidism

ASCITES

DEFINITION

Ascites is the accumulation of free fluid within the peritoneal cavity. It can be due to the accumulation of a:
- transudate – due to hypoalbuminaemia (< 15 g/L)
- modified transudate – due to portal hypertension
- exudates – due to septic and non-septic inflammation

or it may contain:
- bile
- blood

- chyle
- urine

CLINICAL SIGNS

- Abdominal distension
- Pleural effusion and subcutaneous oedema if hypoalbuminaemic
- Respiratory embarrassment if massive ascites
- Signs related to primary cause of fluid accumulation, e.g. jaundice in liver failure

COMMON CAUSES

Transudate (hypoalbuminaemia)
Hepatic failure
- Congenital PSS

Protein-losing enteropathy
- Inflammatory bowel disease

Protein-losing nephropathy
- Glomerulonephritis

Modified transudate (portal hypertension)
Cardiac tamponade (pericardial effusion)
- Idiopathic pericardial haemorrhage
- Right atrial haemangiosarcoma

Hepatic failure
- Chronic hepatopathy/cirrhosis

Right-sided heart failure
- Dilated cardiomyopathy
- Valvular heart disease

Exudate – inflammatory
Blood
- Generalised bleeding disorder
- Ruptured haemangiosarcoma
- Traumatic splenic or hepatic rupture

Non-septic
- Carcinomatosis
- Diaphragmatic rupture and liver entrapment
- Pancreatitis

Septic
- GI perforation
- Ruptured pyometra

Urine
- Ruptured bladder

UNCOMMON CAUSES

Transudate (hypoalbuminaemia)
Hepatic failure
- Chronic hepatopathy/cirrhosis

Protein-losing enteropathy
- Alimentary lymphosarcoma
- Lymphangiectasia

Protein-losing nephropathy
- Amyloidosis

Modified transudate (portal hypertension)
Cardiac tamponade
- Heart-base tumour
- Restrictive pericarditis

Caudal vena cava compression/obstruction
- Caval syndrome (dirofilariasis)
- Cor triatrium dexter
- 'Kinked' CVC
- CVC thrombosis

Liver disease
- Idiopathic hepatic fibrosis

Post-hepatic obstruction
- *Angiostrongylus*
- Budd-Chiari syndrome
- *Dirofilaria* (not in UK)

- Intra-cardiac neoplasia
- Veno-occlusive disease

Exudate – inflammatory
Bile
- Gallstones causing spontaneous rupture of biliary tract
- Perforated proximal duodenal ulcer
- Traumatic rupture of gallbladder or extrahepatic biliary tree

Chyle (lymphatic obstruction or leakage)
- Intestinal obstruction
- Lymphangiectasia
  - Idiopathic
  - Obstruction
    - Right heart failure
    - Phaeochromocytoma

Non-septic
- Pansteatitis

Septic
- Mycotic
- *Nocardia/Actinomyces*
- Penetrating wound
- Ruptured abscess
- Volvulus/infarction of GI tract

Urine
- Ruptured kidney and/or ureters

DIAGNOSTIC APPROACH

1   Distinguish free fluid from other causes of abdominal enlargement (pp. 87–9) by ballottement ± ultrasound examination.
2   Abdominocentesis for fluid collection, and classification based on laboratory analysis, cytological examination and culture.

Fluid characteristics
(See Table 2)

3   Investigation of relevant organ system depending on specific type of fluid and other clinical signs:
    - For transudate, check causes of hypoalbuminaemia
    - For modified transudate, check for right-heart failure, cardiac tamponade, liver disease
    - For exudate, perform bacterial culture, and look for source of inflammation

CLINICAL CLUES

Predisposition
- Cardiac tamponade in large/giant breed dogs
- Chronic liver disease in certain pure bred dogs, e.g. Dobermann, Cocker spaniel, GSD
- DCM in giant breed dogs
- IBD in GSD, Shar pei
- Lymphangiectasia in toy breeds and Rottweiler

History
- GI signs consistent with PLE

Table 2

	Transudate	Modified transudate	Exudate
SG	<1.017	1.017–1.025	>1.025
Protein (g/L)	<25	25–60	>25
Nucleated cells/mm^3	<1000	<7000	>7000
Cytology			Neutrophils

- Intermittent weakness/collapse consistent with recurrent haemorrhage from bleeding haemangiosarcoma or idiopathic pericardial haemorrhage
- Previous trauma
- Signs consistent with liver disease – anorexia, encephalopathy, jaundice, etc.

Physical examination
Observation
- Dyspnoea if massive ascites
- Jaundice if bile peritonitis
- Right-heart failure
  - Extended jugular pulse
  - Hepatojugular reflex

Inspection
- Abdominal enlargement

Palpation
- Fluid wave on ballottement
- Weak peripheral pulse if DCM or cardiac tamponade

Auscultation
- Muffled heart sounds if cardiac tamponade
- Murmur if valvular disease or advanced DCM

LABORATORY FINDINGS

Haematology
- Regenerative anaemia if recurrent bleeding from haemangiosarcoma

- Inappropriate numbers of nucleated RBCs suggest splenic pathology
- Leukocytosis, and perhaps a degenerative left shift, if septic peritonitis

Serum biochemistry (See Table 3)
- Azotaemia and hyperkalaemia if uroperitoneum
- Hyperbilirubinaemia if liver disease or ruptured biliary tree
- Hypocalcaemia secondary to hypoproteinaemia
- Hypoproteinaemia
- Serum bile acids to assess hepatic function

IMAGING

Radiographs
Plain
- Abdominal films generally unhelpful due to loss of detail by free abdominal fluid
- Chest radiographs to evaluate pleural effusion, heart silhouette and lung patterns

Contrast
- Barium can outline position of stomach and hence indicate liver size

Ultrasound examination
- Abdominal masses
- Free fluid
- Heart function
- Hepatic and splenic abnormalities
- Pericardial effusion

PHYSICAL ABNORMALITIES

Table 3

	Albumin	Globulin
Protein-losing enteropathy	Low	Low (raised if severe inflammatory disease)
Protein-losing nephropathy	Low	Normal
Liver disease	Low	Normal/raised

SPECIAL TESTS

- Abdominal fluid analysis
  - Cell count
  - Cholesterol < serum, and triglyceride > serum if chyloabdomen
  - Cytology – sepsis, neoplasia
  - Creatinine > serum indicates uroperitoneum
  - Glucose < plasma indicates sepsis
  - Gram's stain for septic peritonitis
- PCV/RBC count for haemoperitoneum
- Protein
- Specific gravity
- Coagulation times
- Knott's and occult heartworm test
- Endoscopic intestinal biopsy
- Exploratory laparotomy and hepatic or intestinal biopsy
- Pericardiocentesis
- FNA of intra-abdominal mass

BRADYCARDIA

DEFINITION

Bradycardia is a slow heart rate, usually below 60 beats per minute.
- Atrioventricular (AV) nodal block (first, second and third)
- Sick sinus syndrome
- Persistent atrial standstill
- Sinus pause/arrest (sinoatrial (SA) nodal block)
- Idioventricular rhythm

CLINICAL SIGNS

- Bradycardia and slow pulse rate
- May be asymptomatic
- If symptomatic – often during exercise or stress
  - Lethargy/weakness
  - Collapse/syncope
- Other signs related to underlying disease, e.g. vomiting in hypoadrenocorticism

COMMON CAUSES

Excessive vagal tone
- Gastrointestinal disease

Myocardial lesions affecting the conduction tissue
- Idiopathic fibrosis

Myocardial or pacemaker depression
Drugs
- Cardiac glycosides

Metabolic disturbance
- Hyperkalaemia
- Hypoadrenocorticism
- Urinary obstruction
- Hypothyroidism

UNCOMMON CAUSES

Excessive vagal tone
- Raised intracranial pressure/brainstem disease
- Vagal nerve injury

Myocardial lesions affecting the conduction tissue
- Abscess
- Bacterial endocarditis (usually tachycardia)
- Borreliosis
- DCM (usually tachycardia)
- Neoplasia

- True aortic valve stenosis and reflex bradycardia
- Ventricular septal defects

Myocardial or pacemaker depression
Drugs
- Beta-blockers
- Calcium channel-blockers
- Narcotics
- Procainamide
- Xylazine

Metabolic disturbance
- Hyperkalaemia
  - Urinary rupture and uroperitoneum
- Hypothermia
- Hypothyroidism
- Toxaemia

DIAGNOSTIC APPROACH

1 If bradycardia is detected, an ECG is performed to characterise the brady-dysrhythmia.
2 Some are transient and related to obvious disease states, and can be ignored.
3 A full drug history is important.
4 Laboratory testing to rule out metabolic disturbances.
5 Full cardiac evaluation (radiographs, echocardiography, blood pressure measurement) if underlying disease state not found.

CLINICAL CLUES

Predisposition
- Aortic stenosis in Newfoundland, GSD, Boxer, Golden retriever (German short-haired pointer, Rottweiler, Samoyed, Great Dane, Bull terrier)

- Sick sinus syndrome in Miniature Schnauzer
- Sinus arrest/pause can be normal in brachycephalic breeds
- Sinus bradycardia can be normal in fit dogs, and in some giant breeds

History
- Cold intolerance
- Drug exposure
- Signs of underlying disease
  - GI disease – vomiting and diarrhoea
  - Hypoadrenocorticism – vomiting, diarrhoea, weight loss
  - Hypothyroidism – lethargy, coat changes, weight gain
  - Intracranial disease – neurological deficits
  - Urinary obstruction – vomiting, dysuria
- Tick exposure for borreliosis

Physical examination
Observation
- Episodes of weakness, collapse, or syncope

Inspection
- Hypothermia
- Pyrexia if endocarditis

Palpation
- Altered pulse rate and quality

Auscultation
- Bradycardia
- Murmur

LABORATORY FINDINGS

Haematology
- Often unremarkable
- Normocytic, normochromic anaemia in hypothyroidism and hypoadrenocorticism

PHYSICAL ABNORMALITIES

Serum biochemistry
- Hypocalcaemia (see p. 138)
- Hyperkalaemia and azotaemia if urinary obstruction
- Hyperkalaemia and hyponatraemia if hypoadrenocorticism

IMAGING

Plain radiographs
- Presence of any intrathoracic mass
- Size and shape of heart
- State of pulmonary vasculature

Echocardiography
- Blood flow and turbulence

- Size of heart chambers
- State of cardiac muscle

SPECIAL TESTS

- ACTH stimulation test
- Atropine response test
- Blood cultures
- Blood pressure measurement
- Cardiac catheterisation
- Exercise test
- Lyme serology
- Neurological examination
- Serum digoxin concentration
- Thyroid function tests
- 24-hour Holter ECG

CARDIOMEGALY

See Cardiovascular system, Section 4, pp. 199–226.

CYANOSIS

DEFINITION

A bluish colour, most visible in the mucous membranes, nail beds and hairless skin, caused by excessive desaturation of haemoglobin in the blood.

Adequate levels of haemoglobin are present, but inadequate levels of oxygenation.

NB – Anaemia does not cause cyanosis, and oxygen administration is ineffective.

The origin of cyanosis can be:
- Central, from arterial hypoxaemia
  - Due to problems with oxygenation (respiratory disease) or a right to left shunt of blood within the circulation so that deoxygenated blood mixes with oxygenated blood.

- Respiratory disease is a more common cause of cyanosis than cardiac shunts.
- Administration of oxygen alleviates central cyanosis.
- Peripheral due to low tissue oxygenation despite normal arterial oxygen saturation
  - Methaemoglobinaemia
  - Local circulatory problems (vasoconstriction, arterial or venous obstruction)

CLINICAL SIGNS

- Visual detection of cyanosis is notoriously unreliable; severe hypoxaemia can exist without cyanosis

- In general, at least 50 g/L or 5% of haemoglobin must be desaturated for cyanosis to be visible
  - When Hb concentration is normal, the PaO_2 must be below 50 mmHg
  - When Hb concentration is low (anaemia), the PaO_2 must be even lower to produce 50 g/L of reduced-Hb
  - When Hb concentration is high (polycythaemia), cyanosis will occur at a PaO_2 above 50 mmHg, but polycythaemia may also be a consequence of hypoxaemia
- Dyspnoea and tachypnoea
- Exercise intolerance, weakness, syncope
- Extremities cold and cyanotic

COMMON CAUSES

Central
Acquired cardiovascular disease
- Low-output heart failure

Congenital cardiovascular disease
- Pulmonic stenosis

Neurological – depressed respiration
- Anaesthesia

Respiratory disease
- Chronic obstructive airway disease
- Laryngeal paralysis
- Metastatic pulmonary neoplasia
- Pleural effusion
- Pneumothorax
- Pulmonary oedema
- Pulmonary thromboembolism (PTE) probably under-diagnosed

Peripheral
Physiological
- Cold exposure
- Shock (intense peripheral vasoconstriction rather than true cyanosis)

UNCOMMON CAUSES

Central
Congenital cardiovascular disease
- Reverse PDA
- Reverse VSD
- Tetralogy of Fallot

Neurological – depressed respiration
- CNS disease affecting medulla or upper cervical spinal cord
- Increased intracranial pressure
- Neuromuscular weakness

Respiratory disease
- Asthma (rare in dog, cf. cat)
- Atelectasis
  - Compression following ruptured diaphragm
  - Lung lobe torsion
- Collapsing trachea (severe)
- Laryngeal oedema
- Laryngeal neoplasia
- Lung lobe consolidation
- Pneumonia (severe)
- Primary pulmonary neoplasia (extensive)
- Pulmonary fibrosis
- Idiopathic progressive interstitial fibrosis (WHWT)
- Paraquat poisoning

Peripheral
- Arterial obstruction
- Thromboembolism
- Nephrotic syndrome
- Cold agglutinin disease
- Tourniquet application
- Methaemoglobinaemia
- Congenital haemoglobin abnormality
- Paracetamol (rare, cf. cat)

Venous obstruction
- Thrombophlebitis
- Tourniquet

DIAGNOSTIC APPROACH

1 History and physical examination to identify drug exposure and cardiorespiratory disease.
2 If localised cyanosis, examine regional pulse.
3 Arterial blood gas to determine oxygen saturation levels.
4 Chest radiographs for cardiopulmonary disease.
5 ECG and echocardiography.

CLINICAL CLUES

Predisposition
- Congenital cardiovascular disease in puppies
  - Pulmonic stenosis in Cocker spaniel, Miniature Schnauzer, Boxer
  - Tetralogy in Golden retriever, Wirehaired fox terrier, Labrador retriever, Siberian Husky, Toy Poodle
- Idiopathic interstitial pulmonary fibrosis of WHWT

History
- Neurological signs with CNS disease

Physical examination
Observation
- Dyspnoea and tachypnoea
- Stridor (p. 128)

Inspection
- Cyanotic mucous membranes
- Differential cyanosis (pink oral mucous membranes, but cyanotic caudally) in a young animal with a reverse PDA
- Neurological deficits

Palpation
- Weak pulses in heart failure
- Absent pulses in thromboembolism

Auscultation
- Muffled heart sounds with pneumothorax
- Murmurs (pp. 199–226)
- Pulmonary adventitious sounds (p. 122)
- Stridor (p. 128)

LABORATORY FINDINGS

Haematology
- Brown discoloration of blood that does not turn red on shaking with air suggests methaemoglobinaemia
- Polycythaemia secondary to hypoxaemia

Serum biochemistry
- Hypoalbuminaemia and hypercholesterolaemia in nephrotic syndrome

Urinalysis
- Proteinuria in nephrotic syndrome

IMAGING

Plain radiographs
- Cardiac silhouette to assess generalised or localised cardiomegaly (see pp. 205–6)
- Pleural effusion
- Pneumothorax
- Pulmonary parenchymal disease

Echocardiography
- Acquired and congenital cardiac defects

SPECIAL TESTS

- Angiography
- Blood gas analysis
  - Calculate alveolar-arterial oxygen difference
  - Measure PaO_2
- Coombs' test for cold agglutinin
- Knott's and occult heartworm test
- Scintigraphy – ventilation perfusion scans for PTE

PHYSICAL ABNORMALITIES

HEPATOMEGALY

DEFINITION

Hepatomegaly is enlargement of the liver.
- The normally sized liver lies within the costal arch and is generally not palpable
- An enlarged liver is palpable and/or visible on radiographs (see liver, p. 272)

NB – Young animals have relative hepatomegaly normally.

CLINICAL SIGNS

- Enlarged liver may cause abdominal enlargement
- May be asymptomatic
- Rapid, shallow breathing through chest compression if massive
- Signs related to underlying endocrine, heart or liver disease

COMMON CAUSES

Generalised
Congestion
- Pericardial disease
- Right-heart failure

Infiltrative disease
- Extramedullary haematopoiesis
- Hepatic lipidosis
  - Diabetes mellitus
- Primary or metastatic neoplasia
- Reticuloendothelial hyperplasia (chronic infectious/inflammatory diseases)
  - IMHA
  - ITP

Drugs
- Barbiturates
- Steroid hepatopathy
  - HAC
  - Iatrogenic steroid administration

Focal
- Nodular hyperplasia
- Primary or metastatic neoplasia

UNCOMMON CAUSES

Generalised
Congestion
- Bile duct obstruction
- Caudal vena caval obstruction
  - Caval syndrome (dirofilariasis)
  - Cor triatrium dexter
  - 'Kinked' CVC
  - CVC thrombosis

Infiltrative disease
- Amyloidosis
- Cholangiohepatitis
- Chronic hepatitis (microhepatica more common)
- Reticuloendothelial hyperplasia (chronic infectious/inflammatory diseases)
  - Systemic bacterial, fungal and rickettsial diseases

Inflammation
- Acute hepatitis
- Drug reaction

Neoplasia
- Advanced primary or metastatic neoplasia

Focal
- Abscess(es)
- Cyst(s)

DIAGNOSTIC APPROACH

1   Determine from history and clinical signs whether drug administration, endocrinopathy or cardiac disease is likely, and investigate accordingly.

PHYSICAL ABNORMALITIES

PHYSICAL ABNORMALITIES

2   If anaemic or thrombocytopenic, investigate causes other than liver disease first.
3   Investigate primary liver disease by laboratory testing, ultrasound examination and biopsy.

CLINICAL CLUES

Predisposition
- Acute hepatitis in unvaccinated dogs
- Barbiturate usage in epileptic dogs
- DCM and pericardial disease in large/giant breeds
- Diabetes mellitus in older, unspayed bitches
- HAC in older dogs
- IMHA in Cocker spaniel, English Springer spaniel, poodles, OESD, Collies
- ITP in Cocker spaniel, Miniature and Toy poodles, OESD
- Nodular hyperplasia in dogs aged > 8 years

History
- Anorexia or polyphagia
- Drug administration
- PU/PD
- Treated epilepsy
- Weakness/collapse

Physical examination
- Enlarged liver
- Findings related to underlying disease

LABORATORY FINDINGS

Haematology
- Changes related to underlying disease

Serum biochemistry
- Changes related to underlying disease
  - e.g. hyperglycaemia in diabetes mellitus
- Increases in liver enzymes are non-specific
  - Primary liver disease
  - Reactive hepatopathy

Urinalysis
- Glycosuria ± ketonuria in diabetes mellitus
- Hyposthenuria in HAC

IMAGING

Plain radiographs
- Cardiac silhouette
- Enlarged liver
- Primary or metastatic neoplastic disease

Ultrasound examination
- Adrenal glands
- Echocardiography
- Liver architecture

SPECIAL TESTS

- Knott's and occult heartworm test
- Dynamic cortisol testing
- Coombs' test
- Bone marrow examination
- Liver biopsy

HYPERTHERMIA AND PYREXIA

DEFINITION

- *Hyperthermia* is an increase in body temperature resulting from excessive exercise, excessive environmental temperature, or a pathological increase in endogenous heat production (i.e. pyrexia/fever or exercise-induced hyperthermia or malignant hyperthermia).
- *Heat exhaustion* occurs when the body temperature is normal but exercise and environmental conditions cause significant dehydration resulting in clinical signs of dysfunction.
- *Heat stroke* occurs when there is a marked increase in body temperature with simultaneous dysfunction of normal control of body temperature. It is more serious than heat exhaustion, as cell damage will occur with excessive temperatures (>108°F, 42.2°C).
- *Exercise-induced hyperthermia* occurs when the body temperature rises excessively in response to moderate exercise; the cause is unknown.
- *Malignant hyperthermia* is caused by abnormal cellular calcium metabolism, most often triggered by drugs/anaesthetics, causing a rapid – and often fatal – increase in body temperature through uncoupled metabolic heat production.
- *Pyrexia* or true fever is an increase in body temperature because of a resetting of the hypothalamic thermoregulatory set point. The increase in set point is mediated by cytokines and exogenous and endogenous pyrogens released by inflammatory disease.

CLINICAL SIGNS

- Raised core body (rectal) temperature

- Pyrexic dogs may be depressed, lethargic and inappetent

COMMON CAUSES

Heat exhaustion and heat stroke
- Excessive exertion
- High environmental temperature
- High environmental humidity, e.g. shut in a car

Hyperthermia
- Exercise-induced hyperthermia in Collies

Pyrexia
Immune-mediated disease
- Immune-mediated haemolytic anaemia (IMHA)
- Immune-mediated thrombocytopenia (ITP)
- Immune-mediated polyarthritis
- Steroid-responsive meningitis-arteritis (SRMA)

Infection – bacterial
- Abscesses and cellulitis
- Discospondylitis
- Inhalation pneumonia (secondary to oesophageal disease)
- Kennel cough (*Bordetella*)
- Migrating foreign bodies (grass awns), e.g. retroperitoneal abscess
- Prostatitis/prostatic abscess

Infection – viral
- Kennel cough (Parainfluenza)
- Parvovirus

Neoplasia
- Large solid tumours with necrotic centres
- Lymphosarcoma

PHYSICAL ABNORMALITIES

Sterile inflammatory disease
- Pancreatitis

UNCOMMON CAUSES

Heat exhaustion and heat stroke
- Anxiety
- Excessive exertion
- Increased respiratory effort
- Repeated seizures/status epilepticus

Malignant hyperthermia
- Halothane anaesthesia

Pyrexia
Immune-mediated disease
- Glomerulonephritis
- Granulomatous meningoencephalitis (GME)
- Polymyositis
- Systemic lupus erythematosus (SLE)
- Vasculitis

Infection – bacterial
- Actinomycosis
- Bacteraemia/septicaemia
- Bacterial bronchopneumonia
- Bacterial cholangiohepatitis
- Bacterial peritonitis
- Borreliosis (Lyme disease)
- Brucellosis
- Catheter-related phlebitis
- Endocarditis
- Leptospirosis
- Nocardiosis
- Orchitis
- Pyelonephritis
- Pyothorax
- Septic arthritis

Infection – fungal
- Aspergillosis (disseminated)
- Blastomycosis (not in UK)
- Coccidioidomycosis (not in UK)
- Cryptococcosis
- Histoplasmosis (not in UK)

Infection – parasitic
- Babesiosis (imported dogs)
- Cytauxzoonosis (not in UK)
- Dirofilariasis (imported dogs)
- Ehrlichiosis
- Hepatozoonosis (not in UK)
- Leishmaniasis (imported dogs)
- Neosporosis
- Rocky Mountain Spotted Fever (not in UK)
- Toxoplasmosis

Infection – viral
- Distemper
- Canine infectious hepatitis

Neoplasia
- Myeloproliferative disease

Sterile inflammatory disease
- Nodular panniculitis
- Pansteatitis
- Post-surgical – falciform fat necrosis, suture reaction

Miscellaneous
- Drug reaction
- Hyperthyroidism
- Hypocalcaemic tetany
- Phaeochromocytoma
- Splenic torsion
- Testicular or uterine torsion

DIAGNOSTIC APPROACH

- In heat exhaustion, heat stroke and exercise-induced or malignant hyperthermia, the approach is towards the treatment of the raised body temperature rather than diagnosis.
- In pyrexia, the body temperature is raised by resetting of the thermoregulatory set point and is not usually life-threatening. Therefore, attempts to reduce the fever with anti-inflammatories, whilst making the dog more

comfortable, may mask signs and delay the diagnosis.

- Thus, the aim is to identify the primary cause of pyrexia, through history, physical examination, minimum database, imaging and special tests.

CLINICAL CLUES

Predisposition

- Autoimmune disease in females
- Occult neoplasia in older dogs
- Steroid-responsive meningitis arteritis (SRMA) in young dogs

History

- Current drug therapy
- Exposure to other animals
- Past and current geographic locations
- Previous illness or surgery
- Previous wounds – entry of migrating foreign body
- Tick exposure for some arthropod borne diseases (Lyme disease, ehrlichiosis)
- Other signs will vary with the primary cause:
  - Diarrhoea in parvovirus and distemper
  - Migrating foreign body
  - Multifocal neurological signs in GME
  - Neck pain in SRMA
  - Pain with discospondylitis, septic arthritis
  - Petechiation in ITP
  - Respiratory infections will usually present with coughing
  - Shifting lameness/stiffness in polyarthritis and endocarditis
  - Weakness, lethargy and pale mucous membranes in IMHA

Physical examination

Observation

- Hunched/stiff in polyarthritis, discospondylitis, SRMA

Inspection

- Neurological deficits in GME, SRMA
- Ocular manifestations (meningitis, infectious disease)
- Pale mucous membranes in IMHA
- Petechiation in ITP

Auscultation

- Abnormal lung sounds in pneumonia
- Diastolic aortic murmur is characteristic of endocarditis, but any new or changing murmur may be significant
- Flow murmur in anaemia

Palpation

- Joint effusion and reduced range of movement in polyarthritis
- Local areas of pain or swelling
- Lumbosacral pain if discospondylitis or retroperitoneal abscess/migrating foreign body
- Lymphadenopathy
- Neck pain in SRMA
- Organomegaly

LABORATORY FINDINGS

Haematology

- Intracellular organisms in babesiosis; *Ehrlichia* morulae in WBCs
- Leukocytosis suggestive of inflammation, of which infection may be the cause
- Marked anaemia ± spherocytosis in IMHA

Serum biochemistry

- May show various abnormalities that may help to localise the disease

PHYSICAL ABNORMALITIES

Urinalysis
- Active sediment if infection (i.e. presence of bacteria and/or WBCs)
- A urine culture should be performed if there are signs or findings of urinary infection, endocarditis or discospondylitis

IMAGING

Plain radiographs
- Chest and abdomen to show mass(es), organ enlargement or displacement, or the presence of fluid
- Skeletal survey for joint effusions and erosions, and metastatic, lytic lesions

Ultrasonography
- Abdomen to show mass, organ enlargement or displacement, or the presence of fluid
- Echocardiography to show vegetative lesions in endocarditis

SPECIAL TESTS

- ANA (and LE cell preparation) for SLE
- Arthrocentesis and RF for polyarthritis
- Blood cultures – aerobic and anaerobic
- Bone marrow aspirate
- Bronchoscopy
- Coombs' test for IMHA
- CSF tap for SRMA, GME and infectious meningoencephalitides
- Exploratory laparotomy
- Faecal examination
- Fine needle aspirates of enlarged lymph nodes and masses
- Gastroscopy/colonoscopy
- Knott's test
- Peritoneal lavage
- Prostatic wash
- Scintigraphy with labelled leukocytes to localise site of infection/inflammation
- Serology for *Toxoplasma*, *Neospora*, *Ehrlichia*, occult *Dirofilaria*
- Serum protein electrophoresis
- Thyroid function

ICTERUS/JAUNDICE

DEFINITION

Jaundice (syn. icterus) is the yellow discoloration of tissues caused by hyperbilirubinaemia. Jaundice can be caused by:
- massive haemolysis (pre-hepatic jaundice)
- liver dysfunction (hepatic jaundice)
- failure of biliary flow into the intestine (post-hepatic jaundice) because of either biliary obstruction or biliary rupture and leakage leading to bile peritonitis.

CLINICAL SIGNS

- Elastic tissues are most discoloured, but jaundice is more easily recognised in the sclera then the mucous membranes or skin.
- Jaundice in the plasma can be detected when serum bilirubin concentrations exceed 25 µmol/L, but tissue jaundice cannot be detected until serum concentrations exceed 40–50 µmol/L.

COMMON CAUSES

Prehepatic jaundice
- IMHA

Hepatic jaundice
- Chronic hepatitis/cirrhosis

Post-hepatic jaundice
- Acute pancreatitis
- Pancreatic carcinoma

UNCOMMON CAUSES

Prehepatic jaundice
- Babesiosis
- Dirofilariasis
- Haemobartonellosis (usually only after splenectomy and not in UK)
- Onion poisoning
- Resorption of large haematoma or haemoperitoneum (hypothetical, probably does not cause jaundice)
- Septicaemia
- Zinc toxicosis

Hepatic jaundice
- Acute hepatitis (ICH, leptospirosis)
- Bacterial cholangiohepatitis
- Drugs
- Hepatic neoplasia (primary, infiltrative, metastatic)
- Juvenile hepatic fibrosis
- Lobular dissecting hepatitis
- Sepsis

Post-hepatic jaundice
- Chronic fibrosing pancreatitis
- Gallstones
- Intestinal foreign body obstructing major duodenal papilla
- Ruptured gallbladder or extrahepatic bile ducts

DIAGNOSTIC APPROACH

1   The three forms of jaundice are distinguished by history, clinical signs, laboratory analysis and ultrasound examination, and investigated and treated accordingly.
2   If jaundice is pre-hepatic, the dog must be anaemic; normal or mildly decreased haematocrit rule out haemolytic disease.
3   Distinguishing the type of jaundice by determining the relative amounts of unconjugated and conjugated bilirubin (Van den Bergh test) is unreliable, and should not be attempted.
4   Investigate hepatic and post-hepatic causes by ultrasound examination.
5   Liver biopsy if the cause of jaundice is hepatic.

CLINICAL CLUES

Predisposition
- Chronic hepatitis in Cocker spaniel, Retrievers, Standard poodle
- Copper-associated chronic hepatitis in Bedlington terrier, WHWT, Dobermann, Skye terrier
- IMHA in Cocker spaniel, English Springer spaniel, Poodles, OESD, Collies

History
Prehepatic
- Dark urine from hyperbilirubinaemia ± haemoglobinuria if intravascular haemolysis

Hepatic
- Dark urine from hyperbilirubinaemia
- Often have other signs of liver disease (PU/PD, ascites, hepatoencephalopathy)

Post-hepatic
- May have signs of the primary disease, e.g. vomiting and pain in acute pancreatitis, or remarkably few signs if there is a chronic progressive obstruction (e.g. chronic pancreatitis, pancreatic carcinoma)
- Dark urine from hyperbilirubinaemia
- Pale, acholic faeces if biliary obstruction
- Previous episodes of pancreatitis if chronic fibrosing pancreatitis

- Trauma if ruptured biliary tree (may have occurred > 1 week previously)

Physical examination
Observation
- Distended abdomen if ascites, hepatomegaly or bile peritonitis
- Weakness

Inspection
- Pale/jaundiced mucous membranes

Palpation
- Ascites
- Hepatomegaly
- Pancreatic mass

Auscultation
- Haemic murmur if anaemic
- Tachycardia if anaemic

LABORATORY FINDINGS

Haematology
- Inflammatory leukogram in acute hepatitis, pancreatitis
- Leukocytosis in regenerative anaemia
- Mild normocytic, normochromic anaemia if liver disease or post-hepatic
- Severe anaemia if haemolysis ± spherocytosis, autoagglutination

Biochemistry
- Amylase and lipase sometimes increased in pancreatitis
- Hypercholesterolaemia in biliary obstruction
- Hypoglycaemia, hypoalbuminaemia, hypocholesterolaemia, raised ALT + ALP in liver disease
- Raised ALP > ALT in biliary obstruction
- Raised serum bilirubin

Urinalysis
- Absence of urobilinogen in biliary obstruction
- Bilirubinuria > 2+
- Dilute or isosthenuric urine in severe hepatic disease
- Haemoglobinuria in IMHA
- Urate crystals in chronic liver disease

IMAGING

Radiography
- Hepatomegaly if neoplasia
- Hepatosplenomegaly if IMHA, lymphosarcoma
- Loss of detail if ascites or bile peritonitis
- Microhepatica if chronic hepatitis/cirrhosis

Ultrasound
- Ascites
- Diffuse change in echogenic density (cf. spleen and kidney) if infiltrated (e.g. lymphosarcoma)
- Dilated extrahepatic biliary tree if post-hepatic obstruction
- Disorganised or nodular echogenicity if primary or metastatic neoplasia
- Irregular outline and echogenicity in chronic hepatitis/cirrhosis
- Obstructive mass in pancreas

SPECIAL TESTS

- Abdominocentesis if ascitic
- Coombs' test for IMHA
- Dark-field urine examination for *Leptospira*
- Exploratory laparotomy ± pancreatic biopsy
- Liver biopsy + culture

LYMPHADENOPATHY

DEFINITION

Any change in the size or consistency of a lymph node or a group of lymph nodes.

CLINICAL SIGNS

- Decreased appetite
- Lethargy
- Lymph nodes usually are enlarged, firm, painless and without adherence to other tissues. This suggests hyperplasia or infiltrative disease.
  - In lymphadenitis they may be softer, tender, warmer and adherent to adjacent tissues.
- Polydipsia/polyuria (e.g. hypercalcaemia associated with lymphosarcoma)
- Weight loss

COMMON CAUSES

- Haemolymphatic neoplasia
  - Lymphosarcoma
- Mineral-associated lymphadenopathy
- Reactive hyperplasia
  - Post vaccination
  - Secondary to skin disease/pyoderma and superficial/localised wounds

UNCOMMON CAUSES

- Haemolymphatic neoplasia
  - Acute or chronic lymphocytic leukaemia, chronic myeloid leukaemia
- Metastatic neoplasia
  - Squamous cell carcinoma, malignant melanoma
- Inflammatory lymphadenopathy/lymphadenitis
- Pyogenic
  - Juvenile pyoderma (puppy strangles),
  - Bacterial, e.g. mycobacteria, *Nocardia*, *Actinomyces*
- Granulomatous
  - Systemic fungal and bacterial (rickettsial) and protozoal diseases, e.g. *Cryptococcus*, *Ehrlichia*, *Leishmania*, *Babesia*

DIAGNOSTIC APPROACH

1 Assess whether lymph node enlargement is:
  - solitary
  - regional
  - generalised
2 Lymph node FNA or biopsy to determine cause, if local disease not found

CLINICAL CLUES

History
- Duration and type of associated signs
- Duration of lymph node enlargement
- History of previous 'lump' removal
- Travel history/geographical location, e.g. systemic mycoses not currently recognised in UK
- Vaccination history

Physical examination
Inspection
- Oral cavity for gingivitis/periodontal disease that may be responsible for mandibular lymphadenopathy

Palpation
- Hepatosplenomegaly
- Lymph nodes – all palpable nodes should be assessed for size, consistency, mobility and pain

PHYSICAL ABNORMALITIES

LABORATORY FINDINGS

Haematology

- Abnormalities of RBCs and platelets with neoplastic disease affecting the bone marrow or systemic infectious disease, e.g. rickettsial diseases
- Evidence of circulating abnormal cells/blasts in leukaemic patients
- Leukocytosis = inflammatory white cell picture may be seen in systemic inflammatory or infectious diseases
- Look for blood-borne parasites
- Lymphocytosis may be seen with chronic lymphocytic leukaemia or ehrlichiosis
- Non-regenerative anaemia secondary to chronic disease (inflammatory/infectious/neoplastic)
- Pancytopenia is common with acute leukaemias, ehrlichiosis

Biochemistry

- Hyperglobulinaemia
  - Monoclonal gammopathy recognised in dogs with multiple myeloma and also lymphosarcoma and ehrlichiosis
  - Polyclonal gammopathy recognised in lymphosarcoma, ehrlichiosis and systemic mycoses
- Serum calcium (total or ionised)
  - Hypercalcaemia associated with lymphosarcoma, multiple myeloma, some infectious disease, e.g. severe granulomatous reaction

Urinalysis

- Look for abnormal proteinuria if suspect multiple myeloma

IMAGING

Plain radiographs

- Abdominal radiography to assess for other organomegaly, e.g. hepatosplenomegaly, iliac lymphadenopathy (ventral deviation of colon)
- Thoracic and abdominal radiographs to assess for non-palpable lymph node enlargement, e.g. sternal/hilar nodes, mediastinal mass

Ultrasonographic examination

- To assess lymph node enlargement (e.g. mesenteric, aortic or iliac) and other organ involvement particularly the liver and spleen
- Ultrasound-guided biopsies

SPECIAL TESTS

- Bone marrow aspirate/core biopsy indicated if:
  - haematological abnormalities, e.g. cytopenias, circulating blast cells
  - suspect haematological neoplasia
  - unexplained hypercalcaemia
- Perform serum protein electrophoresis to identify if hyperglobulinaemia is monoclonal or polyclonal
- Lymph node aspirate for cytological evaluation:
  - Large soft nodes often have necrotic/haemorrhagic centre so aspiration of a smaller node may be more diagnostic
  - Mandibular nodes usually have a degree of reactive hyperplasia secondary to periodontal disease – aspirate other nodes if generalised lymphadenopathy
- Lymph node biopsy for histopathology ± culture

MALABSORPTION

Malabsorption is not strictly a physical problem, but a syndrome recognised by a combination of diarrhoea and weight loss in the face of increased appetite.

DEFINITION

Malabsorption is the defective absorption of nutrient(s) due to a failure in the digestive or absorptive phases of that (those) molecule(s).

- Malabsorption may lead to weight loss if there is generalised inability to digest and absorb food
- Malabsorption may lead to specific deficiency states if only a single nutrient is malabsorbed, e.g. cobalamin
- Malabsorption typically causes diarrhoea
- Occasionally, there is significant malabsorption without diarrhoea

CLINICAL SIGNS

- Diarrhoea
- Polyphagia including coprophagia
- Weight loss

COMMON CAUSES

Normal to increased food intake
- EPI
- Mild IBD
- SIBO

Normal to decreased food intake
- Severe IBD

UNCOMMON CAUSES

Normal to increased food intake
- Deficiency of cobalamin absorption

- Lactase deficiency (suspected, but never proven in dogs)
- Lymphangiectasia

Normal to decreased food intake
- Alimentary lymphosarcoma

DIAGNOSTIC APPROACH

1. Rule out EPI by TLI test.
2. Minimum data base to screen for PLE.
3. Folate and cobalamin to screen for indication of malabsorption.
4. Absorptive function tests (e.g. xylose absorption) generally unhelpful.
5. Intestinal biopsy.

CLINICAL CLUES

Predisposition
- Cobalamin malabsorption in Border Collie, Giant Schnauzer, Shar pei
- EPI in GSDs
- IBD in GSDs
- Lymphangiectasia in Lundehund, Rottweiler, Yorkshire terrier
- PLE ± PLN in Soft-coated wheaten terrier

History
- Abnormal faeces
- Increased appetite
- Weight loss

Physical examination
Inspection
- Weight loss

Palpation
- Occasionally, thickened bowel loops palpable

LABORATORY FINDINGS

Haematology
- Lymphopenia in lymphangiectasia
- Neutrophilia sometimes in IBD

Serum biochemistry
- Hypoproteinaemia suggestive of PLE
- Hypocholesterolaemia

IMAGING

Radiographs
Plain
- Usually unremarkable except for lack of detail due to loss of fat

Contrast
- Irregular mucosa with infiltrative disease

Ultrasound examination
- Thickened bowel wall

SPECIAL TESTS

- Folate and cobalamin
- Intestinal biopsy
- Intestinal permeability tests (e.g. lactulose/rhamnose)
- Serum TLI
- Xylose absorption (obsolete)

MICROHEPATICA

DEFINITION

Microhepatica is a small liver size.
- As the normal liver is not palpable, a small liver can only be detected indirectly by imaging.
- In some deep-chested breeds the normal liver appears relatively small because of an upright gastric axis.

CLINICAL SIGNS

- Related to liver dysfunction (see pp. 271–2)

COMMON CAUSES

- Chronic hepatitis
- Cirrhosis
- Congenital portosystemic shunt

UNCOMMON CAUSES

- Idiopathic hepatic fibrosis
- Lobular dissecting hepatitis

DIAGNOSTIC APPROACH

1 Confirm significance of apparent microhepatica by dynamic bile acid testing.
2 Ultrasound examination for:
  - PSS and lack of intrahepatic portal vasculature
  - Hepatic parenchymal abnormalities
3 Portovenography for PSS
4 Liver biopsy for chronic hepatopathies

CLINICAL CLUES

Predisposition
- Chronic hepatitis
  - Certain breeds – Dobermann, WHWT
  - Epileptics on barbiturates

- Copper-associated chronic hepatitis in Bedlington, Skye terrier
- Lobular dissecting hepatitis in young GSD, Standard poodle
- Congenital PSS in:
  - Young animals
  - Certain breeds – Border collie, Golden retriever, Irish setter, Irish wolfhound, Lhasa Apso, Shih Tzu, terriers
- Idiopathic hepatic fibrosis in young GSD, Rottweiler

History
- Signs consistent with hepatic dysfunction

Physical examination
- See Liver disease (p. 272)

LABORATORY FINDINGS

- See Liver disease (p. 272)

IMAGING

- See Liver disease (p. 272)

SPECIAL TESTS

- Liver biopsy (p. 273)

MURMUR

See Cardiovascular system, Section 4 (pp. 199–226)

ORAL MASS

DEFINITION

Abnormal proliferative tissue in the oral cavity.

CLINICAL SIGNS

- Drooling
- Dysphagia
- Halitosis
- Oral bleeding
- Tooth loss
- May be asymptomatic

COMMON CAUSES

Benign hyperplasia
- Benign gingival hyperplasia

Benign neoplasia
- Epulides
  - Acanthomatous
  - Fibromatous
  - Ossifying

Malignant neoplasia
- Squamous cell carcinoma
- Malignant melanoma
- Fibrosarcoma

UNCOMMON CAUSES

- Eosinophilic granuloma (very rare, cf. cat)
- Salivary mucocoele in mouth (ranula)

Benign neoplasia
- Papilloma

Malignant neoplasia
- Odontogenic tumours
- Osteosarcoma

DIAGNOSTIC APPROACH

1 Head and chest radiographs to assess invasion and metastasis.
2 Biopsy of mass lesion.
3 FNA of mandibular lymph nodes.
4 Attempt complete surgical excision if not performed when biopsied initially.

CLINICAL CLUES

Predisposition
- Gingival hyperplasia and epulides in brachycephalic breed, especially Boxer
- Gingival hyperplasia associated with periodontal disease
- Papillomatosis in young dogs

Physical examination
- Displacement and/or loss of teeth
- Mandibular lymphadenopathy
- Oral mass itself

LABORATORY FINDINGS

- Usually unremarkable

IMAGING

Plain radiographs
Head
- Soft tissue mass
- Local bone destruction

Chest
- Metastatic disease

SPECIAL TESTS

- Biopsy
- FNA

PERIPHERAL OEDEMA

DEFINITION

Peripheral oedema is an excess of interstitial fluid in body tissues, and may be either localised or generalised.

CLINICAL SIGNS

- Ascites, hydrothorax, hydropericardium, and pulmonary oedema are specific areas of oedema discussed elsewhere that often occur before peripheral oedema
- Generalised peripheral oedema will appear as symmetrical swelling that 'pits' under light pressure, i.e. depression caused by pressure dissipates only slowly
- Localised oedema affects only one part of the body

COMMON CAUSES

Generalised
Decreased capillary oncotic pressure (hypoalbuminaemia)
- Protein-losing enteropathy
- Protein-losing nephropathy
- Severe chronic liver disease

Increased capillary hydrostatic pressure
- Cardiac tamponade
  - Idiopathic pericardial haemorrhage
  - Right atrial haemangiosarcoma
- Over-zealous fluid administration
- Right-heart failure

Increased vascular permeability
- Urticarial angio-oedema

Localised
Increased capillary hydrostatic pressure
- Tourniquet, e.g. bandage, collar
- Venous obstruction
  - Thrombophlebitis

Increased vascular permeability
- Insect bite
- Local infection/cellulitis

UNCOMMON CAUSES

Generalised
Decreased capillary oncotic pressure (hypoalbuminaemia)
- Severe burns

Increased capillary hydrostatic pressure
- Dirofilariasis
- Restrictive pericarditis

Increased vascular permeability
- Vasculitis

Localised
Increased capillary hydrostatic pressure
- Abscess/granuloma
- Arteriovenous fistula
- Neoplasia
- Venous thrombosis

Increased vascular permeability
- Mast cell tumour
- Severe burns
- Snake bite
- Vasculitis

Lymphatic obstruction (variable localisation)
- Congenital lymphoedema – aplasia or hypoplasia
- Lymphangiectasia
- Lymphangioma/sarcoma
- Lymphangitis/lymphadenitis
- Lymphocysts
- Neoplasia
  - Mediastinum – oedema of head
  - Pelvis – oedema of hindlimbs

DIAGNOSTIC APPROACH

1   Determine whether localised or generalised by physical examination.
2   If localised, investigate local lymphatic system and evidence for insect bite, tumours, etc.
3   With generalised peripheral oedema, check serum albumin, and investigate any cause of hypoalbuminaemia.
4   If normal serum proteins, rule out right-heart and pericardial disease, before investigating lymphatic and vascular systems.

CLINICAL CLUES

Predisposition
- Idiopathic pericardial haemorrhage in large/giant breed dogs
- Right-atrial haemangiosarcoma in GSD

History
- Gradual/fluctuating oedema with neoplasia and congenital lymphoedema
- Sudden onset of oedema with right-heart failure, pericardial disease

Physical examination

Observation
- Swelling of limbs and head

Palpation
- Pitting oedema

LABORATORY FINDINGS

Haematology
- Inflammatory leukogram suggests inflammation ± infection

Biochemistry
- Hypoalbuminaemia
- Increased liver enzymes and bile acids suggests liver disease

Urinalysis
- Proteinuria suggests protein-losing nephropathy

IMAGING

- Radiography to demonstrate mass, increase in organ size, or body fluid
- Ultrasonography to demonstrate fluid in various body cavities

SPECIAL TESTS

- Abdominocentesis, thoracocentesis, pericardiocentesis
- Angiography
- Biopsy
- Lymphangiography

PLEURAL EFFUSION

DEFINITION

An accumulation of fluid in the pleural space. It can be the accumulation of a:

- transudate (hydrothorax) due to hypoalbuminaemia
- modified transudate
- exudate due to septic (pyothorax) or non-septic inflammation

or it may contain

- blood (haemothorax)
- chyle (chylothorax)

NB – The same condition can sometimes cause either an exudate or modified transudate.

CLINICAL SIGNS

- Cyanosis
- Exercise intolerance/lethargy
- Varying degrees of dyspnoea and tachypnoea

COMMON CAUSES

Chylothorax (can be modified transudate or exudate)
- Idiopathic
- Traumatic thoracic duct rupture

Exudate
Neoplasia
- Mediastinal
  - Lymphosarcoma
- Pulmonary masses

Pyothorax
- Migrating foreign body
- *Nocardia*, *Actinomyces*

Haemothorax
- Bleeding disorder
- Neoplasia
- Trauma

Modified transudate
- Neoplasia
- Ruptured diaphragm with organ entrapment

Transudate (hydrothorax)
- Hypoalbuminaemia
  - PLE
  - PLN

Chylothorax
- Congenital
- Dirofilariasis
- Jugular vein thrombosis (after cannulation)
- Neoplasia
- Right-heart failure (rare, cf. cat)

Exudate
Neoplasia
- Heart base
- Mediastinal
  - Thymoma
- Mesothelioma
- Rib chondrosarcoma, osteosarcoma

Pyothorax
- Penetrating wound (chest wall or oesophagus)
- Parapneumonic effusion, i.e. extension of pulmonary infection

Sterile inflammation
- Dirofilariasis
- Lung lobe torsion – can occur secondary to other primary cause of effusion
- Pulmonary infiltrates with eosinophils
- Ruptured diaphragm with organ entrapment
- Pancreatitis (small volume)
- Walled-off abscess

Haemothorax
- Lung lobe torsion – when lung lobe becomes necrotic
- Necrotic neoplasm
  - Mesothelioma
  - Thymus

Modified transudate
- Right-heart failure (rare, cf. cat)
- Vasculitis

Small volume
- Post-partum
- PTE
- Pyometra
- Secondary to abdominal surgery

Transudate (hydrothorax)
- Hepatic failure
- Pericardial effusion and cardiac tamponade
- Right-heart failure (rare, cf. cat)

1. Confirm clinical suspicion of pleural effusion by imaging.
2. Obtain sample of effusion for analysis after ruling out generalised bleeding disorder.
3. Repeat imaging after drainage, having used chest drain if large volume.
4. Identify underlying cause – neoplasia, heart failure, pyothorax, etc. from fluid analysis and imaging results.

PHYSICAL ABNORMALITIES

CLINICAL CLUES

Predisposition
- Idiopathic chylothorax in Afghan hound, Borzoi
- Migrating foreign body (e.g. grass awn) in working spaniels

History
- Access to anticoagulant
- Coughing
- Jugular catheterisation
- Previous trauma causing penetrating wound or ruptured diaphragm
- Signs of underlying GI or liver disease

Physical examination
Observation
- Dyspnoea, tachypnoea
- Evidence of generalised bleeding

Palpation
- Chest wall mass
- Displacement of apex beat by intrathoracic mass
- Displacement of trachea from midline of thoracic inlet by intrathoracic mass
- Jugular thrombosis

Auscultation
- Muffled lung sounds ventrally – fluid line may be discernible

Percussion
- Dull ventrally; fluid line discernible

LABORATORY FINDINGS

Haematology
- Inflammatory leukogram if pyothorax or necrotic tumour

Serum biochemistry
- Changes characteristic of underlying systemic disease

Urinalysis
- Proteinuria if PLN

IMAGING

Plain radiographs
- DV (and standing lateral) preferred if lateral recumbency causes dyspnoea
- Lateral recumbent radiograph taken after thoracocentesis
- Lung lobe torsion causes displacement of mainstem bronchi
- Mediastinal mass
  - Soft tissue density cranial to heart and displacing trachea dorsally
  - Associated effusion may obscure mass
- Pleural fluid
  - 50–100 ml is the minimum amount of fluid that can be detected
  - Pleural fissure lines
  - Retraction of lung lobes from thoracic wall
  - Obscured cardiac and diaphragmatic outline

NB – Intrathoracic fat or skin fold may mimic effusion.

Ultrasound examination
- Better contrast between fluid and soft tissue if performed before thoracocentesis
- Echocardiography
- Identification of mass
- Used to guide thoracocentesis, FNA and needle biopsy

SPECIAL TESTS

- ANA test
- Analysis of pleural fluid
  - Cell numbers and morphology
    - Lymphocytes (chylothorax)
    - Neoplastic cells
    - Neutrophils

- Degenerate – pyothorax
- Non-degenerate – neoplasia
- Cholesterol < serum and triglyceride > serum if chylothorax
- Gram's stain for pyothorax
- PCV
- Protein
- SG

- Coagulation profile
- Exploratory thoracotomy
- FNA and needle biopsy
- Lymphangiography
- Serum amylase and lipase
- Thoracocentesis
  - May be negative if loculated or thick exudate

PROSTATOMEGALY

DEFINITION

Enlargement of the prostate gland.
- As the normal prostate size is related to the dog's size, enlargement is defined by:
  - Abdominal position
  - Relationship to height of pelvic canal on rectal examination; normal ≤ one-third
  - Ultrasonographic measurement
- An enlarged prostate may also demonstrate on palpation:
  - Abnormal shape – asymmetric, loss of median raphé
  - Abnormal texture – fluctuant, hard, irregular
  - Adherence to pelvic floor
  - Pain

CLINICAL SIGNS

- Caudal abdominal pain
- Constipation
- Deformed stool (ribbon-shape)
- Dripping blood from penis
- Dysuria
- Fever
- Haematuria
- Hindlimb lameness
- Hindlimb oedema
- Intermittent haemorrhage from penis, not associated with urination

- Urinary and/or faecal tenesmus

COMMON CAUSES

- Acute prostatitis
- Benign prostatic hypertrophy (BPH)
- Chronic prostatitis
- Prostatic abscess
- Prostatic neoplasia
  - Carcinoma

UNCOMMON CAUSES

- *Brucella canis* (not yet in UK)
- Paraprostatic cyst
- Prostatic neoplasia
  - Lymphosarcoma
  - Metastatic disease
- Prostatic cyst
- Squamous metaplasia

DIAGNOSTIC APPROACH

1 Assess prostate size and structure by abdominal/rectal palpation.
2 Image prostate by ultrasound and/or positive contrast retrograde urethrogram.
3 Urine culture.
4 Biopsy: FNA, prostatic wash, catheter suction biopsy, needle biopsy.

PHYSICAL ABNORMALITIES

CLINICAL CLUES

Predisposition
- *Brucella canis* in imported stud dog
- BPH in older intact dog
- Prostatic carcinoma is seen in castrated dogs

History
- Signs of urinary tract infection, dysuria and tenesmus

Physical examination
Observation
- Dysuria
- Tenesmus

Inspection
- Blood may drip from penis between urination
- Haematuria
- Pyrexia if prostatitis or prostatic abscess, or brucellosis
- Signs of feminism and testicular tumour if squamous metaplasia

Palpation
- Enlarged prostate ± abnormal structure
- Pain on rectal palpation if prostatitis or prostatic abscess
- Orchitis, epididymitis or lymphadenopathy in brucellosis

LABORATORY FINDINGS

Haematology
- Inflammatory leukogram if prostatitis or prostatic abscess
- Usually unremarkable

Serum biochemistry
- Azotaemia if urinary obstruction
- Usually unremarkable

Urinalysis
- Abnormal cells in prostatic carcinoma
- Haematuria sometimes in BPH, prostatic cyst
- Pyuria in prostatitis

IMAGING

Radiographs
Plain
- Caudal abdominal mass – prostate, paraprostatic cyst or distended bladder
- Sublumbar lymph node enlargement with periosteal reaction on lumbar vertebral bodies if neoplastic
- Thoracic radiographs for metastatic disease

Contrast
- Asymmetric position of urethra if neoplasia or cyst
- Extravasation of contrast on retrograde urethrogram if prostate is diseased

Ultrasound examination
- Cysts, abscess, neoplasia
- Prostate size and changes in echoarchitecture

SPECIAL TESTS

- Prostatic wash or ejaculate for culture and cytology
- (Ultrasound-guided) FNA and Tru-cut biopsy

PULMONARY ADVENTITIOUS SOUNDS

See Respiratory system, Section 4, pp. 291–6

PULMONARY ALVEOLAR PATTERN

DEFINITION

An alveolar pattern is a radiographic description of pulmonary parenchymal disorders where there is an accumulation of fluid or cells causing a soft tissue density.
- The pattern is characterised radiographically by increased soft tissue density and the presence of air bronchograms.
- On auscultation, there may be moist crackles or râles.
- It can be caused by:
  - Haemorrhage
  - Inflammatory exudate
  - Neoplastic infiltrate
  - Oedema
- Pulmonary oedema is the accumulation of fluid within the alveolar and interstitial spaces.

CLINICAL SIGNS

- Coughing
- Cyanosis
- Dyspnoea, tachypnoea
- Exercise intolerance
- Signs of underlying disease

COMMON CAUSES

Haemorrhage
- Trauma – pulmonary contusion

Neoplasia
- Metastatic disease – often nodular

Pulmonary oedema
Cardiogenic
- Acquired mitral insufficiency
- DCM
- Over-zealous fluid administration

Hypoalbuminaemia
- Liver failure
- PLE
- PLN

Respiratory
- Airway obstruction
  - Brachycephalic airway disease (only common in brachycephalics)
  - Laryngeal paralysis
- Bacterial pneumonia
- Inhalation pneumonia
- PIE (eosinophilic bronchopneumopathy)
- Pulmonary foreign body
- PTE

UNCOMMON CAUSES

Haemorrhage
- DIC
- Generalised bleeding disorder

Infiltration/neoplasia
- Lymphomatoid granulomatosis
- Pulmonary carcinoma

Pulmonary oedema
Cardiogenic
- Aortic stenosis (rare)
- PDA

Infection
- *Angiostrongylus*
- Blastomycosis (not in UK)
- Canine distemper
- Coccidioidomycosis (not in UK)
- *Dirofilaria* (not in UK)
- Histoplasmosis (not in UK)
- Toxoplasmosis

Neurogenic
- Electrocution
  - Biting electric cord
  - Cardioversion

PHYSICAL ABNORMALITIES

- Head trauma
- Seizures, especially status epilepticus

Respiratory
- Acute respiratory distress syndrome
  - Anaphylaxis – drug and blood transfusion reactions
  - Endotoxaemia
  - Inhalation of gastric acid
  - Pancreatitis
  - Parvovirus
  - Sepsis
  - Uraemia
- Exogenous toxins
  - alpha-naphthyl thiourea (ANTU)
  - Paraquat
  - Snake venom (monocrotaline)
- Near-drowning
- Smoke inhalation

DIAGNOSTIC APPROACH

1 After identification of alveolar pattern by radiographs, patients should be evaluated for cardiac disease by assessment of clinical signs (tachycardia, pulse deficits, murmur, arrhythmia, jugular distension) and evaluation of cardiac silhouette.
2 Perform echocardiography if clear cardiac disease or if suspicion remains.
3 Any signs of upper airway disease or neurological disease investigated appropriately.
4 Rule out bleeding disorder.
5 Pulmonary parenchymal changes investigated by bronchoscopy and BAL.

CLINICAL CLUES

Predisposition
- Acquired valvular disease in CKCS and other small breeds

- Brachycephalics may have obstructive upper-airway disease
- DCM in large/giant breeds
- Laryngeal paralysis
  - Acquired in medium/large breeds, e.g. Labrador retriever, Afghan hound, Irish setter
  - Congenital in Bouvier des Flandres, Siberian Husky
- Megaoesophagus and inhalation pneumonia in Great Dane, GSD, Irish setter

History
- Evidence of electrocution
- Exposure to anticoagulants
- Exposure to fire/smoke
- Primary tumour diagnosed previously
- Regurgitation leading to inhalation pneumonia
- Signs of underlying disease – GI, liver, renal
- Trauma

Physical examination
Observation
- Dyspnoea and tachypnoea
- Upper-airway stridor

Inspection
- Halitosis
- Pyrexia with infectious/inflammatory disease

Auscultation
- Heart murmur
- Upper-airway stridor

Palpation
- Pain/crepitus if fractured ribs

LABORATORY FINDINGS

Haematology
- Eosinophilia sometimes present with PIE

Serum biochemistry
- Changes reflecting underlying diseases – GI, liver, renal
- Usually unremarkable if cardiogenic

IMAGING

Plain radiographs
- Alveolar pattern
  - Cardiogenic oedema starts as interstitial and spreads to perihilar alveolar pattern
  - Non-cardiogenic oedema is patchy and often not perihilar
- Fractured ribs may not be readily detected

- Left-sided or generalised cardiomegaly suggests cardiogenic oedema
- Right-heart enlargement alone probably secondary to pulmonary disease (*cor pulmonale*)

Ultrasound examination
- Echocardiography

SPECIAL TESTS

- BAL
- Coagulation profile
- Knott's test or heartworm serology
- Neurological examination

SPLENOMEGALY

DEFINITION

Enlargement of the spleen; the enlargement may be either focal or generalised.

CLINICAL SIGNS

It is unusual for the splenomegaly to be the presenting complaint.
- Abdominal enlargement
- Intermittent weakness/collapse from splenic haemorrhage or torsion
- Non-specific signs
  - Anorexia
  - Lethargy
- Signs related to underlying cause

COMMON CAUSES

Congestive
- Barbiturates
- Portal hypertension

Hyperplastic
- Haemolytic disease
- Nodular hyperplasia

Infiltrative
Neoplastic
- Lymphosarcoma

Non-neoplastic
- Extramedullary haematopoiesis

Splenic mass (usually focal)
- Haemangioma
- Haemangiosarcoma
- Haematoma
- Nodular hyperplasia

UNCOMMON CAUSES

Congestive
- Phenothiazines
- Splenic torsion

Hyperplastic
- Bacterial endocarditis

- Discospondylitis
- Pyometra
- SLE

Infiltrative
Neoplastic
- Acute and chronic leukaemias
- Systemic mastocytosis
- Malignant histiocytosis
- Metastatic disease (rare)
- Multiple myeloma

Non-neoplastic
- Amyloidosis

Inflammatory
Eosinophilic
- Eosinophilic enteritis

Lymphoplasmacytic
- Brucellosis
- Ehrlichiosis

Necrotising
- Chronic splenic torsion
- Salmonellosis
- Splenic infarction
- Splenic tumour

Pyogranulomatous
- Blastomycosis
- Sporotrichosis

Suppurative
- Acute infectious canine hepatitis
- Bacterial endocarditis
- Migrating foreign body
- Penetrating wound
- Septicaemia
- Toxoplasmosis

DIAGNOSTIC APPROACH

1   Confirm palpable cranial abdominal
    organomegaly as splenic in origin by
    imaging.

2   Identify underlying infectious/
    inflammatory diseases causing reac-
    tive splenomegaly by laboratory test-
    ing.
3   Rule out bleeding disorders.
4   FNA.
5   Exploratory laparotomy and biopsy
    or removal.

CLINICAL CLUES

Predisposition
- Haemangiosarcoma in middle-aged
  GSDs
- Nodular hyperplasia in old dogs
- Malignant histiocytosis in Bernese
  Mountain dog
- Splenic torsion in large/giant dogs

History
- Barbiturate administration
- Intermittent weakness/collapse from
  splenic haemorrhage or torsion
- Signs related to underlying disease

Physical examination
Observation
- Abdominal enlargement
- Haemoglobinuria sometimes seen in
  splenic torsion

Palpation
- Ascites if portal hypertension or rup-
  tured spleen
- Splenomegaly
  - Focal
  - Generalised

LABORATORY FINDINGS

Haematology
- Anaemia
  - Inappropriate number of normo-
    blasts

- Microangiopathic haemolytic anaemia (presence of schistocytes) in primary splenic pathology
- Regenerative due to haemorrhage
- Leukocytosis if inflammatory/infectious disease

Serum biochemistry
- Changes reflecting underlying disease
- No specific changes for primary splenic disease

Urinalysis
- Haemoglobinuria sometimes seen in splenic torsion

IMAGING

Plain radiographs
- Splenomegaly
- Metastatic disease

Ultrasound examination
- Splenic parenchymal changes
  - Altered echogenicity and homogeneity
  - Mass(es)
  - Vasculature
- Hepatic metastasis
- Lymphadenopathy
- Peritoneal fluid

SPECIAL TESTS

- Exploratory laparotomy
- FNA

STOMATITIS

DEFINITION

Stomatitis is inflammation of the oral mucosa.

It may be generalised or localised to one area of the mouth or to one structure within the mouth, e.g. glossitis is inflammation of the tongue.

CLINICAL SIGNS

- Blood-stained saliva
- Drooling
- Dysphagia
- Halitosis

COMMON CAUSES

Local
- Foreign object
- Periodontal and dental disease

Systemic
- Uraemia

UNCOMMON CAUSES

Local
- Candidiasis
- Lymphoplasmacytic stomatitis (rare, cf. cat)

Contact stomatitis
- Caustic ingestion
- Electrical burns
- Thermal burns

Systemic
- Canine distemper
- Cyclic neutropenia
- Diabetes mellitus

PHYSICAL ABNORMALITIES

- Drug reaction
- Eosinophilic stomatitis
- Heavy metal toxicity
- Pemphigus – pemphigus vulgaris, bullous pemphigoid
- SLE
- Toxic epidermal necrolysis
- Vasculitis

DIAGNOSTIC APPROACH

1 Laboratory testing for underlying systemic disease – crucial if uraemia suspected.
2 Complete oral examination – may require GA.
3 Remove any obvious cause (e.g. foreign body) or biopsy any suspect lesions.
4 Radiograph teeth and tooth roots to diagnose dental disease.
5 Radiograph skull if suspected bone involvement.
6 Appropriate dental care if no other cause detected.

CLINICAL CLUES

Predisposition
- Cyclic neutropenia in grey collies
- Distemper in unvaccinated dogs
- Electrical burns in puppies chewing electric cords
- Prolonged antibiosis and/or immunosuppression for candidiasis

History
- Drug administration
- Known electrocution
- Vaccination status

Physical examination
Inspection
- Foreign body
- Lesions at other mucocutaneous junctions in pemphigus
- Small white plaques characteristic of candidiasis
- Ulceration

LABORATORY FINDINGS

Haematology
- Usually unremarkable

Serum biochemistry
- Azotaemia in uraemia
- Hyperglycaemia in diabetes mellitus

IMAGING

Plain radiographs
- Usually unremarkable unless significant dental disease

SPECIAL TESTS

- ANA
- Biopsy

STRIDOR

DEFINITION

Stridor is a noise associated with turbulent airflow in the upper airways.
- Stertor (snoring) originates in the nasal cavity or nasopharynx – see Nasal discharge, p. 51
- Stridor (harsh, high-pitched, reverberating sound) arises in the oro-nasopharynx and larynx

CLINICAL SIGNS

- Airway noise arising in the upper airway
  - Will be loudest during inspiration
  - May only be evident at increased respiratory rate, e.g. during exercise, when panting
- Cyanosis if severe obstruction
- Dysphonia
  - Loss of bark
  - Altered pitch
- Inspiratory dyspnoea (may only be evident at increased respiratory rate)
- Syncope

COMMON CAUSES

- Brachycephalic airway disease (common in brachycephalic dogs, especially Bulldog)
  - Stenotic nares
  - Everted laryngeal saccules
  - Laryngeal collapse
  - Over-long soft palate
  - Tracheal hypoplasia
- Laryngeal/tracheal foreign body
- Laryngeal paralysis
- Tonsillar hypertrophy

UNCOMMON CAUSES

- Acromegaly (excess pharyngeal soft tissue)
- Laryngeal oedema
- Laryngeal tumour
  - Chondrosarcoma
  - Lymphosarcoma
  - Squamous cell carcinoma
- Laryngitis
- Nasopharyngeal polyps (rare, cf. cat)
- *Oslerus* granuloma
- Pharyngeal/laryngeal/cervical trauma
- Squamous cell carcinoma of tonsil

DIAGNOSTIC APPROACH

1 Localise noise to upper airway by physical examination.
2 Chest radiography.
3 Laryngeal ultrasound (if available).
4 Laryngoscopy under GA – light plane to observe vocal fold abduction during inspiration – then nasopharyngoscopy/tracheoscopy.

CLINICAL CLUES

Predisposition
- Brachycephalic breeds
- Laryngeal paralysis
  - Acquired in medium/large breeds, e.g. Labrador retriever, Afghan hound, Irish setter
  - Congenital in Bouvier des Flandres, Siberian Husky

History
- Change in phonation
- Trauma
- Worse on exercise or in hot weather

Physical examination
Observation
- Audible inspiratory noise
- Dyspnoea

Inspection
- Cyanosis in severe cases
- Subcutaneous emphysema with penetrating trauma

LABORATORY FINDINGS

- Mild polycythaemia if chronic upper-airway obstruction
- Usually unremarkable

IMAGING

Plain radiographs
- Laryngeal radiographs difficult to interpret unless hyoid fracture
- Tracheal hypoplasia

Ultrasound examination
- Laryngeal masses
- Vocal fold movement

SPECIAL TESTS

- Biopsy
- Upper-airway endoscopy

SYSTEMIC HYPERTENSION

DEFINITION

Elevation of the systolic and/or diastolic blood pressures in the region of greater than 180 and 100 mmHg, respectively.

CLINICAL SIGNS

- May be asymptomatic

Vascular accident related to hypertension
- Epistaxis
- Retinal detachment/haemorrhage and consequent blindness
- Seizures, syncope, paresis or collapse

Related to underlying disorder
- Ascites
- Oedema
- PU/PD
- Weight loss

COMMON CAUSES

Secondary
- Diabetes mellitus
- Glucocorticoid excess
- Renal disease

UNCOMMON CAUSES

Primary
- Idiopathic

Secondary
- Alpha-agonists
  - Phenylpropanolamine
- Cardiac disease
- CNS disease
- Hyperaldosteronism (Conn's syndrome – not yet documented in dogs)
- Hypercalcaemia
- Hyperviscosity syndrome
  - IgM myeloma
  - Ehrlichiosis
- Liquorice toxicity
- Phaeochromocytoma
- Polycythaemia
- Pregnancy toxaemia
- Thyrotoxicosis
  - Iatrogenic
  - Functional tumour (very rare, cf. cat)

DIAGNOSTIC APPROACH

1 Measure blood pressure on several occasions.
2 Look for underlying disease by history, physical examination, laboratory testing and imaging.
3 Primary hypertension is a diagnosis of exclusion.

CLINICAL CLUES

Predisposition
- HAC in older dogs
- Older male dogs?

History
- Sudden-onset blindness
- Drug administration

Physical examination
Inspection
- Retinal detachment and haemorrhage
- Tachycardia and weight loss if hyper-thyroid

Palpation
- Thyroid mass

Auscultation
- Systolic murmur

LABORATORY FINDINGS

Serum biochemistry
- Azotaemia if renal disease
- Raised ALP, cholesterol in HAC

Urinalysis
- Proteinuria

IMAGING

Ultrasound examination
- Adrenal glands
- Echocardiography
  - Left ventricular hypertrophy

SPECIAL TESTS

- Blood pressure measurement
  - Direct – arterial puncture
  - Indirect – Doppler preferred over oscillometric
- Dynamic cortisol testing
- Resting T4 level
- 24-hour urinary catecholamines

TACHYCARDIA

DEFINITION

- *Tachycardia* is a rapid heartbeat.
- Heart rates greater than 160 bpm are generally considered abnormal, although rates up to 180 bpm may be normal in small dogs and puppies.
- *Tachydysrhythmias* are excessively fast ± irregular heart rhythms.
- Specific dysrhythmias are discussed in Section 4, Cardiovascular system (pp. 215–17)
- Sinus tachycardia
- Supraventricular (atrial, junctional) premature contractions
- Supraventricular tachycardia
- Atrial fibrillation and flutter
- Ventricular premature contractions
- Ventricular tachycardia
- Ventricular flutter and fibrillation

CLINICAL SIGNS

- Asymptomatic
- Intermittent collapse
- Signs of heart failure
  - Coughing
  - Dyspnoea
  - Exercise intolerance

PHYSICAL ABNORMALITIES

COMMON CAUSES

Cardiovascular disease
- Chronic valvular disease
- DCM
- Pericardial disease

Drugs affecting myocardium
- Digoxin

Metabolic
- Acidosis
- Hypercalcaemia
- Hypokalaemia
- Hypoxia

Others
- Hypotension
- Infection
- Pain
- Pyrexia
- Renal failure
- Splenic disease

UNCOMMON CAUSES

Drugs/toxins affecting autonomic nervous activity
- Atropine
- Glycopyrrolate
- Theobromine (in chocolate)
- Thyroxine

Cardiovascular disease
- Cardiac tumour
- Hypertrophic cardiomyopathy (very rare, cf. cat)
- Lyme myocarditis (borreliosis)

Drugs affecting myocardium
- Doxorubicin

Metabolic
- Alkalosis

- Hyperthyroidism
- Hypocalcaemia
- Hypokalaemia
- Hypomagnesaemia

Others
- CNS disease
- Phaeochromocytoma

DIAGNOSTIC APPROACH

1 Characterise tachycardia by ECG.
2 Treat tachycardia if it is causing clinical signs.
3 Look for and treat underlying cause.

CLINICAL CLUES

See Section 4, Cardiovascular system (pp. 199–207)

LABORATORY FINDINGS

- Changes reflecting any underlying metabolic abnormality
- Unremarkable in primary cardiac disease

IMAGING

See Section 4, Cardiovascular system (pp. 203–6)

SPECIAL TESTS

- ECG
- Exercise test
- Lyme serology
- 24-hour Holter monitoring
- 24-hour urinary catecholamines

SECTION 3
LABORATORY ABNORMALITIES

AMYLASE AND LIPASE

Common causes for elevation
Marked increase
- Pancreatic disease
  - Necrosis
  - Pancreatitis

Mild increase
- Decreased glomerular filtration
- Hyperadrenocorticism or exogenous glucocorticoids (lipase)
- Non-specific GI disease

Uncommon causes
Marked increase
- Pancreatic disease
  - Neoplasia
  - Pancreatic duct obstruction

Mild increase
- Liver disease

Diagnostic significance
- Increases of amylase more than three times the reference range and lipase more than four times the reference range are considered significant.
- Amylase and lipase increases are often considered specific for pancreatitis, but neither is pancreas-specific.
  - Decreased GFR (with azotaemia) is likely in any dog with acute vomit-ing, and then raised activities must be interpreted with caution.
  - Use of glucocorticoids and HAC should be assessed if signs are not typical of pancreatitis.
- Raised amylase and lipase merely support the diagnosis of pancreatitis in dogs with typical signs

Adjunctive tests
- Canine pancreatic lipase immunoreactivity (cPLI) is the most sensitive and specific test for pancreatitis reported so far
  - It is a new immunoassay for pancreas-specific lipase, and therefore avoids the complication of non-pancreatic lipase activity measured by conventional enzyme assays
- Canine trypsin-like immunoreactivity (cTLI) is specific but not as sensitive for pancreatitis, as an early rise is transient
- Exploratory laparotomy and pancreatic biopsy
- Urinary trypsinogen activation peptide (TAP)
  - TAP is a peptide cleaved when trypsinogen is activated
  - Increased TAP in urine appears to be specific, but not very sensitive, test for pancreatitis
- Ultrasound examination of pancreas

AZOTAEMIA (ELEVATED UREA AND CREATININE)

Azotaemia is an increased concentration of nitrogenous substances (urea, nitrogen and creatinine) in the plasma.

Uraemia is the clinical sign, and biochemical and haematological abnormalities associated with marked azotaemia.

Common causes
Pre-renal
- Increased ammonia production leading to increased urea production
  - High protein meal (mild increase)
- Any cause of dehydration, hypovolaemia or decreased renal perfusion
  - Congestive heart failure

LABORATORY ABNORMALITIES

- Hypoadrenocorticism
- Osmotic diuresis in diabetes mellitus
- Pyometra
- Vomiting and diarrhoea

Renal – primary, intrinsic renal disease
(see Section 4, pp. 315–19)
- Acute renal failure
- Chronic renal failure

Post-renal (see Section 4, pp. 330–33)
- Obstruction of bladder neck or urethra by calculi

Uncommon causes
Pre-renal
- Increased ammonia production leading to increased urea production
  - GI bleeding
  - Increased catabolism
    - Fever
    - Tetracyclines
- Any cause of dehydration, hypovolaemia or decreased renal perfusion
  - Diabetes insipidus with water restriction
  - Excess diuretics
  - Excess glucocorticoids
  - Haemorrhagic shock

Post-renal
- Rupture of ureters, bladder or intrapelvic urethra with development of uroabdomen

Diagnostic significance
- Mildly azotaemic patients are unlikely to show clinical signs of uraemia.
- Urea and creatinine will not rise until more than 75% of the glomeruli are non-functional.
- Dogs with azotaemia and concentrated urine should be investigated for causes of pre-renal azotaemia. Pre-renal azotaemia responds well to i/v fluid therapy and carries a good prognosis as long as intrinsic acute renal failure (ARF) has not occurred secondary to renal ischaemia.

- Azotaemia in dogs producing no urine suggests heart failure, anuric renal failure or post-renal causes.
- Isosthenuric urine (SG 1.007–1.016) in a dehydrated dog with azotaemia suggests renal failure.
- Elevations in urea are always significant, but the magnitude of elevations cannot be used to distinguish among pre-renal, renal and post-renal causes.

Urea
- Increases with decreased GFR
- Increases with gastrointestinal haemorrhage, catabolic states and high-protein meal
- Decreased with liver disease and prolonged starvation
- Dehydrated patients – urea is reabsorbed by renal tubules – may overestimate renal functional impairment in dehydrated patients, i.e. pre-renal azotaemia

Creatinine
- Creatinine is more accurate reflection of GFR than urea
- It is less affected by diet and non-renal factors
- It is produced at constant rate from muscle breakdown, freely filtered by the glomerulus and excreted in the urine
- Cachectic animals produce less creatinine, and so can underestimate renal disease
- Male dogs can excrete small amount of creatinine via renal tubules in advanced renal failure, and so can underestimate renal disease
- Some creatinine may be metabolised in the large intestine and so can underestimate renal disease

Artefactual
- Creatinine assay unreliable in presence of icterus

Adjunctive tests for renal function
- Serum phosphate

- Urine protein:creatinine ratio
- Urinary tract imaging
- Urine SG

NB – Renal biopsy is rarely justified if a dog is already azotaemic.

BILE ACIDS

Bile acids are produced in the liver, secreted in bile, and then undergo enterohepatic recycling, being removed from the portal circulation by the liver. Therefore, finding elevated bile acids in the peripheral circulation is indicative of hepatic dysfunction or portosystemic shunting, or both. The sensitivity of the test is improved by taking a sample 2 hours after a meal, where gallbladder contractions will have increased the bile acid pool being recycled.

Common causes for elevations
Marked
- Cholestatic disease
- Portosystemic shunting
  - Congenital PSS
  - Microvascular dysplasia
  - Secondary PSS: acquired shunts due to primary hepatopathy
- Severe hepatocellular disease

Moderate
- Non-icteric hepatocellular disease

Mild
Secondary hepatic disease
- Steroid hepatopathy
  - HAC, iatrogenic
- Vacuolar hepatopathy
  - Inflammatory or neoplastic disease elsewhere

Artefactual
- Haemolysis
- Icterus

Diagnostic significance
- Bile acid testing is superfluous if the patient is icteric, as bilirubin will interfere with the assay, even if there is only prehepatic jaundice.
- By assay methods currently in use in the UK, bile acid levels <25 µmol/L are not significant.
- Bile acids levels >30 µmol/L are always associated with hepatic pathology, but this can be primary hepatic disease or a secondary (vacuolar) hepatopathy.
- Marked increases in bile acids (>100 µmol/L) are always associated with significant (usually primary) hepatic dysfunction, but the concentrations correlate poorly with the degree of dysfunction and do not allow progression of disease to be evaluated.
- Portosystemic shunting typically causes a low/normal resting bile acid concentration and markedly increased postprandial values.
- Hepatocellular and cholestatic disease more typically produces elevated resting concentrations, with less increase post-prandially.

Adjunctive tests for hepatic disease
- Hepatic ultrasound
- Liver biopsy
- Serum proteins and liver enzyme activities

BILIRUBIN

See Icterus/jaundice, Section 2 (p. 108)

CALCIUM

HYPERCALCAEMIA

Total serum calcium concentration may appear increased if serum albumin concentration is also raised, as the proportion of bound calcium (physiologically inactive) is increased. An increase in ionised calcium has greater significance.

Common causes
Marked
- Malignancy (associated with production of parathyroid-related protein, PTH-rp)
  - Anal sac adenocarcinoma
  - Lymphosarcoma, Lymphosarcoma, Lymphosarcoma!

Mild
- Dehydration/haemoconcentration
- Physiological in young growing dogs

Uncommon causes
Marked
- Granulomatous disease, e.g. blastomycosis (not in UK)
- Malignancy (PTH-rp production)
  - Mammary tumours
  - Sarcomas
- Primary hyperparathyroidism
- Vitamin D toxicosis
  - Calcipotriene ointment
  - Cholecalciferol rodenticide
  - Jasmine toxicosis
  - Over-supplementation

Mild/moderate
- Dietary excess
- Hypoadrenocorticism
- Osteolytic disease
  - Multiple myeloma
  - Septic osteomyelitis
- Renal failure

Diagnostic significance
- Unless ionised calcium can be measured, adjustments should be made for the albumin concentration.
- If there is no history of vitamin D overdose, and the anal sacs are normal on palpation, the most likely diagnosis is lymphosarcoma.
- Lytic bone disease is usually obvious clinically or at least radiographically.
- If lymphosarcoma cannot be proven and/or a parathyroid mass can be demonstrated by ultrasound, measurement of PTH to assess primary hyperparathyroidism is appropriate.
- Marked hypercalcaemia in the presence of azotaemia is more likely cause than effect.

Adjunctive tests
- FNA and/or biopsy of lymph nodes
- Ionised calcium
- Radiographs for lymphadenopathy and bone lesions
- Serum albumin to indicate true calcium
- Serum phosphate
- Serum PTH
- Serum PTH-rp
If all other tests negative:
- Bone marrow aspirate

HYPOCALCAEMIA

Total serum calcium concentration may appear to be decreased if serum albumin concentration is also decreased, as the proportion of bound (physiologically inactive) calcium is decreased.

A decrease in ionised calcium has greater significance.

Common causes
- Eclampsia
- Hypoproteinaemia (hypoalbuminaemia)

Uncommon causes

- Acute or chronic renal failure
- Alkalosis
- Ethylene glycol toxicity
- Excess dietary phosphate
- Fanconi's syndrome and renal tubular acidosis
- Hypovitaminosis D
- Intravenous phosphate administration
- Malabsorption
- Muscle necrosis
- Necrotising pancreatitis
- Parathyroidectomy
- Primary hypoparathyroidism
- Renal secondary hyperparathyroidism
- Thyroid C cell tumour

Artefactual

- EDTA contamination
- Oxalate contamination

Diagnostic significance

Unless ionised calcium can be measured, adjustments should be made for the albumin concentration.

- Clinical signs of hypocalcaemia include tremors, twitching and tetanic muscle contraction.
- Eclampsia occurs during peak lactation, a few weeks after parturition.
- Hypocalcaemia in the presence of azotaemia is likely secondary to primary renal disease.

Adjunctive tests

- Creatinine and urea to assess renal function
- Ionised calcium to assess physiological calcium concentration
- Serum albumin to indicate true calcium
- Serum phosphate elevated in renal failure and vitamin D toxicosis
- Tests for pancreatitis

GLUCOSE

HYPERGLYCAEMIA

Causes

Marked
- Diabetes mellitus

Mild
- Acromegaly
- Acute pancreatitis
- Drugs
- Ethylene glycol toxicosis
- Exogenous corticosteroids
- Glucose-containing fluids
- HAC
- Progestagens
- Stress
- Xylazine

Diagnostic significance

- Elevation above the renal threshold (~10 mmol/L) is associated with osmotic diuresis and the consequent clinical signs of diabetes mellitus, i.e. PU/PD, polyphagia and weight loss.
- Glycosuria is not proof of hyperglycaemia, as a reduced renal threshold is seen in renal glycosuria and Fanconi's syndrome.
- Mild increases in serum glucose are secondary and not of clinical significance.

Adjunctive tests

- Urinalysis
- Serum fructosamine
- Serum glycosylated haemoglobin

HYPOGLYCAEMIA

Hypoglycaemia is a low blood glucose concentration. It causes clinical signs of neuroglycopenia (weakness, lethargy, seizures, coma), depending both on how low the concentration is, and how rapidly it declines.

Common causes
Artefactual
- Delayed separation of RBCs and serum, failure to use fluoride-oxalate tube

Hyperinsulinism
- Insulin overdose in diabetic
- Insulinoma

Uncommon causes
- End-stage liver disease
- Hypoadrenocorticism
- Glycogen storage diseases
- Juvenile hypoglycaemia
- Hunting dog hypoglycaemia (may be glucocorticoid deficient?)
- Septicaemia

- Massive tumour burden
  - Hepatoma
  - Leukaemia and polycythaemia
- Pregnancy

Diagnostic significance
- If samples have been correctly handled, hypoglycaemia sufficient to cause clinical signs of neuroglycopenia is, in adult dogs, almost exclusively due to hyperinsulinism.
- Other causes are very rare and usually readily obvious from the history, physical examination or minimum database.

Adjunctive tests
- ACTH stimulation test
- Haematology for sepsis, leukaemia
- Serum insulin
- Radiographs for neoplasia

LIPIDS/CHOLESTEROL

HYPERLIPIDAEMIA/ HYPERCHOLESTEROLAEMIA

Common causes
- Diabetes mellitus
- Dietary content
- Exogenous glucocorticoid
- HAC
- Hypothyroidism
- Pancreatitis
- Post-prandial lipaemia

Uncommon causes
- Biliary obstruction
- Nephrotic syndrome
- Primary hyperlipidaemia

Diagnostic significance
- Lipaemia of a blood sample may indicate inadequate fasting before sampling. This is of no clinical significance,

except lipaemia interferes with other assays.
- A persistent lipaemia after fasting is significant.
- Lipaemia is commonly secondary to underlying endocrine or cholestatic disease.
- Repeatable finding after prolonged fast (12–24 hours), in the absence of other diseases, in the absence of other abnormalities suggests primary hyperlipidaemia.

Adjunctive tests for endocrine/ metabolic disease
- Adrenal and thyroid hormone status
- Blood glucose
- Lipid profile
- Serum triglycerides

HYPOCHOLESTEROLAEMIA

Common causes
- Hypoadrenocorticism
- Starvation

Malabsorption
- Exocrine pancreatic insufficiency
- Intestinal disease, especially lymph-angiectasia

Liver failure
- Hepatocellular disease
- PSS

Uncommon causes
- Dietary deficiency

Diagnostic significance
- No clinical significance *per se*, but a marker for other conditions.
- Low serum cholesterol is indicative of low intestinal uptake or impaired hepatic metabolism.

Adjunctive tests
- Bile acids for liver disease
- Intestinal biopsy for malabsorption
- TLI

POTASSIUM

HYPERKALAEMIA

Potassium is largely intracellular, and hyperkalaemia occurs if there is failure of intracellular uptake and/or increased leakage, or if there is failure of urinary excretion.

Common causes
Marked
- Anuric/oliguric acute renal failure
- Diabetic ketoacidosis (although total body potassium is actually depleted)
- Hypoadrenocorticism
- Rupture of urinary tract
- Urinary tract obstruction

Mild
- Acidosis
- Chronic renal failure
- Dehydration

Artefactual
- Prolonged exposure of serum to clot

Uncommon causes
- Acute tumour lysis
- Chylothorax with repeated thoracocentesis
- Diffuse tissue damage (crush injury)
- Drugs
  - ACE inhibitors
  - Propranolol
- GI perforation
- Haemolysis in Akitas and individual dogs with high intracellular potassium
- Hypoaldosteronism
- Reperfusion injury
- *Trichuris* infestation

Artefactual
- Marked leukocytosis or thrombocytosis
- Collection in K-EDTA or K-heparin

Diagnostic significance
- Marked elevation is clinically significant causing serious bradydysrhythmia.
- Mild increases are often artefactual or insignificant.

Adjunctive tests
- Sodium: low in hypoadrenocorticism
- Urea and creatinine for azotaemia

HYPOKALAEMIA

Common causes
- Anorexia
- Vomiting
- Diarrhoea
- Chronic renal failure
- Potassium-deficient fluid therapy
- Insulin therapy
- Loop-diuretic therapy

Uncommon causes
- Alkalosis
- Post-obstructive diuresis
- Hyperadrenocorticism (mild)
- Renal disease

- Fanconi's syndrome
- Renal tubular acidosis
- Primary hyperaldosteronism

Diagnostic significance
- Recognition of hypokalaemia is important so that correction can be made by potassium supplementation.
- Signs of hypokalaemia include weakness.

Adjunctive tests
- Creatinine and urea
- Other serum electrolytes
- Urinary fractional excretion

SODIUM

HYPERNATRAEMIA

Common causes
Dehydration
Hypotonic water losses
- Diarrhoea (sodium-poor fluid)
- HAC (mild)
- Osmotic diuresis (glucose, mannitol)
- Post-obstructive diuresis
- Renal failure
- Salt gain
- Vomiting (especially if GI obstruction)

Insensible water loss
- Panting
- Fever, hyperthermia

Restricted intake (especially if associated with polyuria)
- Water withheld accidentally/deliberately

Uncommon causes
Hypotonic water losses
- Diabetes insipidus (with water restriction)

Insensible water loss
- Burns
- Third space effect

Restricted intake
- Primary hypodipsia or adipsia
- CNS disease

Salt gain
- Increased dietary intake
- Hypertonic saline
- Hyperaldosteronism

Diagnostic significance
- Hypernatraemia is usually secondary to obvious dehydration.
- Occasionally, in animals with CNS disease, profound hypernatraemia develops because of a decline in thirst and failure to drink.

Adjunctive tests
- Potassium may be low
- Urea and creatinine to assess renal function

HYPONATRAEMIA

Common causes
Increased plasma osmolality
- Diabetes mellitus

Reduced plasma osmolality
Hypovolaemic
- GI loss (vomiting and diarrhoea, especially if obstruction)
- Hypoadrenocorticism

Normovolaemic
- 5% dextrose infusion

Hypervolaemic
- CHF
- Severe liver disease

Uncommon causes
Increased plasma osmolality
- Mannitol infusion

Reduced plasma osmolality
Hypovolaemic
- Burns
- Third space effect (peritonitis)

Normovolaemic
- Inappropriate ADH release
- Myxoedematous coma in hypothyroidism
- Psychogenic polydipsia

Hypervolaemic
- Advanced renal failure
- Nephrotic syndrome

Artefactual
- Pseudohyponatraemia if sodium measured by flame photometry in lipaemic sample. Does not occur with ion-selective electrode

Diagnostic significance
- The rate of reduction is more important than the magnitude.
- Rapid onset more likely to cause lethargy, depression, vomiting, seizures and coma, and should be corrected gradually with isotonic saline.
- If slow onset, signs are related to underlying disease.

Adjunctive tests
- Glucose
- Potassium
- Thyroid function
- Urea and creatinine

TOTAL PROTEIN (ALBUMIN AND GLOBULIN)

HYPOPROTEINAEMIA (HYPOALBUMINAEMIA)

Hypoproteinaemia can be due to hypoalbuminaemia, hypoglobulinaemia, or both.

Common causes
- External haemorrhage
- Hepatic dysfunction
  - Hepatocellular disease
  - PSS
- Protein-losing enteropathy (PLE)
  - Inflammatory bowel disease (IBD)
  - *Ancylostoma* hookworms (not in UK)
- Protein-losing nephropathy (PLN)
  - Glomerulonephritis
- Starvation (mild)

Uncommon causes
- Exocrine pancreatic insufficiency (mild)
- Burns

LABORATORY ABNORMALITIES

Table 4

	Albumin	Globulin
PLE	Low	Low (raised if severe inflammatory disease)
PLN	Low	Normal
Liver disease	Low	Normal/raised

- GI ulceration
- PLE
  - Lymphosarcoma
  - Lymphangiectasia
- PLN
  - Amyloidosis

Diagnostic significance

- Mild hypoalbuminaemia is seen in most sick dogs as a negative acute-phase reaction in response to increased globulins.
- More severe hypoproteinaemia is related to either increased losses or decreased synthesis.

(See Table 4.)

Adjunctive tests

- Liver function test (bile acids)
- Intestinal biopsy
- Urine protein:creatinine ratio to quantify proteinuria

HYPERGLOBULINAEMIA

Common causes

- Dehydration/haemoconcentration
- Chronic inflammatory/infectious diseases

Uncommon causes

- Multiple myeloma (monoclonal)
- Ehrlichiosis (mono- or polyclonal)

Diagnostic significance

- Isolated increases in globulin occur in inflammatory and neoplastic disease, and are often associated with a mild/moderate decrease in serum albumin.
- Raised serum globulin concentrations are seen with increased serum albumin when there is haemoconcentration.
- Mild increases are most typical of dehydration; typical clinical signs and increased albumin should be noted.
- Serum protein electrophoresis can help classify the cause:
  - Monoclonal increases indicate multiple myeloma, lymphosarcoma (occasionally) or ehrlichiosis (rarely)
  - Polyclonal increases in globulin suggest a chronic inflammatory or neoplastic process

Adjunctive tests

- *Ehrlichia* serology, PCR for infectious agents
- Radiographs for lytic lesions of multiple myeloma
- Serum protein electrophoresis
- Urine protein electrophoresis (Bence-Jones proteins, etc.)

LIVER ENZYME ALTERATIONS

Common causes
- Primary liver disease
- Secondary hepatopathy

Diagnostic significance
- Increases more than twice reference range are considered significant, but give no indication of primary or secondary hepatic disease, disease progression, or prognosis.
- Increases may indicate primary hepatopathy, or may be a reactive hepatopathy, secondary to disease elsewhere.

Alanine aminotransferase (ALT)
This is a very sensitive marker of hepatocellular damage and repair, but it is also elevated in many systemic diseases.

Causes
- Isoenzyme induction by:
  - Barbiturates
  - Glucocorticoids
- Primary liver disease
- Secondary hepatopathy
  - Any local inflammatory or neoplastic disease
  - Any systemic inflammatory or immune-mediated disease
  - Diabetes mellitus
  - Endocrinopathy
  - HAC
  - IMHA
  - Sepsis

Aspartate aminotransferase (AST)
This is a relatively sensitive marker of hepatocellular damage and repair, so any increases indicate more severe damage than if only ALT is increased. Muscle isoenzyme also occurs.

Causes
- Liver damage
- Muscle damage

Alanine aminotransferase (ALP) and GGT
These are sensitive markers of cholestatic disease.

Causes
Cholestasis
- Bile duct obstruction
- Cholangitis
- Choleliths
- Nodular hyperplasia
- Pancreatic tumour
- Pancreatitis
- Primary liver disease

Isoenzymes induced by
- Anticonvulsants
- Glucocorticoids
  - HAC
  - Iatrogenic

Bone growth (usually mild and no GGT isoenzyme)
- Bone neoplasia
- Diabetes mellitus
- Fractures
- Hyperparathyroidism
- Osteomyelitis
- Young growing dog

Adjunctive tests
- History, physical examination, minimum data base and imaging to identify cause of secondary hepatopathy
- Bile acid to test hepatic function
- Liver ultrasound
- Liver biopsy

LABORATORY ABNORMALITIES

PANCYTOPENIA

Pancytopenia is a decrease in the total numbers of circulating RBCs, WBCs and platelets as a result of bone marrow disease.

Bicytopenia and some monocytopenias may be present initially, since many conditions do not affect all cell lines to the same extent or at the same rate because of differences in cell longevity.

Common causes
• Parvovirus (neutropenia most marked because of shortest cell lifespan)
• Stage V lymphosarcoma

Oestrogen toxicity
• Exogenous (misalliance injection)
• Sertoli cell tumour

Uncommon causes
• Ehrlichiosis

• Leukaemia
• Malignant histiocytosis
• Myelo-aplasia
• Myelodysplasia
• Myelofibrosis
• Myeloma
• Myelonecrosis

Diagnostic significance
• Pancytopenia is an indication of bone marrow disease.

Adjunctive tests
• Bone marrow aspirate and core biopsy
• *Ehrlichia* serology
• Evaluate lymph node involvement (radiographs, FNAs) for lymphoma
• Radiographs for lytic lesions of multiple myeloma

POLYCYTHAEMIA

An increase in the number of RBCs in the circulation.

A haematocrit > 0.65 is considered abnormal except in sight hounds (e.g. greyhounds), which naturally have a higher haematocrit than other breeds.

Common causes
Dehydration
• Hypotonic water loss (renal and GI losses)
• Isotonic volume depletion, e.g. Addisonian crisis

Drugs
• Glucocorticoids (mild)

Hypoxia
• Cardiac disease
• Pulmonary disease

• Obesity causing poor ventilation (Pickwickian syndrome)
• Upper-airway obstruction (brachycephalic dogs)

Physiological
• Splenic contraction

Uncommon causes
Hypoxia
• High altitude (not in UK!)

Pathological
• Erythropoietin-secreting renal tumour
• Polycythaemia vera (primary)

Drugs
• Androgens
• Erythropoietin

Diagnostic significance

- Splenic contraction can be marked in some dogs, especially in GSD.
- Relative polycythaemia is associated with signs of dehydration and possible electrolyte abnormalities.
- Absolute polycythaemia may be secondary to hypoxia, when signs of dyspnoea, etc. are present or excess endogenous or exogenous EPO. True polycythaemia is rare.

Adjunctive tests

- Blood gas analysis to check for hypoxia
- Chest radiographs to assess cardiorespiratory disease
- Renal ultrasound to look for renal neoplasia
- Serum erythropoietin

PROTEINURIA

Excessive loss of protein in urine can be assessed semi-quantitatively by judging the protein concentration on dipstick (1 to 4 +) in relation to urine SG.

- Proteinuria can arise from many sources in the urinary tract. In the lower urinary tract it is usually associated with an inflammatory sediment (RBCs, WBCs).
- Massive proteinuria is associated with glomerular disease:
  - More objective data is given by the urine protein:creatinine ratio:
    - normal   < 1.0
    - uncertain 1.0–2.0
    - abnormal   > 2.0
- Early glomerular disease is often not associated with azotaemia

Common causes
Marked (pathological)
- Glomerulonephritis
- Haemoglobinuria (IMHA)
- Pyelonephritis

Mild-moderate (physiological)
- Extreme heat or cold
- Hypertension
- Pyrexia
- Strenuous exercise

Uncommon causes
- Bence-Jones proteins (multiple myeloma)
- Myoglobinuria
- Renal amyloidosis
- SLE (glomerulonephritis)

Diagnostic significance
The presence of inflammatory urinary tract disease must be ruled out first by examining the urine sediment.
- Check urinary tract for infection, uroliths, neoplasia by imaging.
- Heavy proteinuria indicates glomerular damage.
- If no underlying disease can be found, idiopathic glomerulonephritis is most likely.

Adjunctive tests
- Antithrombin III if hypercoagulable
- Blood pressure
- Serum urea and creatinine, and urine SG to assess renal function

THROMBOCYTOPENIA

Definition
A decrease in the blood platelet count below $150 \times 10^9/L$.

It is most commonly caused by immune-mediated thrombocytopenia (ITP), where the platelet count is usually $< 10 \times 10^9$/L.

Common causes
Decreased platelet production
- Bone marrow infiltration/neoplastic proliferation
- Myelosuppressive drugs

Disorders with increased sequestration/use/destruction

Increased platelet consumption or use
- Adherence to tumour endothelium due to abnormal endothelial development
- Blood loss
- DIC

Increased platelet destruction
- Immune-mediated thrombocytopenia (IMT)
  - Primary/autoimmune
  - Secondary
    - Associated with neoplasia
    - Drugs adsorbed to platelets
    - Systemic infectious agents
    - Viral infections – herpesvirus, parvovirus, ICH, distemper

Uncommon causes
Decreased platelet production
- Aplasia/hypoplasia bone marrow
- Ineffective platelet production
- Myelosuppressive drugs
- Rickettsial organisms (*Ehrlichia*) – not common in UK

Disorders with increased sequestration/use/destruction
Increased sequestration
- Splenic torsion

Increased platelet consumption or use
- Severe vasculitis

Increased platelet destruction
- Direct damage to platelets by bacterial toxins
- IMT
  - Secondary
    - Systemic infectious agents
    - Bacterial infections – leptospirosis, salmonellosis, bacteraemia
    - Fungal disease
    - Protozoal/Babesia infections
    - Rickettsial infections – ehrlichiosis, Rocky Mountain spotted fever

Diagnostic significance
- Platelet count between 50 000 and 150 000/mm^3 is not a cause of bleeding unless platelet function is abnormal, but it is a potential marker of consumption by an underlying disease.
- Spontaneous bleeding is not usually seen until the platelet count is $< 50\,000$/mm^3.
- The platelet count in IMT is often $< 10 \times 10^9$/L.

Artefacts
- Undetected clot in sample
- Macrothrombocytes in CKCS are not counted by automated analyser

Adjunctive tests
- Coagulation screen for DIC
- Bone marrow biopsy
- Platelet factor 3 (PF$_3$) release test not reliable for IMT
- Platelet antibody tests not reliable for IMT
- Coombs' test, ANA test to evaluate for immune-mediated disease
- Blood cultures, fungal titres, rickettsial disease serology for infectious causes

UREA

Definition
Urea is produced by the urea cycle in the liver, where ammonia (produced from amino acid metabolism and GI bacterial fermentation) is detoxified. Urea is excreted in the urine.
- An increase in serum urea is defined as azotaemia (see p. 135)
- A decrease in urea occurs through either decreased production or increased excretion.

Causes of low urea
Diuresis
- Aggressive fluid therapy
- Diabetes insipidus
- Glucocorticoids
- HAC
- Haemodialysis
- Liver failure
- Polydipsia

Liver dysfunction
- Cirrhosis
- PSS
- Urea cycle enzyme deficiency

Neonates

Nutritional
- Low-protein diet
- Malnutrition/low muscle mass

Diagnostic significance
There are no clinical signs associated directly with a low serum urea concentration; it is merely a marker for other conditions.

Adjunctive tests
- Bile acids
- Dynamic cortisol testing
- Serum creatinine

WHITE BLOOD CELLS

LEUKOCYTOSIS

This is an increase in the total circulating WBC count.

It is most commonly caused by an increase in the total number of neutrophils (neutrophilia) and is found in many dogs, partly as a stress response, as well as an inflammatory response.

Diagnostic significance
The WBC response is defined by both independent changes in individual cell lines, and by the pattern of changes in all cell lines. For example, a stress leukogram is defined as neutrophilia, lymphopenia and eosinopenia.

EOSINOPHILIA

Common causes
Hypersensitivity/immune-mediated reactions
- Atopy
- Flea allergy

Parasitism
- *Angiostrongylus vasorum* (limited geographically in UK)
- *Trichuris vulpis*

Uncommon causes
Hypersensitivity/immune-mediated reactions
- Food allergy
- PIE/eosinophilic bronchopneumopathy

LABORATORY ABNORMALITIES

Parasitism
- *Ancylostoma caninum* (not in UK)
- *Dirofilaria immitis* (not in UK)
- *Oslerus osleri* (rarely)
- *Toxocara* (common infection, but rarely causes eosinophilia)
- *Uncinaria stenocephala*

Other
- Eosinophilic gastroenteritis
- Eosinophilic myositis
- Panosteitis (GSD)
- Eosinophilic leukaemia
- Hypoadrenocorticism
- Oestrus in some bitches

LYMPHOCYTOSIS

Common causes
Age-related
- Young animals higher counts than adults
- Increased particularly after vaccination

Other
- Chronic infections (particularly those which elicit an antibody response)
- Hypoadrenocorticism
  - ± Eosinophilia

Physiological
- Response to exercise, excitement or forceful handling

Uncommon causes
Neoplasia
- Acute lymphoblastic leukaemia
- Chronic lymphocytic leukaemia
- Lymphosarcoma

MONOCYTOSIS

Common causes
- Glucocorticoid therapy or HAC

- Inflammatory disease especially pyo-granulomatous, suppurative, or necrotic inflammatory disease
- Immune-mediated disease
- Neoplasms with necrotic centres

Uncommon causes
- Monocytic/myelomonocytic leukaemia

NEUTROPHILIA

Common causes
Physiological
- Adrenaline release
- Stress (endogenous or exogenous corticosteroids)

Reactive
- Acute inflammation
- Chronic inflammation

Infectious
- Localised
  - Abscess
  - Pyometra
- Systemic

Non-infectious/inflammatory
- Acute pancreatitis
- Haemorrhage/haemolysis
- Immune-mediated disease
- Tissue necrosis

Neoplasia
- Large necrotic tumour

Uncommon causes
Non-infectious/inflammatory
- Early oestrogen toxicity
- Surgery

Neoplasia
- Myeloproliferative disorder

LEUKOPENIA

This is a decrease in the total circulating WBC count caused by a decrease in one or all of the white cell lines.

EOSINOPENIA

Common causes
- Acute inflammation and infection (endogenous corticosteroid release)
- Stress leukogram: neutrophilia, monocytosis, lymphopenia and eosinopenia
  - Stress
  - HAC
  - Exogenous steroid

Uncommon causes
- Tissue inflammation with production of eosinophilic chemotactic substances leading to eosinopenia

LYMPHOPENIA

Common causes
- Impaired production
  - Prolonged corticosteroid use
- Loss of lymph
  - Lymphangiectasia
- Neoplasia
- Part of stress leukogram (see eosinopenia above)
- Viral disease
  - Parvovirus

Uncommon causes
- Impaired production
  - Chemotherapy
  - Irradiation
- Loss of lymph
  - Repeated drainage of chylothorax
- Septicaemia/endotoxaemia (? part of stress response)
- Viral disease
  - Distemper
  - Infectious hepatitis

NEUTROPENIA

Lack of neutrophils means that with infection the classical signs may not be evident, e.g. lack of pus formation.

Neutropenia is usually followed by rebound neutrophilia with left shift due to release of cells from maturation and storage pools.

Common causes
Excessive demand/consumption
- Infectious disease

Reduced production – bone marrow disease
- Neoplasia
- Parvovirus infection
- Toxic and drug reactions

Sequestration in marginating pool
- Anaesthesia

Uncommon causes
Excessive demand/consumption
- Drug-induced
- Hypersplenism
- Immune-mediated neutropenia
- Paraneoplastic

Ineffective production
- Most often a result of myeloid leukaemia or myelodysplasia.
- Myelodysplasia often has anaemia, neutropenia and thrombocytopenia associated to varying degrees and is often associated with maturation arrest.

Reduced production – bone marrow disease
- Cyclic neutropenia in grey collie

Sequestration in marginating pool
- Anaphylactic shock
- Endotoxic shock

SECTION 4
ORGAN SYSTEMS

ALIMENTARY SYSTEM

Problems
Presenting complaints (see Section 1)
- Abdominal discomfort
- Anorexia
- Constipation
- Diarrhoea
- Drooling
- Dysphagia
- Dyspnoea
- Faecal incontinence
- Haematemesis
- Halitosis
- Melaena
- Polyphagia
- Regurgitation
- Tenesmus
- Vomiting
- Weight loss

Physical abnormalities (see Section 2)
- Abdominal enlargement
- Ascites
- Oral mass
- Stomatitis

Laboratory abnormalities (see Section 3)
- Amylase/lipase
- Sodium/potassium
- Total protein/albumin

Diagnostic approach
In general, signs of GI disease reflect the anatomical region affected
- Constipation – large intestine
- Diarrhoea – small intestine, large intestine, pancreas
- Regurgitation – oesophagus
- Vomiting – stomach, intestine

However:
- GI diseases can affect more than one part of the GI tract simultaneously
- Non-GI diseases can cause typical GI signs

- Diarrhoea can usually be localised to the SI or LI by the nature of diarrhoea and defecation (see Table 1, p. 29), but can also be due to concurrent SI and LI disease.
- Thus, the overall diagnostic approach is to rule out non-GI causes of GI signs first, before specific investigations.

Diagnostic methods
History
- Reflects the anatomical region affected

Physical examination
- See individual diseases below

Laboratory findings
- No pathognomonic haematological or biochemical changes in GI disease
- Normal results help rule out non-GI causes of GI signs
- Faecal parasitology may give specific diagnosis
- Identification of dehydration
- Panhypoproteinaemia in PLE

Imaging
Plain radiographs
- Abnormal distension of organs
- Abnormal position of organs
- Foreign bodies
- Masses

Contrast radiographs
- Highlight structural abnormalities
- Investigate GI motility

Ultrasound examination
- Investigate organ structure – size and wall thickness
- Normal layering
  - Lumen-mucosa-submucosa-muscularis-serosa

ORGAN SYSTEMS

ORGAN SYSTEMS

Empirical treatment
- Scientifically unsatisfactory method of diagnosis

Special investigative techniques
- Pancreas specific enzymes – See Pancreas, p. 194
- Serum folate and cobalamin – See SI, p. 182
- Intestinal inspection and biopsy
  - Endoscopy
    - Minimally invasive
    - No wound healing or convalescence
    - Anaesthetic risk
    - Jejunum largely inaccessible
    - Small biopsies
  - Exploratory laparotomy
    - Can biopsy all levels of GI tract
    - Full-thickness biopsies
    - Can inspect/biopsy extra-intestinal organs
    - Anaesthetic risk
    - Surgical risk
    - Wound healing and convalescence

NB – Biopsies **MUST** always be taken, even if GI tract looks grossly normal.

ORAL CAVITY

The mouth and its associated structures are responsible for prehending, chewing and swallowing food.

Presenting complaints (see Section 1)
- Bleeding
- Drooling
- Dysphagia
- Halitosis
- Nasal discharge
- Pain
- Regurgitation

Physical abnormalities (see Section 2)
- Lymphadenopathy (mandibular)

- Oral mass
- Stomatitis

Laboratory abnormalities (see Section 3)
- Azotaemia in uraemia
- Otherwise generally unremarkable

Diagnostic approach
- Laboratory testing for underlying systemic disease – crucial if uraemia suspected
- Complete oral examination – may require GA
- Remove any obvious cause (e.g. foreign body) or biopsy any suspect lesions
- Radiograph teeth and tooth roots to diagnose dental disease
- Radiograph skull if suspected bone involvement
- Investigation of neuromuscular causes of dysphagia
- Appropriate dental care if no other cause detected

Diagnostic methods
History
- See presenting complaints above
- Nasal discharge if oro-nasal fistula

Physical examination
- See Physical abnormalities above

Laboratory findings
- Usually no significant abnormalities

Imaging
Plain radiographs
- Look for dental disease
- Look for bone involvement – abscess/osteomyelitis, tumour

Special investigative techniques
- Neurological examination
- EMG of temporal muscles
- 2M antibody for temporal myositis
- Fluoroscopic assessment of swallowing motion

ORAL NEOPLASIA
Aetiology
- Spontaneous tumour
- See Oral mass (Section 2)

Major signs
- Dysphagia
- Drooling

Minor signs
- Bleeding
- Halitosis
- Pain

Potential sequelae
- Uncontrollable haemorrhage
- Recurrence after surgical excision
- Metastatic spread

Predisposition, Historical clues, Physical examination
- See Oral mass (Section 2)

Laboratory findings
- Usually unremarkable
- Anaemia if profuse, prolonged haemorrhage

Imaging, Special investigations
- See Oral mass (Section 2)

Treatment
- Radical excision for rostral tumours
- Surgery plus chemotherapy for malignant melanoma
- Surgery plus radiotherapy for squamous cell carcinoma

Monitoring
- Visual inspection
- FNA of mandibular lymph nodes
- Chest radiographs

Prognosis
- Good for benign lesions

Fibrosarcoma
- Guarded, depending on whether radical excision can achieve wide margins

Squamous cell carcinoma
- Guarded, but curable if wide margin of excision
- Respond to radiation therapy

Osteosarcoma, malignant melanoma
- Guarded to grave
- High metastatic potential

STOMATITIS
Aetiology
- See Stomatitis (Section 2)

Major signs
- Drooling
- Halitosis

Minor signs
- Dysphagia
- Blood-stained saliva

Potential sequelae
- Gingival recession
- Loss of teeth

Predisposition, Historical clues, Physical examination, Laboratory findings
- See Stomatitis (Section 2)

Imaging
- Usually unremarkable unless significant dental disease

Special investigations
- See Stomatitis (Section 2)

Treatment
- Remove inciting cause, e.g. foreign body
- Remove diseased teeth
- Scaling and polishing teeth
- Antibacterials

ORGAN SYSTEMS

- Chlorhexidine mouth wash
- Metronidazole and spiramycin for anaerobes

Monitoring
- Visual inspection

Prognosis
- Good, but preventative measures must be taken to prevent recurrence of dental disease

TEMPORAL MYOSITIS
Aetiology
- Immune-mediated
- Eosinophilic infiltrate, followed by muscle atrophy and fibrous tissue formation

Major signs
- Dysphagia

Minor signs
- Drooling
- Weight loss through inability to eat

Potential sequelae
- Permanent closure of jaw

Predisposition
- None

Historical clues
- Gradual onset of signs
- Dog drops food during prehension

Physical examination
- Temporal muscle swelling initially, which may be painful
- Ultimately atrophy and fibrosis, so it is physically impossible to open the mouth

Laboratory findings
Haematology
- Eosinophilia in some, but not all, cases

Serum biochemistry
- Usually unremarkable except increased creatine kinase

Imaging
Skull radiographs
- Unremarkable
- Rule out temporomandibular joint disease

Special investigations
- EMG
- 2-M antibody
- Temporal muscle biopsy

Treatment
- Prednisolone at up to 2 mg/kg/day, then weaning whilst checking jaw opening
- Breaking down of fibrous tissue under GA in severe cases
- Tube feeding if dog cannot eat

Monitoring
- Measure size of oral bite

Prognosis
- Guarded
- Some cases need prolonged steroid therapy

SALIVARY GLANDS

- The salivary glands [mandibular, orbital (zygomatic), parotid and sublingual] produce saliva.
- A sialocoele is a ruptured salivary duct and is treated surgically.
- Medical conditions of the salivary gland are rare:
  - Adenocarcinoma
  - Hypersialosis
  - Salivary gland infarction
  - Sialoadenitis

Presenting complaints (see Section 1)
- Anorexia
- Drooling
- Dysphagia
- Pain
- Vomiting

Physical abnormalities (see Section 2)
- Pyrexia
- Lymphadenopathy (mandibular)
- Stridor
- Swollen salivary gland

Laboratory abnormalities (see Section 3)
- Azotaemia (pre-renal)
- Leukocytosis

Diagnostic approach
- Examine salivary glands by palpation
- Imaging generally unrewarding; sialography technically difficult
- FNA or biopsy

Diagnostic methods
History, Physical examination,
Laboratory findings, Imaging
- See diseases below

Special investigative techniques
- FNA
- Biopsy

HYPERSIALOSIS/SALIVARY GLAND INFARCTION/ SIALOADENITIS
Aetiology
May be same or related conditions, as all have been reported to improve with phenobarbitone.

Hypersialosis
- Hypertrophy and increased saliva production possibly due to overstimulation by CNS

Salivary gland infarction
- Spontaneous infarction of gland

Sialoadenitis
- Inflammation of the salivary gland
  - Commonly spontaneous, possibly immune-mediated
  - Occasionally caused by paramyxovirus (mumps)

Major signs
- Dysphagia
- Drooling
- Pain

Minor signs
- Halitosis
- Vomiting

Potential sequelae
- Death in severe cases
  - Euthanasia may be necessary if pain cannot be controlled

Predisposition
- Salivary gland infarction reported in Jack Russell terrier

Historical clues
- Sudden onset of clinical signs

Physical examination
- Drooling saliva
- Dull and depressed
- Swollen painful salivary glands
- Pyrexia

Laboratory findings
- Leukocytosis

Imaging
- Generally unhelpful

Special investigations
- FNA and biopsy

Treatment
- Antibiotics in case of infection
- Immunosuppression with prednisolone
- Phenobarbitone at anti-epileptic doses

Monitoring
- Clinical response
- Salivary gland size

Prognosis
- Guarded

OESOPHAGUS

Presenting complaints (see Section 1)
- Regurgitation is the cardinal sign
- Anorexia
- Drooling
- Dysphagia
- Polyphagia (re-eats regurgitated food)
- Secondary signs may develop from inhalation of inadequately swallowed food
  - Cough
  - Dyspnoea
  - Halitosis
  - Nasal discharge
- Weight loss

Physical abnormalities (see Section 2)
- Pyrexia secondary to inhalation pneumonia
- Pulmonary alveolar pattern

Laboratory abnormalities (see Section 3)
- Leukocytosis if inhalation pneumonia
- Otherwise generally unremarkable

Diagnostic approach
- Distinguish regurgitation from vomiting
- Investigate first by:
  - plain radiographs; and/or
  - endoscopy
- Fluoroscopic assessment of swallowing motion

Diagnostic methods
History
- See Presenting complaints above

Physical examination
- See Physical abnormalities above

- Palpate cervical oesophagus for dilatation or foreign body

Laboratory findings
- Usually no significant abnormalities

Imaging
Plain radiographs
- Oesophagus not visible normally
- Radiodense foreign bodies

Contrast radiographs
- Fluoroscopic assessment of swallowing motion
- Radiolucent foreign bodies
- Strictures

Special investigative techniques
- Endoscopy
- Manometry (not available in practice)
- Serum acetylcholine receptor antibody – see Megaoesophagus below

FOREIGN BODY
Aetiology
Accidental ingestion
- Stick injury

Deliberate ingestion
- Bones
- Fish hooks
- Others

Major signs
- Regurgitation
- May still be able to swallow liquids if irregular foreign body
  - Solids regurgitated immediately

Minor signs
- Agitation if foreign body causes discomfort
- Depression from dehydration, perforation
- Drooling saliva
- Odynophagia (pain on swallowing)
- Retching/gulping

Potential sequelae
- Oesophagitis
- Oesophageal stricture
- Perforation of oesophageal wall
  - Broncho-oesophageal fistula (rare)
    - Chronic cough
  - Mediastinitis
  - Pleural effusion

Predisposition
- WHWT are vastly over-represented
- More common in young and greedy dogs

Historical clues
- Acute onset in previously healthy animal
- Ingestion may have been observed

Physical examination
- Outwardly unremarkable in most cases
- Occasionally, foreign body will be palpable in pharynx or cervical oesophagus
- Occasionally, stick will be protruding from mouth

Laboratory findings
- No significant changes
- Leukocytosis if perforation and subsequent mediastinitis
- Pre-renal azotaemia if ingestion of fluids impaired

Imaging
Radiographs
Plain
- Radiodense foreign body
- If perforated:
  - Mediastinitis
  - Pneumothorax or pleural effusion
  - SC emphysema

Contrast
- Should *not* be given *before* plain radiographs, as radiodense foreign body will be obscured

- Use iodinated contrast if perforation suspected
  - Identify radiolucent foreign body
  - Rule out other differential diagnoses

Special investigations
Oesophagoscopy
- Identification of foreign body
- Possible removal of foreign body
- Evaluation of post-traumatic oesophagitis, perforation

Treatment
Removal of foreign body
- Endoscopically
- Forceps under fluoroscopic guidance
- Surgical removal if:
  - significant perforation
  - stick injury requiring exploration of soft tissues
  - other removal methods unsuccessful

Treat oesophagitis – see below

Monitoring
- Check for clinical signs of persistent oesophagitis or stricture formation
- Repeat endoscopy if signs persist

Prognosis
- Excellent if foreign body removed quickly with no perforation
- Guarded if surgical removal required
- Poor if perforation and mediastinitis and pyothorax develops

MEGAOESOPHAGUS (MO)
Aetiology
Primary
- Acquired-idiopathic MO
- Congenital-idiopathic MO
- Focal myasthenia gravis
- Generalised myasthenia gravis

Secondary
NB – Signs of underlying disease are usually as important as regurgitation.

ORGAN SYSTEMS

Myopathies
- Dermatomyositis
- Dystrophin deficiency
- Polymyositis
- Systemic lupus erythematosus (SLE)
- Toxoplasmosis

Neuropathies/junctionopathies
- Bilateral vagal damage
- Brainstem disease
  - Hydrocephalus
  - Meningoencephalitis
- Botulism
- Dysautonomia (rare in dogs)
- Giant axonal neuropathy
- Polyradiculoneuritis
- Tick paralysis

Toxins
- Anticholinesterase
- Acrylamide
- Lead
- Thallium

Miscellaneous
- Distemper
- Glycogen storage disease Type II
- Hypoadrenocorticism
- Hypothyroidism?
- Thymoma

Localised
- Localised dilatation, and ultimately a dilated, dysfunctional segment oesophagus can arise
  - Diverticulum
  - Persistent right aortic arch
  - Stricture
  - Tumour

NB – Not true megaoesophagus as distal oesophagus is normal.

Major signs
- Regurgitation
- Inhalation pneumonia
  - Coughing
- Dyspnoea/tachypnoea
- Pyrexia

Minor signs
- Appetite
  - Initially increased
  - Later decreased if pneumonia develops
- Ballooning of cervical oesophagus
- Halitosis
- Lethargy
- Nasal discharge
- Weight loss

Potential sequelae
- Cachexia
- Sepsis
- Severe inhalation pneumonia leading to death

Predisposition
- Idiopathic megaoesophagus
  - Congenital and acquired MO are most common in GSD, Great Dane and Irish setter

NB – PRAA also seen in GSD and Irish setter.

Historical clues
- Regurgitation is the major sign, but is sometimes mistaken for vomiting
- Acquired MO most common at 5–7 years
- Congenital MO causes signs at weaning (as does PRAA)
- Coughing is common sign
- Lethargy/weakness if generalised MG

Physical examination
Observation
- Depressed and dyspnoeic
- Halitosis

Inspection
- Ballooning of cervical oesophagus
- Nasal discharge and coughing
- Weight loss

ORGAN SYSTEMS

Palpation
- Gag reflex may be absent if pharynx also affected

Auscultation
- Moist lung sounds if inhalation pneumonia
- 'Slopping' sounds from fluid in oesophagus

Laboratory findings
Haematology
- Low-grade inflammatory leukogram if inhalation pneumonia

Serum biochemistry
- Usually unremarkable
- Pre-renal azotaemia if ingestion of fluids impaired

Imaging
Plain radiographs
- Entire oesophagus dilated and gas-filled from neck extending to diaphragm

NB – Beware over-interpretation of passive dilatation under GA.

Barium swallow
- Usually not required for diagnosis
- Assess oesophageal dysmotilty – dilated, hypomotile
- Danger of inhalation

Special investigations
Manometry
- Not available in practice

Oesophagoscopy
- Dilated oesophagus often difficult to assess endoscopically
- Pooling of swallowed and refluxed material
- Danger of aspiration on recovery from GA

Focal myasthenia gravis (MG)
- Acetylcholine receptor antibody titre
- Tensilon test ineffective as any response is too weak/transient to detect

Generalised MG
- Acetylcholine receptor antibody titre
- Tensilon test

Hypothyroidism
- Thyroid function tests

Polymyositis
- Creatine kinase
- EMG

Systemic lupus erythematosus
- Anti-nuclear antibody
- Evidence of multi-organ disease – see p. 270

Treatment
Idiopathic megaoesophagus
No specific therapy
- Postural feeding
  - Empirically try different food textures, e.g. gruel versus kibble
  - Use gravity to deliver food to stomach
- Antibiotics for inhalation pneumonia
  - Need to be given parenterally as oral delivery suspect
- Prokinetics
  - It is suggested that cisapride worsens signs
  - No evidence that metoclopramide or bethanecol help
- Gastrostomy feeding
  - Maintains nutritional intake
  - Does not stop inhalation of saliva

Myasthenia gravis
Anticholinesterase inhibitors
- Pyridostigmine @ 1–3 mg/kg PO BID
- Avoid over-dosing and causing cholinergic crisis

Immunosuppression

There is a danger of immunosuppression when pneumonia is present.

- Prednisolone
  - Start at low dose and increase to avoid muscle weakness
  - Ultimately give @ 2 mg/kg/day
- Azathioprine
  - Give @ 2 mg/kg PO SID
  - Monitor haematology
- Mycophenalate mofetil
  - Give @ 5–10 mg/kg PO BID

Monitoring

- Anti-acetylcholine receptor antibody titre
  - Stop immunosuppression when titre becomes negative
- Clinical response

Prognosis

- Guarded to poor
  - Congenital disease sometimes resolves spontaneously
  - Idiopathic disease potentially manageable, but not curable
  - MG potentially curable
- Death from inhalation pneumonia and malnutrition common

OESOPHAGITIS
Aetiology

Gastric reflux – acid, pepsin and intestinal proteases

- Acute and persistent vomiting
- During anaesthesia
- Hiatal hernia
- Natural reflux oesophagitis

Ingestion

- Foreign bodies
- Caustics
- Drugs acting locally if not swallowed fully
  - NSAIDs

- Doxycycline? (only reported in cats so far)
- Hot liquids and food

Major signs

- Anorexia
- Drooling
- Odynophagia
- Regurgitation is less common than in other oesophageal disorders

Minor signs

- Blood in regurgitated material
- Lethargy
- Weight loss

Potential sequelae

- Stricture formation – see below

Predisposition

- No age or sex predisposition
- Oesophageal foreign body in WHWT
- Reflux under GA more likely if:
  - Not fasted
  - Operating table tilted head-down
  - Prolonged recovery, e.g. after OHE for pyometra

Historical clues

- A recent history of:
  - Ingestion of caustics
  - Foreign body removal
  - GA (with presumed reflux)
- Because of pain, the dog may appear uncomfortable and regurgitate actively

Physical examination

- Dull/depressed/anxious

Laboratory findings

- No significant changes

Imaging

- Usually no significant findings on plain or static contrast studies
- Dysmotility and/or spontaneous reflux may be seen if fluoroscopy is available

Special investigations
Oesophagoscopy
- Bleeding
- Inflammation
- Erosions
- Mucosa very friable on contact with endoscope
- Ulcers

Treatment
Prevent further damage by gastric reflux
- Cisapride or metoclopramide to increase pressure in lower oesophageal sphincter
- Acid blockade, e.g. H$_2$ antagonist, proton pump inhibitor – see Gastric ulcer, pp. 174–5

Rest oesophagus
- Soft, liquidised food
- Gastrostomy tube feeding

Treat oesophageal inflammation
- Sucralfate
  - To coat ulcers
  - Give @ 5–10 ml PO up to six times daily
- Local anaesthetic gels to aid swallowing
- Prednisolone?

Monitoring
- Clinical response
- Repeat oesophagoscopy

Prognosis
- Good if treated aggressively
- Guarded to poor if stricture develops

STRICTURE
Aetiology
- Healing of severe ulceration by fibrosis
- Following severe oesophagitis, or foreign body removal

Major signs
- Regurgitation
- Other signs of oesophagitis

Minor signs
- Lethargy
- Weight loss

Potential sequelae
- Inhalation pneumonia
- Cachexia
- Euthanasia if treatment unsuccessful

Predisposition
- See Oesophagitis above
- Stricture usually develops within 3 weeks of severe post-GA oesophagitis

Historical clues
- Progressively smaller pieces of food can be swallowed
- Small volumes of liquids can still be swallowed

Physical examination
- Outwardly unremarkable initially
- Weight loss, and ultimately cachexia with time

Laboratory findings
- Unremarkable

Imaging
Radiographs
Plain
- Unremarkable unless remnants of food trapped

Contrast
- Liquid barium suspension may pass stricture
- Barium mixed with food (barium meal) will highlight obstruction

Special investigations
Oesophagoscopy
- Observation of stricture
- Proximal oesophagitis
- Treatment by dilatation

Treatment
Dilate stricture
- May need to be done twice weekly for between 1 and 20 times before stricture abolished

Bougienage
- Progressively larger diameter rubber-tipped probes passed
- Danger of tearing from shear forces

Balloon dilatation
- Balloon catheter passed alongside or through endoscope
- Radial stretching force produces less tearing

Treat oesophagitis
- As above
- Gastrostomy tube feeding to rest the oesophagus if severe oesophagitis
- No evidence that prednisolone or colchicine prevent stricture from reforming

Monitoring
- Clinical response
- Repeat oesophagoscopy

Prognosis
- Guarded
- Danger of oesophageal tearing
  - Stricture tends to reform

STOMACH

Problems
Presenting complaints (see Section 1)
- Abdominal discomfort/pain
- Anorexia
- Drooling
- Haematemesis
- Halitosis
- Melaena
- Vomiting
- Weight loss

Physical abnormalities (see Section 2)
- Abdominal enlargement
- Anaemia

Laboratory abnormalities (see Section 3)
- Usually unremarkable
- Azotaemia from dehydration

Diagnostic approach
- Vomiting is the cardinal sign of gastric disease but:
  - non-GI diseases can cause vomiting
  - intestinal diseases can cause vomiting
- Thus, the overall diagnostic approach is to:
  - rule out non-GI causes of vomiting first
  - investigate stomach and intestine

Diagnostic methods
History
- The cardinal sign is vomiting

Physical examination
- Often unremarkable
- Cranial abdominal discomfort if ulcerative disease
- Cranial abdominal mass if large tumour

Laboratory findings
- Frequently normal, but helps rule out non-GI diseases
- No pathognomonic changes
- Secondary electrolyte abnormalities
- Dehydration and hypochloraemic metabolic alkalosis if loss of gastric acid
- Dehydration and metabolic acidosis if vomiting of intestinal and gastric contents
- Hypoglycaemia in young animals not eating

Imaging
Plain radiographs
- Normal right lateral
  - Gas fills fundus

- Fluid in pylorus – do not mistake for circular foreign body
- Normal left lateral
  - Gas in pylorus
- Free abdominal gas (gastric perforation)
- Gastric dilatation-volvulus (GDV)
  - Reverse of gas pattern
  - Compartmentalisation of stomach
- Gastric mass
- Radiopaque foreign body

Contrast radiographs
- Low yield if vomiting and diarrhoea
  - Only indicated if unremarkable plain films and supportive laboratory studies are non-diagnostic and endoscopy is unavailable
- Identify obstruction
- Irregular mucosa/rugal folds
- Monitor GI motility and delayed emptying
- Fluoroscopic assessment of gastric emptying
- Radiolucent foreign body

Ultrasound examination
- Foreign body
- Abnormal gastric wall layering and thickness
  - Gastric tumour
  - Gastric ulcer

Special investigative techniques
- Gastroscopy
  - Inspection
  - Biopsy
  - Foreign body removal
- Serum pepsinogen
  - Test for gastric damage
  - Not commercially available for testing dogs yet
- Sucrose permeability
  - Not commercially available for testing dogs yet
- Exploratory laparotomy

ACUTE GASTRITIS
Aetiology
See Acute vomiting for non-gastric causes, pp. 75–6.
- Dietary indiscretion (change in diet, overindulgence)
- Gastric foreign body
- Haemorrhagic gastroenteritis*
- NSAIDs
- Parvovirus infection*
- Toxins
- GDV – ineffective attempts to vomit

*NB – Diarrhoea is major concurrent sign.

Major signs
- Vomiting
  - Bile
  - Blood
  - Foreign material
  - Mucus

Minor signs
- Bloating
- Eructation
- Lethargy/anorexia/depression
- Polydipsia
- Pyrexia

Potential sequelae
- Dehydration
- Hypochloraemic metabolic alkalosis if pyloric obstruction
- Metabolic acidosis if intestinal contents refluxed and vomited as well

Predisposition
- HGE in toy breeds
- Parvovirus in unvaccinated dogs
- Young dogs more likely to scavenge

Historical clues
- Exposure to toxins, drugs, scavenging
- Sudden onset of vomiting in previously healthy dog
- Concurrent diarrhoea if generalised GI inflammation

Physical examination
- Unremarkable in mild cases
- Anorexia/lethargy/depression in severe cases
- Dehydration
- Cranial abdominal discomfort

Laboratory findings
- Largely to rule out non-GI diseases, especially hypoadrenocorticism

Haematology
- Haemoconcentration
- Rarely an inflammatory leukogram

Serum biochemistry
- Pre-renal azotaemia
- Raised serum proteins

Urinalysis
- Hypersthenuria is appropriate if dehydrated
- Isosthenuria indicates renal cause of azotaemia

Imaging
Radiographs
Plain
- Usually unremarkable
- Foreign body

Contrast
- Rarely indicated in acute disease

Ultrasound examination
- Foreign body

Special investigations
- ACTH stimulation test if suspicion of hypoadrenocorticism

Treatment
- Usually self-limiting with symptomatic support
- Parenteral fluid therapy
- Antibiotic cover if pyrexic or haematemesis

- Acid blockade (H_2 antagonist, PPi) and sucralfate only indicated if marked haematemesis; see Gastric ulcers, pp. 174–5
- Anti-emetic (metoclopramide @ 0.5 mg/kg PO TID) only *after* obstruction ruled out

Monitoring
- Clinical response
- Hydration status

Prognosis
- Excellent for complete recovery

CHRONIC GASTRITIS
Aetiology
- Chronic gastritis of unknown aetiology
  - Auto-antigen?
  - Food allergy
  - *Helicobacter* infection?
  - Part of idiopathic IBD complex
    - Eosinophilic gastritis
    - Hypertrophic gastritis
    - Lympho-plasmacytic gastritis most common
- Drugs
  - NSAIDs
  - Corticosteroids: probably do not cause gastritis, but impair healing of any damage to the gastric mucosal barrier
- Increased HCl production
  - Gastrinoma (very rare)
  - Mast cell tumour
- Persistent foreign body
- *Physaloptera* (not in UK)

Major signs
- Chronic vomiting
  - Bile
  - Blood
  - Food

Minor signs
- Abdominal discomfort
- Borborygmi

- Diarrhoea if part of inflammatory bowel disease or gastrinoma
- Inappetence
- Lethargy/depression
- Weight loss

Potential sequelae
- Gastric ulceration
- Progression to gastric carcinoma, as in man, has not been described in dogs

Predisposition
- None

Historical clues
- Chronic vomiting, with little progression of signs
- Often vomit bile in the morning, and seem better if fed early

Physical examination
- Usually unremarkable
- May be dull and have lost weight

Laboratory findings
Haematology
- Often unremarkable
- Occasional blood loss anaemia

Serum biochemistry
- Often unremarkable
- Normal results rule out extra-intestinal diseases
- Occasional low protein through blood loss

Imaging
Radiographs
Plain
- Usually unremarkable
- Foreign body

Contrast
- Irregular mucosa sometimes
- Rule out outflow obstruction if fluoroscopy available

Ultrasound examination
- Thickening of gastric wall possible, but wide variation in thickness normally

Special investigations
Gastroscopy
- Erosions
- Incomplete emptying of the stomach
- Irregular friable mucosa
- Occasional spontaneous haemorrhages
- Biopsies always taken, even if grossly normal

Histology
- Eosinophilic gastritis
- Hypertrophic gastritis
- Lympho-plasmacytic gastritis

Treatment
Acid blockade (see Gastric ulcers, pp. 174–5)
- H_2 antagonists
- Proton-pump inhibitors

Anti-emetics
- Metoclopramide

Dietary modification
- Exclusion diet trial in case gastritis is a dietary sensitivity
- Low-fat, highly digestible food speeds gastric emptying

Immunosuppression
- Judicious use of steroid as it may impair the mucosal barrier
- Prednisolone @ 1–2 mg/kg/day

Triple therapy
- To treat *Helicobacter* infection
- Combination of two antibiotics (e.g. amoxycillin and metronidazole) plus an acid blocker (see below)
- No evidence that *Helicobacter* are pathogenic and that triple therapy is indicated

ORGAN SYSTEMS

Monitoring
- Clinical response
- Repeat gastroscopy and biopsy

Prognosis
- Guarded – often manageable, but not curable

GASTRIC CARCINOMA
Aetiology
- Spontaneous neoplasm
- No evidence to incriminate *Helicobacter*, unlike in man

Major signs
- Anorexia
- Haematemesis
- Vomiting
- Weight loss

Minor signs
- Drooling saliva
- Dull/depressed

Potential sequelae
- Cachexia
- Metabolic alkalosis
- Death

Predisposition
- Age 7–9 years
- Collies (especially Rough collie), Bull terrier, Belgian shepherd

Historical clues
- Insidious onset of chronic vomiting
- Fresh or changed blood in vomitus
- Gradual decline in appetite

Physical examination
- Pale mucous membranes if anaemic
- Tachycardia if active bleeding
- Rarely a palpable abdominal mass

Laboratory findings
Haematology
- Anaemia from blood loss and chronic illness
  - Regenerative or non-regenerative
  - Microcytic if long course

Serum biochemistry
- Hypoproteinaemia from blood loss

Imaging
Radiographs
Plain
- Cranial abdominal mass occasionally obvious
- Interpretation of thickening of gastric wall notoriously unreliable
- Chest radiographs should be taken, but visible lung metastasis unusual

Contrast
- Delayed gastric emptying
- Irregular mucosal outline
- Poorly distensible stomach

Ultrasound examination
- Mass lesion or thickening of gastric wall
- Loss of normal layering
- Gastric ulceration
- Gastric and hepatic lymph node enlargement
- Liver metastasis

Special investigations
Endoscopy and biopsy
- Ulcerated mass visible
- Biopsies may be too superficial to reach a diagnosis

Exploratory laparotomy and biopsy
- Full-thickness biopsies more diagnostic
- Opportunity for resection

Treatment
- Surgical resection
- Chemotherapy not shown to be effective

Monitoring
- Clinical response
- Repeat endoscopy

Prognosis
- Grave
- Most cases are euthanased because of advanced disease at time of diagnosis

GASTRIC DILATATION-VOLVULUS (GDV)
Aetiology
- Unknown cause, but numerous epidemiological risk factors identified
- Accumulation of gas and frothy ingesta, combined with inability to eructate, causes dilatation of stomach
- Dilatation causes torsion of stomach around its long axis, usually 360° in a clockwise direction (pylorus lies left-dorsal)
- Splenic torsion may also occur
- Stretching of gastric wall ± tearing of short gastric arteries causes gastric ischaemia and ultimately gastric wall necrosis
- Obstruction of caudal vena cava and venous return from viscera causes hypovolaemic shock
- Endotoxins and inflammatory mediators cause cardiac arrhythmias

Major signs
- Abdominal discomfort
- Bloating
- Retching and unproductive attempts to vomit
- Weakness/collapse

Minor signs
- Dyspnoea
- Pale mucous membranes with prolonged CRT
- Tachycardia

Potential sequelae
- Gastric rupture and septic peritonitis
- Shock
- Ventricular tachycardia
- DIC
- Death

Predisposition
- Large/giant breed dogs: Great Dane, GSD, Irish setter
- Deep-chested breeds
- 'Anxious' personality
- Following excitement, car ride
- Feeding single variety of food
- Feeding from raised bowl
- Possible relationship to weather/season
- No association with:
  - dry food
  - exercise

Historical clues
- Sudden onset of bloating, sometimes following excitement/car journey

Physical examination
- Distended tympanitic cranial abdomen
- Tachypnoea
- Weak thready pulses and tachycardia
- Weak/collapsed

Laboratory findings
Haematology
- Usually not performed as presumptive diagnosis made on clinical signs
- Haemoconcentration

Serum biochemistry
- Usually not performed as presumptive diagnosis made on clinical signs
- Pre-renal azotaemia

Imaging
Plain radiographs
- Dilated stomach
- Volvulus confirmed by:
  - reverse of normal gas pattern
  - compartmentalisation of stomach
- GDV is a continuum, and presence or absence of volvulus on radiographs is irrelevant to treatment

Special investigations
ECG
- VPCs or ventricular tachycardia

Treatment
- Surgical intervention, either acutely to correct a torsion, or later to perform an elective gastropexy, is always indicated.

Emergency stabilisation
Correction of shock
- Aggressive fluid therapy
  - Hartmann's
  - Colloid
  - Hypertonic saline?
- Corticosteroids – no proof of efficacy

Gastric decompression
- Orogastric tube
- Needle gastrocentesis
- Temporary flank gastrostomy

Definitive
Surgery
- Gastric derotation
- Removal of devitalised fundic wall if necessary
  - Inversion – quicker and safer
  - Partial resection
- Gastropexy
  - Belt-loop – strongest gastropexy
  - Circumcostal – risk of pneumothorax
  - Incisional
  - Incorporation of stomach in abdominal wall closure: not commonly practised in UK
  - Tube gastrostomy – allows postoperative decompression

Supportive
- Anti-arrhythmics
- Antibiotic cover
- Correction of electrolyte abnormalities

Monitoring
- Signs of bloating

- Haematemesis indicating gastric necrosis
- TPR for signs of sepsis
- ECG

Prognosis
- Variable (full recovery or death) depending on:
  - speed of treatment
  - need for partial gastric resection
  - ventricular arrhythmias
- Recurrence rate significantly decreased if gastropexy performed

GASTRIC OUTFLOW OBSTRUCTION
Aetiology
Delayed gastric emptying and vomiting of gastric contents is caused by:
- alterations in gastric motility, i.e. not a true outflow obstruction
- anatomical obstruction of pylorus

Altered motility
- Acidosis
- Diabetic neuropathy
- Gastritis
- Hypoadrenocorticism
- Hypokalaemia
- Idiopathic gastric hypomotility
- Malabsorption causing physiological delay in gastric emptying
- Neoplastic infiltration
- Pain
- Uraemia

Anatomical obstruction
- Chronic hypertrophic pylorogastropathy (CHPG); also known as antral mucosal hypertrophy
- Foreign body acting as a 'ball-valve'
- Hypertrophic gastritis
- Neoplasia
  - Antral polyp
  - Carcinoma
  - Lymphoma
  - Leiomyoma/sarcoma

- Pyloric stenosis – congenital muscular hypertrophy

Major signs
- Vomiting

Minor signs
- Abdominal distension
- Reduced appetite
- Weight loss

Potential sequelae
- Dehydration
- Hypochloraemic metabolic alkalosis

Predisposition
- CHPG in male, toy breed dogs
- Congenital pyloric stenosis in brachycephalic dogs
- Hypertrophic gastritis in Basenji and Boxer

Historical clues
- Vomiting of food occurs hours/days after eating
- Known ingestion of foreign body

Physical examination
- Usually unremarkable except mild dehydration and weight loss
- Distended stomach sometimes palpable

Laboratory findings
Haematology
- Usually unremarkable
- Haemoconcentration if dehydrated

Serum biochemistry
- Usually unremarkable
- Raised proteins and pre-renal azotaemia if dehydrated

Imaging
Radiographs
Plain
- Distended stomach
- Radiodense foreign body

- Stomach contains mixture of gas and ingesta

Contrast
- Delayed gastric emptying
  - Normal emptying begins within 2 hours and is complete by 8 hours
    - Great individual variation
    - Dependent on nature of contrast agent: time for iodine < barium suspension < barium meal
- Radiolucent foreign body
- Persistent 'beak' of contrast at pylorus consistent with stenosis and CHPG

Ultrasound examination
- Gas and ingesta in stomach
- Thickening of pyloric muscle or mucosa

Special investigations
- Gastroscopy
- Exploratory laparotomy

Treatment
- Removal of foreign body
- Fredet-Ramstedt pyloromyotomy
- Heineke-Mikulicz pyloroplasty
- Y-U pyloroplasty

NB – Altered motility causing delayed gastric emptying is treated by:

- Correcting underlying cause, e.g. potassium supplementation
- Dietary modification
- Prokinetics
  - Cisapride: product withdrawn from market
  - Metoclopramide @ 0.5 mg/kg TID/QID
  - Erythromycin @ 1–2 mg/kg TID
  - Ranitidine @ 2 mg/kg TID (also blocks acid secretion)
  - Nizatidine @ 1 mg/kg BID (also blocks acid secretion)

Monitoring
- Clinical response

Prognosis
- Excellent if foreign body removed
- Good if pyloroplasty successful

GASTRIC ULCERS
Aetiology
- Ulcer(s) extending through the mucosa
- Potentially caused by anything damaging the gastric mucosal barrier:
  - NSAIDs – most important cause in dogs
  - Abrasive gastric foreign body
  - Acute and chronic gastritis – see pp. 167–70
  - Acute neurological disease or trauma
  - Gastric carcinoma – see p. 170
  - Gastric leiomyoma/sarcoma
  - Gastric lymphosarcoma
  - Gastrinoma
  - Mast cell tumour – see p. 268
  - Portal hypertension in end-stage liver disease
  - Uraemic gastritis

Major signs
- Vomiting
- Haematemesis

Minor signs
- Abdominal discomfort
- Anorexia
- Melaena
- Weight loss

Potential sequelae
- Anaemia
- Gastric perforation and septic peritonitis
- Death from blood loss

Predisposition
- Gastric carcinoma – see p. 170
- NSAIDs more commonly used to treat osteoarthritis in older dogs

- Renal and liver failure more common in older dogs

Historical clues
- Administration of NSAIDs
- Cutaneous mast cell tumour
- Icterus and other signs of liver failure
- PU/PD and other signs of renal failure

Physical examination
- Cranial abdominal pain
- Dull/depressed
- Pale mucous membranes
- Tachycardia

Laboratory findings
Haematology
- Regenerative anaemia
- Microcytic anaemia if chronic bleeding

Serum biochemistry
- Hypoproteinaemia

Imaging
Radiographs
Plain
- Usually unremarkable
- Pneumoperitoneum if gastric perforation

Contrast
- Occasionally ulcerated mucosa is highlighted
- Leakage of contrast indicates perforation

Ultrasound examination
- Irregular mucosa
- Sometimes loss of layering
- Minimal thickening, cf. neoplasia

Special investigations
- Gastroscopy
- Exploratory laparotomy if perforated or major haemorrhage

Treatment
Remove underlying cause
- e.g. stop NSAIDs

Chemical diffusion barrier
- Sucralfate
  - Complex of aluminium and sucrose octasulphate
  - Binds ulcerated tissue and prevents acid attack
  - Give @1 g PO QID

Acid blocker
Antacids
- Aluminium, magnesium hydroxide or carbonate
- Need to be given at least six times daily

H_2 antagonists
- Block histamine-mediated acid secretion
  - Cimetidine @ 5 mg/kg QID
  - Famotidine @ 1 mg/kg SID
  - Nizatidine @ 1 mg/kg BID
  - Ranitidine @ 2 mg/kg BID/TID

Proton-pump inhibitor (PPi)
- Completely block gastric epithelial pump that secretes hydrogen ions
  - Omeprazole @ 0.7 mg/kg SID

Surgery
- If perforating ulcer

Monitoring
- Clinical response
- Haematology
- Repeat gastroscopy

Prognosis
- Good if underlying cause can be removed

SMALL INTESTINE

Problems
Presenting complaints (see Section 1)
- Abdominal discomfort/pain
- Anorexia
- Diarrhoea
- Haematemesis
- Haematochezia (more commonly LI)
- Halitosis
- Melaena
- Polyphagia
- Pruritus
- Vomiting
- Weight loss

Physical abnormalities (see Section 2)
- Abdominal enlargement
- Anaemia
- PLE
  - Ascites
  - Peripheral oedema
  - Pleural effusion
- Pyrexia

Laboratory abnormalities (see Section 3)
- Amylase and lipase
- Hypocalcaemia (secondary to hypoproteinaemia)
- Hypocholesterolaemia
- Hypokalaemia
- Hyponatraemia
- Hypoproteinaemia (hypoalbuminaemia)
- Leukocytosis
- Leukopenia
- Total protein

Diagnostic approach
- Diarrhoea is the cardinal sign of small intestinal disease – see p. 23
- Diarrhoea can also be caused by extra-intestinal diseases
- Thus, the overall diagnostic approach is first to rule out the extra-intestinal causes

- The extent of investigations and the rapidity with which they are performed depends on:
  - how acute or chronic the problem is; and
  - how severe the problem is.

Diagnostic methods
- Depends on whether acute or chronic SI disease

ACUTE SMALL INTESTINAL DISEASES
Diagnostic approach
- Acute diarrhoea is most often self-limiting, but can be life-threatening, and has many causes – see p. 23.
- It is often not restricted to the SI, but affects the whole GI tract.
- Differentiate between primary (GI) and secondary (non-GI) disease by history, physical examination and laboratory findings.
- If primary GI disease present, determine whether the patient requires:
  - symptomatic support only
  - aggressive medical therapy
  - surgical intervention

Diagnostic methods
History
- Diarrhoea - see p. 23
  - Varies from soft to profuse and watery
  - ± Haemorrhagic
- Borborygmi
- Vomiting, see p. 75
- Weight loss is not a feature

Physical examination
- Dehydration
- Palpation for pain, foreign body, masses or intussusception

Laboratory findings
- see Acute diarrhoea, p. 23

Haematology
- Often unremarkable except for haemo-concentration

Serum biochemistry
- Often unremarkable except for dehydration
  - Pre-renal azotaemia
  - Raised proteins
- Rule out non-GI causes

Urinalysis
- Hypersthenuria in the face of dehydration is appropriate

Faecal examination
- Identify parasites

Imaging
- Identify:
  - Pancreatitis
  - Surgical conditions (e.g. intussusception, foreign body)

Special investigative techniques – see Acute diarrhoea, p. 23
- ACTH stimulation test
- Gastroscopy rarely indicated in acute disease
- Exploratory laparotomy

ACUTE ENTERITIS
Aetiology
Dietary
- Dietary indiscretion
  - Change in diet
  - Overindulgence
  - Scavenging
  - Sudden change in diet
- Food intolerance
- Toxins, especially garbage

Infection – bacterial
- *Campylobacter*
- *Clostridium*
- *E. coli*

Infection – viral
- Coronavirus (mild)
- Parvovirus – see below

Obstructive (surgical)
- Foreign body
- Intussusception

Major signs
- Diarrhoea
  - Large volume
  - Watery
  - Melaena
- Vomiting if whole GI tract affected

Minor signs
- Abdominal discomfort
- Borborygmi
- Dull/depressed/lethargic
- Tenesmus if associated acute colitis

Potential sequelae
- Dehydration
- Hypovolaemic shock if severe
- Sepsis
- Death if hypoadrenocorticism or un-corrected surgical disease

Predisposition
- Young dogs are more likely to scavenge
- Young dogs more likely to be suscepti-ble to parvovirus

Historical clues
- Opportunity to scavenge
- Known access to inappropriate diet
- Contact with possible infection sources

Physical examination
- Unremarkable in mild cases
- Dehydration
- Dull/depressed
- Mild abdominal discomfort
- No other abnormality on abdominal palpation

Laboratory findings
Haematology
- Often unremarkable except for haemo-concentration

Serum biochemistry
- Often unremarkable except for dehy-dration
  - Pre-renal azotaemia
  - Raised proteins
- Rule out non-GI causes

Urinalysis
- Hypersthenuria in the face of dehydra-tion is appropriate

Faecal examination
- Identify parasites

Imaging
Radiographs
Plain
- Mild ileus quite common
- No sign of obstructive disease

Contrast
- No intestinal obstruction

Ultrasound examination
- No evidence of obstruction/intus-susception

Special investigations
- ACTH stimulation test
- Exploratory laparotomy

Treatment

Nil per os

Parenteral fluid therapy

Symptomatic treatment

Antibiotics
- If haemorrhagic diarrhoea

Anti-emetics
- Only *after* obstruction ruled out
  - Chlorpromazine @ 0.5 mg/kg i/m, s/c TID
  - Metoclopramide @ 0.5 mg/kg PO TID
  - Ondansetron @ 0.5 mg/kg i/v initially, then 0.2 mg/kg s/c TID

Anti-diarrhoeal
- Opioid motility modifiers – if infective cause ruled out
  - Diphenoxylate @ 0.05 mg/kg PO TID
  - Loperamide @ 0.1 mg/kg PO TID
- Antimuscarinics – not the best choice as they cause ileus
  - Butylscopolamine (with metamizole) @ 0.1 ml/kg i/v or i/m
- Protectants – act by absorbing free water and bacterial toxins
  - Kaolin
  - Pectin

Monitoring
- Clinical response
- PCV/TP and other markers of dehydration
- If the dog is not improving after 48–72 hours of symptomatic therapy, the case must be re-assessed

Prognosis
- Excellent for full recovery as long as fluid therapy is adequate

HAEMORRHAGIC GASTROENTERITIS (HGE)
Aetiology
- Uncertain
- Suspected clostridial enterotoxaemia

Major signs
- Vomiting
- Haemorrhagic diarrhoea

Minor signs
- Dull/depressed
- Abdominal discomfort

Potential sequelae
- Hypovolaemic shock
- Death

Predisposition
- Toy breed dogs
  - Miniature Schnauzer, Maltese and Yorkshire terriers
- Tends to recur in individuals
- Has also been seen in large breed dogs

Historical clues
- Sudden onset of signs in previously healthy dog
- Owner may recognise some precipitating 'stress'

Physical examination
- Dull/depressed
- Skin turgor often relatively normal because rapid loss of plasma does not allow for equilibration from intracellular fluid
- 'Raspberry jam'-like faeces on rectal thermometer
- Slow CRT
- Tachycardia

Laboratory findings
Haematology
- Marked haemoconcentration
- PCV > 60 and reaching 90 in severe cases
- No abnormal WBC response

Serum biochemistry
- Often unremarkable initially
- Hypoproteinaemia after fluid therapy

Urinalysis
- Hypersthenuria

Faecal examination
- Negative

Imaging
- Unremarkable

Special investigations
- Stool cultures are unhelpful as *Clostridium* can be a normal commensal

Treatment
- Aggressive fluid therapy at shock doses
  - i.e. up to 90 ml/kg for first hour
    - then reduce rate when PCV below 55, to maintain it
- Antibiotic cover
- Antidiarrhoeals
- Nil *per os*
- Plasma transfusion if hypoproteinaemic

Monitoring
- PCV: keep at < 55 by adjusting fluid rate
- Clinical response

Prognosis
- Mortality is low if aggressive fluid therapy
- Tendency to recurrence in individual dogs

PARVOVIRUS
Aetiology
- Canine parvovirus (CPV2)
- Attacks rapidly dividing tissue
  - Bone marrow, causing leukopenia
  - Intestinal crypt, causing haemorrhagic diarrhoea
  - Myocardium in unprotected neonate, causing sudden death or cardiomyopathy; uncommon now because vaccination or exposure of bitch usually provides maternally derived antibody cover

Major signs
- Vomiting
- Diarrhoea
  - Haemorrhagic in 60% of severe cases

Minor signs
- Dull/weak/lethargic
- Pyrexia

Potential sequelae
- Death from endotoxaemia and/or sepsis

Predisposition
- Young (unvaccinated) dogs

Historical clues
- Acute course after 5–10 days' incubation
  - Day 1 – Off-colour, pyrexia
  - Day 2 – Vomiting
  - Day 3 – Diarrhoea
- Exposure to potential infection
- Unvaccinated

Physical examination
- Dull/depressed
- Dehydration
- Mild abdominal discomfort
- Haemorrhagic diarrhoea on thermometer

Laboratory findings
Haematology
- Haemoconcentration
- Leukopenia, especially neutropenia, in about 50% of cases requiring hospitalisation
- Left shift appears during early recovery as bone marrow starts to release immature cells

Serum biochemistry
- Pre-renal azotaemia
- Increased liver enzymes secondary to intestinal inflammation
- Hypoproteinaemia after fluid therapy

ORGAN SYSTEMS

Urinalysis
- Hypersthenuria

Faecal examination
- No endoparasitic ova

Imaging
Radiographs
Plain and contrast
- Generalised ileus often present
- No specific obstruction

Special investigations
- Serology (haemagglutination inhibition)
  - Rising titre necessary, as single titre merely indicates exposure or vaccination
- Identification of parvo antigen in faeces:
  - Electron microscopy
  - ELISA

Treatment
- Aggressive fluid therapy
- Intravenous antibiotic cover
- Metoclopramide
- Omega-interferon has been shown to shorten the recovery phase

Monitoring
- Clinical response
- Hydration status
- WBC count

Prognosis
- Initially guarded as end-result is variable, i.e.
  - Full recovery
  - Death if overwhelming endotoxaemia/sepsis
- Prognosis depends on:
  - Age
  - Leukopenia
  - Vaccination status

SMALL INTESTINAL OBSTRUCTION
Aetiology
- Foreign body
- Incarceration
  - External
    - Inguinal hernia
    - Umbilical hernia
  - Internal
    - Hernia through mesenteric defect
- Intussusception
  - Neoplasia
  - Adenocarcinoma most common
  - Lymphosarcoma
  - Leiomyoma/sarcoma
  - Mast cell tumour
- Volvulus

Major signs
- Vomiting
  - Large volume of bilious fluid if high obstruction
  - Faecal-like material if low obstruction

Minor signs
- Abdominal discomfort
- Anorexia
- Depression/lethargy
- Diarrhoea
- Haematochezia
- Melaena

Potential sequelae
- Dehydration
- Perforation and peritonitis
- Death from sepsis and hypovolaemic shock

Predisposition
- Intussusception in puppies, perhaps related to helminths
- Foreign bodies more likely in younger dogs
- Tumours in older dogs
- Volvulus in dogs with EPI

Historical clues
- Acute onset of vomiting
- Dog's favourite toy missing
- Intussusception often preceded by diarrhoea

Physical examination
- Dehydration
- Dull and depressed
- Palpation of mass or foreign body
- Rarely, ileo-colic intussusception protrudes from anus

Laboratory findings
Haematology
- Inflammatory leukogram if severe localised inflammation or perforation

Serum biochemistry
- Hyponatraemia and hypokalaemia in prolonged cases

Urinalysis
- Hypersthenuria is appropriate

Imaging
Radiographs
Plain
- Foreign body
- Gravel sign – accumulation of material proximal to obstruction
- Ileus
  - Bowel loop dilatation greater than two ribs width or greater than height of vertebral body generally indicates obstruction
- Mass
- Pneumoperitoneum if perforated

Contrast
- Radiolucent foreign body
- Use iodinated contrast if perforation suspected

Ultrasound examination
- Double-layered structure of intussusception

- Foreign body
- Mass

Special investigations
- Exploratory laparotomy

Treatment
- Surgical correction

Monitoring
- Signs of sepsis and peritonitis
  - Abdominal discomfort
  - Persistence of vomiting
  - TPR

Prognosis
Guarded to good depending on:
- Duration of obstruction
- Water/electrolyte disturbances
- Perforation and sepsis
- Vascular compromise of SI, e.g. infarction in volvulus

CHRONIC SMALL INTESTINAL DISEASES
Diagnostic approach
Having ruled out non-GI causes by history, physical examination and minimum database, and localised to signs to SI by history and faecal characteristics (see Table 1, p. 29):

1. Rule out simple causes, such as diet-induced and parasitism
2. Perform TLI test to diagnose EPI *before* further investigations
3. Suspect PLE from serum proteins – see Ascites, p. 94
4. Faecal culture often unhelpful
5. Folate and cobalamin to screen for SIBO and infiltrative bowel disease – see below
6. Radiographs to screen for masses, partial obstruction
7. Ultrasound examination to examine bowel wall thickness, and identify masses

ORGAN SYSTEMS

8   Endoscopic biopsy
9   Exploratory laparotomy and biopsy if endoscopy unavailable or non-diagnostic, or focal disease found on imaging. Biopsy must always be performed, even if no gross abnormalities are found

Diagnostic methods
History
Diarrhoea
- Infrequent watery diarrhoea is suggestive of SI disease
- Melaena may indicates upper GI haemorrhage, and in association with diarrhoea suggests SI bleeding

Vomiting
- SI disease can reflexly inhibit gastric emptying
- SI disease can stimulate vomiting directly

Physical examination
- Ascites (p. 94) occurs if a PLE causes significant hypoalbuminaemia (< 15 g/L)
- Borborygmi
- Polyphagia in the presence of diarrhoea is suggestive of malabsorption
- Weight loss is characteristic of SI disease

Laboratory findings
Haematology
- Commonly unremarkable in primary, chronic GI disease

Serum biochemistry
- Commonly unremarkable in primary, chronic GI disease
- Panhypoproteinaemia is suggestive of PLE

Urinalysis
- Commonly unremarkable

Faecal examination
- Identify parasites

Imaging
- see Chronic diarrhoea, p. 30

Special investigative techniques
- Faecal alpha$_1$-protease inhibitor (α_1-PI)
  - Endogenous serum protein that is lost into faeces if PLE is present
  - It follows albumin, but is not easily biodegradable in faeces and so persists and can be assayed
  - Marker of PLE even before hypoproteinaemia has developed
- Folate and cobalamin (vitamin B$_{12}$)
  - Principle
    - Serum folate absorbed in proximal jejunum
    - Serum cobalamin absorbed in ileum
    - Bacteria synthesise excess folate
    - Bacteria bind cobalamin
  - Interpretation
    - Low folate suggests folate malabsorption and proximal SI damage
    - Low cobalamin suggests cobalamin malabsorption and distal SI damage
    - Low folate and cobalamin suggests diffuse malabsorption and generalised SI damage
    - High folate *plus* low cobalamin is suggestive of bacterial overgrowth
    - High folate *or* low cobalamin may indicate bacterial overgrowth
    - Low sensitivity and specificity because results affected by:
      - Anorexia
      - Dietary vitamin content
      - Nature, severity and duration of SI disease
- TLI – see Pancreas, p. 194
- Intestinal biopsy – see Alimentary, p. 156

DIETARY SENSITIVITY

Aetiology

- Food intolerance is an adverse food reaction due to non-immunological causes
  - Food causes histamine release via non-immunological mechanisms
  - Food contains non-digestible, osmotically active substance
  - Food contains pharmacologically active substance
- Food allergy is an adverse food reaction due to immunological causes
  - Food hypersensitivity is an adverse food reaction due to a Type I (IgE-mediated) reaction
  - Most GI food allergies are probably Type III or IV

Major signs

- Cutaneous signs are the most common manifestation of food allergy
  - Pruritus
  - Secondary lesions due to self-trauma
- GI signs are non-specific
  - Vomiting
  - Diarrhoea

Minor signs

- Other signs of GI dysfunction

Potential sequelae

- Anaphylaxis

Predisposition

- Allergic food disease possibly more common in WHWT and retrievers
- None for food intolerance, although specific individuals may have an idiosyncratic reaction

Historical clues

- Signs associated with particular foodstuffs
- Combination of GI signs and pruritus

Physical examination

- Signs of self-trauma: erythema, excoriation, scaling, etc.

Laboratory findings

Haematology
- No specific changes noted
- No proof that eosinophilia is a marker for dietary sensitivity

Serum biochemistry
- No specific changes noted

Imaging

- Unremarkable

Special investigations

- Exclusion diet trial
  - Remission on exclusion diet
    - Novel protein source
    - Novel carbohydrate source
    - Fed as sole food for trial period of at least 3 weeks, until remission achieved
  - Relapse when challenged with original diet
  - Rescue by exclusion diet
- Allergy testing
  - Serology unreliable
  - Gastroscopic food sensitivity testing technically demanding, and can only identify Type I reactions

Treatment

- Avoidance of allergen

Monitoring

- Clinical response

Prognosis

- Excellent if offending foodstuff can be eliminated from diet

INFLAMMATORY BOWEL DISEASE (IBD)

Aetiology

There are numerous potential causes of intestinal inflammation (see Chronic diarrhoea, p. 27).

- Food allergy
- Idiopathic
- Many different infections

Inflammatory bowel disease (IBD) is, by definition, idiopathic.

- Suspected immune dysregulation leading to loss of tolerance to bacteria
- Variety of histological types (*most common type)
  - Eosinophilic enteritis (or gastro-enteritis)
  - Granulomatous enteritis
  - Immunoproliferative small intestinal disease (IPSID – Basenji only)
  - Lympho-plasmacytic enteritis* (and/or colitis)

Major signs

- Diarrhoea
  - Infrequent (< 3 times per day) unless concurrent colonic involvement
  - Large volume
  - Watery
- Vomiting
- Weight loss

Minor signs

- Abdominal discomfort
- Altered appetite
  - Anorexia if severe inflammation
  - Polyphagia if malabsorption
- Borborygmi
- Melaena
- Poor hair coat secondary to malabsorption

Potential sequelae

- Protein-losing enteropathy (PLE)
  - Ascites/oedema
  - Hypoproteinaemia
- Thromboembolism
- Lymphosarcoma? (some suggestion IBD undergoes neoplastic transformation)

Predisposition

- All forms of IBD, except histiocytic ulcerative colitis, are rare in dogs aged < 1 year
- Eosinophilic gastroenteritis (EGE): GSD
- Lymphoplasmacytic enteritis (LPE): GSD, Shar pei
- Immunoproliferative small intestinal disease (IPSID): only recorded in Basenji

Historical clues

- Acute initiating event in some cases, e.g. following scavenging
- Chronic intermittent signs for a long period
- Waxing-waning problem that is gradually getting worse or more frequent

Physical examination

- Variable body condition from normal or even overweight to cachexic
- Dull/depressed in severe IBD
- Ascites/oedema if PLE
- Thickened bowel loops sometimes palpable, but interpretation is subjective

Laboratory findings

Haematology

- Often unremarkable
- Anaemia of chronic disease, or blood loss
- Sometimes a mild/moderate neutrophilia
- Eosinophilia is an unreliable marker of EGE, and parasitism should be considered first

Serum biochemistry

- Often unremarkable

- Panhypoproteinaemia typical in PLE, although severe inflammatory disease may cause raised globulins – see p. 143
- Hypocalcaemia, reflecting hypoalbuminaemia
- Hypocholesterolaemia suggestive of malabsorption
- Increased liver enzymes, secondary to intestinal inflammation

Urinalysis
- Proteinuria if secondary immune-complex glomerulonephritis

Faecal examination
- Identification of parasites or pathogenic bacteria may suggest cause of intestinal inflammation, rather than idiopathic IBD

Imaging
Radiographs
Plain
- Usually unremarkable
- Thickening of bowel wall difficult to assess on plain films

Contrast
- Irregular mucosal surface consistent with infiltration (e.g. IBD, lymphosarcoma)

Ultrasound examination
- Increased intestinal wall thickness seen sometimes
- Layering of intestinal wall should be present
- Mesenteric lymphadenopathy present sometimes

Special investigations
- Faecal alpha$_1$-PI as a marker for a PLE
- Folate and cobalamin
  - Decreases suggestive of infiltrative disease (IBD, lymphosarcoma)

- Low serum concentrations indicative of need for supplementation
- Intestinal biopsy
  - Histological classification is applied to IBD
  - However, an underlying cause for the inflammation must be ruled out before confirming idiopathic IBD
  - Endoscopic biopsy preferred, as no convalescence before starting steroids
    - Retained food in stomach due to delayed gastric emptying
    - Irregular mucosa
    - Erosions, ulceration, bleeding
  - Surgical biopsy more likely to be representative of disease

Treatment
Antibiotics
- May reduce the antigenic burden on the mucosal immune system

Metronidazole
- May also modulate immune response
- 10–15 mg/kg PO BID

Oxytetracycline
- May be anti-inflammatory
- 10 mg/kg PO TID

Diet
- Response to exclusion diet suggests food allergy, not idiopathic IBD
- Easily digestible, hypoallergenic is helpful

Immunosuppression
Prednisolone
- First-choice immunosuppressive for IBD
- Start at 2–4 mg/kg PO divided BID
- Reduce after 2–3 weeks to 1–2 mg/kg PO SID
- Then taper every few weeks to find minimum effective dose

Azathioprine
- Adjunctive immunosuppressive given for its steroid-sparing effect
- 2 mg/kg/day initially, reducing to every other day after 4–6 weeks
- Potentially bone marrow-suppressive, so monitor haematology
- Toxicity in individuals is related to activity of degradatory TPMT enzyme

Vitamin supplements
- Oral folic acid
- Vitamin B_{12} by s/c injection

Monitoring
- Clinical response
- Serum protein concentrations
- Side effects of steroids
- Repeat intestinal biopsy

Prognosis
- Guarded
- Potential individual outcomes
  - Weaned off all medication completely
  - Need low-dose continuous therapy
  - Only respond to high-dose therapy
  - Fail to respond
  - Undergo transformation to lymphosarcoma?

LYMPHANGIECTASIA
Aetiology
Abnormal dilatation of the intestinal lymphatics leading to:
- Fat malabsorption
- PLE from lipoprotein loss

- Idiopathic
  - May have associated lymphangitis and lipogranulomas
  - Occasionally there is concurrent chylothorax
- Secondary obstruction
  - Neoplastic infiltration
  - Pericardial disease
  - Right heart failure

Major signs
- Chronic diarrhoea – may occur late in disease after ascites develops
- Weight loss

Minor signs
- Ascites/generalised subcutaneous oedema if PLE
- Polyphagia

Potential sequelae
- PLE
- Thromboembolism
- Severe cachexia

Predisposition
- Breed associations
  - Maltese terrier
  - Norwegian Lundehund
  - Rottweiler
  - Soft-coated Wheaten terrier
    - may have concurrent PLN
    - this may not be a true lymphangiectasia, but IBD and secondary lymphatic dilatation
  - Yorkshire terrier

Historical clues
- Intractable wasting disease

Physical examination
- Underweight
- Ascites/generalised subcutaneous oedema if PLE

Laboratory findings
Haematology
- Lymphopenia

Serum biochemistry
- Panhypoproteinaemia typical of PLE
- Hypocalcaemia, reflecting hypoalbuminaemia
- Hypocholesterolaemia suggestive of fat malabsorption

Imaging
Radiographs
- Often unremarkable

Ultrasound examination
- Bowel wall thickening may be due to tissue oedema

Special investigations
- Faecal alpha$_1$-PI
  - May detect PLE before hypoprotein-aemia develops
  - Potential screening test in predis-posed breeds
- Folate and cobalamin
  - Unchanged, as water- not fat-soluble
- Intestinal biopsy
  - Grossly dilated lymphatics seen on endoscopy if duodenum affected
  - Diagnosis is by histological appear-ance
  - Full-thickness surgical biopsies from several levels of the SI may be needed for an accurate diagnosis
  - Presence of lipogranulomas (multi-ple, small white spots) on mesentery is very suggestive

Treatment
- Prednisolone (up to 2 mg/kg/day) may reduce associated inflammation and produce a clinical improvement
- Low-fat diet reduces fat malabsorption and amount of diarrhoea
  - A reduced-fat, highly digestible diet is indicated
  - A low-fat, weight-reducing diet is contra-indicated
- Anecdotal reports of positive response to dietary glutamine

Monitoring
- Clinical response
- Serum proteins

Prognosis
- Guarded

- Can cause intractable diarrhoea and weight loss
- Can respond to steroids
- Can resolve spontaneously

SMALL INTESTINAL BACTERIAL OVERGROWTH (SIBO)
Aetiology
- SIBO was originally described as an increase in the number of bacteria in the upper SI during the inter-digestive phase
- SIBO was defined by the number of bacteria cultured from duodenal juice:
  - Normal $< 10^5$ total or $< 10^4$ anaerobic colony-forming units/ml
  - These figures are disputed because:
    - The technique has great variability even in individual dogs
    - Greater numbers have been found in healthy dogs
- SIBO is now included in the syndrome of 'antibiotic-responsive diarrhoea' (ARD)
  - SIBO
  - Specific bacterial infection

The cause of SIBO can be:
- Primary, idiopathic
- Secondary
  - EPI
  - Partial intestinal obstruction
  - Redundant, 'blind-loop' of bowel
  - Mucosal disease? e.g. secondary to IBD

SIBO causes malabsorption and diar-rhoea by:
- Competition for nutrients
- Deconjugation of bile salts causing fat malabsorption
- Deconjugated bile salts and hydoxy-lated fatty acids from bacterial fermen-tation stimulate colonic secretion
- Cobalamin sequestration leading to malabsorption and deficiency
- Subtle brush border biochemical changes

ORGAN SYSTEMS

Major signs
- Chronic diarrhoea
  - Continuous or intermittent
  - Varying from soft to very watery
- Coprophagia
- Polyphagia
- Stunting or weight loss

Minor signs
- Borborygmi and flatus
- Greasy hair coat
- Occasionally anorexia
- Occasionally, secondary LI-type diarrhoea
- Vomiting

Potential sequelae
- Cobalamin deficiency
- Ill-thrift
- Permanent stunting
- May transform to IBD?

Predisposition
- Large/giant breeds, especially the GSD
- Young dogs (aged < 2 years)

Historical clues
- Antibiotic-responsive
  - ARD appearing in older dog suggests development secondary to an underlying cause, e.g. partial obstruction due to neoplasia
- Coprophagia is most characteristic of SIBO or EPI
- Some response to dietary manipulation
- Suggestive clinical signs in young dog of predisposed breed

Physical examination
- Thin
- Stunted
- Poor hair coat

Laboratory findings
Haematology
- Usually unremarkable

Serum biochemistry
- Usually unremarkable

Faecal examination
- Parasitology should be performed to eliminate complicating infections

Imaging
Radiographs
- Unremarkable in idiopathic SIBO
- Gravel sign if underlying partial obstruction

Ultrasound examination
- Unremarkable

Special investigations
- TLI
  - EPI must be ruled out as predisposition and signs are very similar
- Folate and cobalamin
  - Classic increased folate, decreased cobalamin is only seen in 5% of dogs with culture proven SIBO
  - Using just increased folate or decreased cobalamin as a marker improves sensitivity but decreases specificity
- Breath hydrogen
  - Test not readily available in practice
- Serum unconjugated bile acids
  - Theoretically will be increased by bacterial deconjugation of bile acids
  - Not proven diagnostically
- Intestinal biopsy
  - Normal or subtle/mild inflammatory changes
- Duodenal juice culture
  - Claimed 'gold standard'
  - Difficult to do in practice
  - Unreliable results

Treatment
Diet
- Fat restriction reduces volume of diarrhoea

- Probiotics and prebiotics (e.g. fructo-oligosaccharides) may modulate the SI flora and/or the mucosal immune response

Antibiotics
- SIBO is partly defined as 'ARD'
- Use broad-spectrum, low-cost, safe antibiotics
  - Oxytetracycline @ 10–20 mg/kg PO TID
  - Metronidazole @ 10–15 mg/kg PO BID
- Some dogs require continuous antibiotics, but may be controlled by lower doses
- Some dogs need single course or intermittent administration of antibiotics

Vitamins
- Parenteral vitamin B_{12} is needed if the dog is cobalamin-deficient

Monitoring
- Clinical response
- Re-testing folate and cobalamin does not appear helpful

Prognosis
- Guarded to good
  - May 'grow out of' condition
  - May only need intermittent antibiotics
  - May need continuous antibiotics to control signs

LARGE INTESTINE

Problems
Presenting complaints (see Section 1)
- Abdominal discomfort/pain
- Constipation
- Diarrhoea
- Faecal incontinence
- Haematochezia
- Pain
- Tenesmus and dyschezia

- Vomiting
- Weight loss

Physical abnormalities (see Section 2)
- Abdominal enlargement

Laboratory abnormalities (see Section 3)
- Anaemia
- Hyperkalaemia
- Hyponatraemia
- Hypoproteinaemia (hypoalbuminaemia)
- Leukocytosis
- Total protein

Diagnostic approach
- Distinguish constipation from diarrhoea by history and physical examination.
- Localise disease to the LI by the nature of diarrhoea and defecation (Table 1, p. 29), but diarrhoea can also be due to concurrent SI and LI disease.
- The extent of investigations and the rapidity with which they are performed depends on:
  - how acute or chronic the problem is
  - how severe the problem is
- Colonoscopy indicated in chronic disease.

Diagnostic methods
History
- Deformation of stool shape by pelvic mass
- Haematochezia with inflammatory or neoplastic disease
- Tenesmus before defecation suggests constipation
- Tenesmus after diarrhoea suggests colitis
- Weight loss is not a feature unless advanced neoplasia or repeated withholding of food

Physical examination
- Abdominal palpation for constipation or mass

Rectal examination
- Constipation
- Diarrhoea
- Haematochezia
- Rectal mass

Laboratory findings
- Usually unremarkable
- Hyponatraemia and hyperkalaemia reported with whipworm infection

Imaging
- Abdominal mass
- Accumulated faecal material in constipation
- Often unremarkable

Special investigative techniques
- Colonoscopy

ACUTE COLITIS
Aetiology
Dietary
- Dietary indiscretion
  - Change in diet
  - Overindulgence
  - Scavenging
  - Sudden change in diet
- Food intolerance
- Toxins, especially garbage

Infection – bacterial
- *Campylobacter*
- *Clostridium*
- *E. coli*

Infection – parasitic
- *Giardia* – lives in SI, but can cause colitis-like signs
- *Trichuris* whipworms

Infection – viral
- Parvovirus – see pp. 179–80

Traumatic
- Abrasions from bone fragments

Major signs
- Diarrhoea
  - Haematochezia
  - Mucus
  - Small volume
- Tenesmus

Minor signs
- Abdominal discomfort

Potential sequelae
- Progression to chronic colitis

Predisposition
- Young dogs are more likely to scavenge

Historical clues
- Opportunity to scavenge
- Known access to inappropriate diet
- Contact with possible infection sources

Physical examination
- Unremarkable in mild cases
- Dull/depressed
- Mild abdominal discomfort
- No other abnormality on abdominal palpation

Laboratory findings
- Often unremarkable

Faecal examination
- *Giardia* oocysts
- *Trichuris* ova

Imaging
Radiographs
- Unremarkable

Special investigations
- ACTH stimulation test if abnormal electrolytes

Treatment
Symptomatic treatment
- Nil *per os*
- Parenteral fluid therapy as necessary

Antibiotics
- If haemorrhagic diarrhoea

Anti-diarrhoeal
- Opioid motility modifiers
  - Diphenoxylate @ 0.05 mg/kg PO TID
  - Loperamide @ 0.1 mg/kg PO TID
- Dietary fibre – acts by absorbing free water and providing colonocyte nutrients

Monitoring
- Clinical response
- If the dog is not improving after 72 hours of symptomatic therapy, the case must be re-assessed

Prognosis
- Good for complete recovery

CHRONIC COLITIS
Aetiology
There are numerous potential causes of colonic inflammation (see Chronic diarrhoea, p. 27).
- Food allergy
- Colonic infection
  - *Clostridium difficile*
  - *Clostridium perfringens*
  - *Histoplasma capsulatum*
- Idiopathic IBD
  - Eosinophilic colitis (or gastro-enterocolitis)
  - Histiocytic ulcerative colitis: rare
  - Lymphoplasmacytic colitis (and enteritis): most common

Major signs
- Diarrhoea
  - Haematochezia
  - Mucus
  - Small volume
- Tenesmus
- Weight loss is not a feature

Minor signs
- Abdominal discomfort

Potential sequelae
- Persistence of problem

Predisposition
- Lymphoplasmacytic colitis in GSD
- Histiocytic ulcerative colitis in Boxer and French bulldog

Historical clues
- Clinical signs
- No weight loss

Physical examination
- Usually unremarkable

Rectal examination
- Blood and mucus
- Thickened irregular mucosa

Laboratory findings
- Usually unremarkable
- Blood loss anaemia is uncommon

Faecal examination
- *Trichuris* ova

Imaging
Radiographs
Plain
- Unremarkable

Contrast
- Not very helpful
- Thickened, irregular, ulcerated mucosa

Special investigations
- Colonoscopy and biopsy
- Folate and cobalamin
  - If abnormal, indicates concurrent SI disease

ORGAN SYSTEMS

Treatment
Antibiotics
- May reduce the antigenic burden on the mucosal immune system
  - Metronidazole
    - Active against colonic anaerobes
    - May also modulate immune response
    - 10–15 mg/kg PO BID/TID

Diet
- Response to exclusion diet suggests food allergy not idiopathic IBD
- Easily digestible, hypoallergenic is helpful
- Fibre:
  - Moderately fermentable for colonocyte nutrition, e.g. ispaghula, beet pulp, chicory
  - Non-fermentable to regulate motility and bind water, e.g. wheat bran

Immunosuppression
Prednisolone and azathioprine
- See SI IBD, pp. 184–6

Sulphasalazine
- 5-Aminosalicylic acid derivative, released in colon
- Direct anti-inflammatory effect
- Dosage 10–20 mg/kg PO BID
- Keratoconjunctivitis is serious side effect; perform periodic Schirmer tear test

Monitoring
- Clinical response
- Repeat colonoscopy

Prognosis
- Excellent for parasitic colitis
- Good for control of lymphoplasmacytic colitis
- Grave for histiocytic ulcerative colitis

CONSTIPATION
Aetiology
- See Constipation – Section 1

Major signs
- Dyschezia
- Failure to pass faeces or small, hard, dry faeces
- Haematochezia if intraluminal cause
- Tenesmus

Minor signs
- Anorexia
- Lethargy
- Paradoxical diarrhoea (scant liquid faeces passed around the sides of constipated mass)
- Vomiting

Potential sequelae
- Progressively worsening constipation leading to:
  - Obstipation
  - Disruption of colonic musculature and development of megacolon

Predisposition, Historical clues, Physical examination, Laboratory findings, Imaging, Special investigations
- See Constipation – Section 1

Treatment
Correct underlying cause
- Rehydration
- Castration for prostatomegaly
- Stop drugs
- Surgery for perineal disease

Dietary modification
- Non-fermentable fibre, e.g. wheat bran
- Moderately fermentable fibre, e.g. ispaghula, psyllium, sterculia
- Poorly digested food, e.g. milk

Laxatives
Osmotic
- Lactulose

Lubricant
- Paraffin paste
- Liquid paraffin (mineral oil); beware of inhalation

Surfactant
- Docusate
- Sodium citrate

Stimulant
- Castor oil
- Glycerol
- Danthron/poloxamer

Enemas
- Warm soapy water
- Docusate
- Phosphate

Monitoring
- Ability to pass faeces naturally

Prognosis
- Good for mild constipation if underlying cause can be addressed
- Poor if severe obstipation or uncorrectable underlying cause

LARGE INTESTINAL NEOPLASIA
Aetiology
- Spontaneous tumour
  - Benign polyps
  - Adenocarcinoma most commonly affecting rectum or caecum

Major signs
- Constipation
- Haematochezia
- Tenesmus

Minor signs
- Deformation of stool
- Diarrhoea
- Dyschezia
- Dysuria
- Weight loss in advanced disease

Potential sequelae
Benign polyps
- May theoretically undergo malignant transformation

Adenocarcinoma
- Metastasis to sublumbar LN, liver, lungs
- Obstruction of colon

Predisposition
- More common in older dogs

Historical clues
- Presence of fresh blood on stool of normal consistency is suggestive of a bleeding mass and not colitis

Physical examination
- Mass or constipation on abdominal palpation

Rectal examination
- Haematochezia
- Mass

Laboratory findings
- Usually unremarkable

Imaging
Radiographs
Plain
- Caudal abdominal mass
- Sublumbar lymphadenopathy
- Pulmonary metastasis

Contrast
- Barium enema may identify mass, but superseded by colonoscopy

Ultrasound examination
- Caudal abdominal mass
- Sublumbar lymphadenopathy

Special investigations
- Colonoscopy and biopsy

Treatment
- Traction and avulsion or submucosal resection of polyp
- Surgical resection of carcinoma, but often inoperable

Monitoring
- Recurrence of haematochezia

Prognosis
- Excellent for polyp, although recurrence quite common
- Grave for carcinoma

PANCREAS

Problems
Presenting complaints (see Section 1)
- Abdominal discomfort/pain
- Anorexia
- Diarrhoea
- Haematemesis
- Haematochezia
- Melaena
- Polyphagia
- Polyuria/polydipsia
- Vomiting
- Weight loss

Physical abnormalities (see Section 2)
- Pyrexia
- Icterus/jaundice
- Malabsorption

Laboratory abnormalities (see Section 3)
- Amylase and lipase
- Azotaemia
- Bile acids
- Bilirubin
- Hypocalcaemia
- Hyperglycaemia
- Hyperlipidaemia/hypercholesterolaemia
- Hypokalaemia

- Hyperglobulinaemia
- Liver enzyme alterations
- Leukocytosis
- Leukopenia

Diagnostic methods
History
- Malabsorption with EPI
- Vomiting with pancreatitis

Physical examination
- Abdominal palpation for masses and pain

Laboratory findings
- See specific conditions below

Imaging
Radiographs
- See specific conditions below

Ultrasound
- Abnormalities of size and echogenicity in pancreas

Special investigative techniques
Serum trypsin-like immunoreactivity (TLI)
- Assay measures circulating trypsinogen and trypsin
  - Decreased in EPI
  - Increased in pancreatitis

Serum pancreatic lipase immunoreactivity (PLI)
- Assay measures circulating pancreatic lipase
  - Decreased in EPI
  - Increased in pancreatitis

Serum or urinary trypsin activation peptide (TAP)
- Assay measures small peptide cleaved when trypsinogen is activated
  - Decreased in EPI
  - Increased in pancreatitis
  - Urinary TAP more reliable if reported as TAP:creatinine ratio

ACUTE PANCREATITIS
Aetiology
- Spontaneous inflammation of pancreas
  - Activation of proteases and phospholipases within pancreas initiates autodigestion
  - Inflammation spreads to cause localised peritonitis and fat necrosis
  - Systemic release of proteases eventually overwhelms circulating anti-proteases and reticuloendothelial system, and then causes systemic problems
- Severity of the condition varies from mild, oedematous pancreatitis to severe necrotising pancreatitis
- Specific cause not known, but risk factors identified
  - High-fat diet/dietary indiscretion
  - Obesity
  - Hyperlipidaemia
    - HAC
    - Primary hyperlipidaemia
  - Pancreatic ischaemia
    - Anaesthesia
    - GDV
    - Hypovolaemia
  - Trauma
  - Drugs
    - Azathioprine
    - L-asparaginase
- Corticosteroids are *not* now considered a risk factor

Major signs
- Abdominal pain
  - May adopt the 'prayer' position
- Diarrhoea
- Icterus if bile duct obstructed by pancreatic inflammation (EHBDO)
- Vomiting

Minor signs
- Anorexia
- Depression
- Haematochezia
- Melaena
- Pyrexia

Potential sequelae
Local
- Pancreatic abscess
- Pseudocyst
- Recurrent episodes

Systemic
- Acute renal failure
- Cardiac arrhythmias
- Pleural effusion

Leading to:
- Shock
- DIC
- Death

Predisposition
- Obese, middle-aged females
- Hyperlipidaemia in Miniature Schnauzer

Historical clues
- Sudden onset of GI signs
  - Abdominal pain in 60% of cases
  - Diarrhoea in 33% of cases
  - Vomiting in 90% of cases
- Episode of dietary indiscretion

Physical examination
- Dull and depressed
- Cranial abdominal discomfort or pain

Laboratory findings
Haematology
- Leukocytosis with neutrophilia and left shift

Serum biochemistry
- Transient hyperglycaemia
- Hyperlipidaemia
- Occasional hypocalcaemia
- Raised liver enzymes
- Hyperbilirubinaemia if extrahepatic bile duct obstruction
- Increased amylase (see Section 3, p. 135)

- low sensitivity and specificity (62% and 71%, respectively)
- Increased lipase (see p. 135)
  - greater sensitivity, but lower specificity (73% and 55%, respectively)

Urinalysis
- Hypersthenuria is appropriate

Imaging
Plain radiographs
- Classic radiographic changes are unreliable and non-specific
  - Lateral displacement of duodenum by pancreatic mass seen on VD view
  - Localised peritonitis giving loss of detail in right cranial quadrant
  - Ileus of adjacent duodenum and transverse colon

Ultrasound examination
- Sensitivity of pancreatic ultrasound is operator-dependent
  - May appear normal
  - Mottled echogenicity
  - Thickened
  - Abscess or pseudocyst

Special investigations
- Increased TLI
  - Low sensitivity and moderate specificity (33% and 65%, respectively)
  - Transient rise early in the disease, then normalises or goes subnormal
- Increased pancreatic lipase immunoreactivity (PLI)
  - Good sensitivity and high specificity (80% and >95%, respectively)
- Urine trypsinogen activation peptide (TAP):creatinine ratio
  - Very low sensitivity but high specificity (26% and 100%, respectively)
- Pancreatic biopsy
  - Definitive diagnosis, but risk of hypotension during anaesthesia and handling of pancreas may make pancreatitis worse

Treatment
- Nil *per os*
- Parenteral fluids
- Plasma transfusion to replace circulating anti-proteases
- Analgesia
  - Pethidine (Demerol)
  - Buprenorphine
- Antibiotic cover
- Partial pancreatectomy if pseudocyst or abscess
- Convalescence on fat-restricted diet

Monitoring
- Clinical response
- Repeat ultrasound examination may not distinguish active from inactive disease

Prognosis
- Good with mild pancreatitis
- Potentially fatal with necrotising pancreatitis

CHRONIC PANCREATITIS
Aetiology
- Repeated attacks of acute pancreatitis
- Smouldering low grade inflammation
- Eventual replacement of acinar tissue with fibrous tissue

Major signs
- Abdominal discomfort
- Vomiting

Minor signs
- Diarrhoea
- Jaundice from EHBDO
- Weight loss

Potential sequelae
- Diabetes mellitus
- EHBDO
- EPI

Predisposition
- As for acute pancreatitis

Historical clues
- Repeated episodes of GI signs

Physical examination
- Cranial abdominal discomfort
- Occasionally, pancreatic mass is palpable

Laboratory findings
Haematology
- Mild inflammatory leukogram

Serum biochemistry
- Increased ALP (tends to be > ALT increase)
- Hyperbilirubinaemia if EHBDO
- Hyperglycaemia if DM develops
- Amylase and lipase even less sensitive

Imaging
Radiographs
Plain
- Same non-specific signs as for acute pancreatitis
- Cranial abdominal mass
- Mass may be calcified

Ultrasound examination
- Abnormal pancreatic mass

Special investigations
- Sensitivity and specificity of TLI, PLI and TAP is unknown
- Pancreatic biopsy

Treatment
- Supportive care as for acute pancreatitis
- Maintenance on fat-restricted diet
- Controlled weight loss
- Oral pancreatic enzymes potentially have negative feedback on pancreas, reducing production of destructive enzymes
- Biliary diversion (e.g. cholecystoduodenostomy) for EHBDO

Monitoring
- Clinical response
- If weight loss occurs
  - Blood and urinary glucose for development of DM
  - TLI for development of EPI

Prognosis
- Guarded for short-term alleviation
- Poor of long-term success; repeated episodes and progression likely

EXOCRINE PANCREATIC INSUFFICIENCY (EPI)
Aetiology
Malabsorption from failure of digestion as a consequence of a lack of pancreatic enzymes.
- Congenital pancreatic hypoplasia
  - Rare
  - May have concurrent DM
- End-stage chronic pancreatitis
- Pancreatic acinar atrophy
  - Heritable trait proven in GSD and Rough collie
  - May be auto-immune, as preceding lymphocytic pancreatitis reported
  - Most common cause of EPI

Major signs
- Diarrhoea
  - Large volume
  - Steatorrhoea
  - Variable consistency ('cow-pat' to watery)
- Polyphagia, including coprophagia
- Weight loss

Minor signs
- Occasional tenesmus
- Poor, greasy coat
- Polydipsia
- Vomiting

ORGAN SYSTEMS

Potential sequelae
- Cachexia
- DM if hypoplasia or chronic pancreatitis
- Intestinal volvulus

Predisposition
Pancreatic acinar atrophy
- Aged 6 months to 6 years
- GSD represent two-thirds of cases
- Collies, Chow chow, CKC spaniel, small terriers

Chronic pancreatitis
- Older dogs

Historical clues
- Signs of malabsorption, i.e. diarrhoea and weight loss despite an increased appetite

Physical examination
- Bright and alert
- Poor body condition
- Poor, greasy coat

Laboratory findings
Haematology
- Usually unremarkable

Serum biochemistry
- Usually unremarkable
- Occasional hypocholesterolaemia

Urinalysis
- May have low urine SG if polydipsic

Imaging
Radiographs
- Unremarkable, except for poor abdominal detail due to loss of fat

Ultrasound examination
- Pancreas cannot be identified, but it is not always visible in normal dogs

Special investigations
- Folate and cobalamin
  - Raised folate and decreased cobalamin are common because of secondary SIBO, and lack of pancreatic intrinsic factor
- TLI
  - Subnormal TLI (0.1–2.5 µg/L; normal 5.0 to 35 µg/L) is diagnostic
  - Very high sensitivity and specificity

Treatment
Exogenous enzyme supplementation
- Fresh pancreas (100–200 g per meal) works best
- Dried, powdered extract can be effective
- Enteric-coated preparations least effective

Diet
- Highly digestible
- Fat restriction is controversial as it reduces secondary bacterial fermentation and hence diarrhoea, but it restricts the calorie intake so the dog cannot gain weight
- Feed two to three meals per day; more frequent meals requires more enzyme, which is expensive

Antibiotics
- Secondary SIBO complicates EPI
- Give 10 mg/kg oxytetracycline PO with each meal

Vitamins
- Parenteral vitamin B_{12}

Monitoring
- Stool consistency
- Weight gain

Prognosis
- Good for control
- Life-long condition

CARDIOVASCULAR SYSTEM

Problems
Presenting complaints (see Section 1)
- Anorexia
- Cough
- Dyspnoea and tachypnoea
- Exercise intolerance
- Weakness-lethargy-collapse/syncope
- Weight gain
- Weight loss

Physical abnormalities (see Section 2)
- Abdominal enlargement
- Ascites
- Bradycardia
- Cardiomegaly – see pp. 203–6
- Cyanosis (uncommon)
- Hepatomegaly
- Murmur – see pp. 201–2
- Peripheral oedema
- Pleural effusion
- Pulmonary adventitious sounds
- Pulmonary alveolar pattern
- Splenomegaly
- Tachycardia

Laboratory abnormalities (see Section 3)
- Azotaemia (pre-renal)
- Polycythaemia

Diagnostic approach
1   Suspect cardiac disease from clinical signs and physical examination
    - Auscultation
    - Capillary refill
    - Palpation of pulses
    - Percussion
2   Radiography
3   ECG
4   Blood pressure
5   Echocardiography
6   Cardiac catheterisation

Diagnostic methods
History
- May be minimal history if cardiac disease is compensated
- Likely presenting complaints and physical findings listed above

Physical examination (see Section 1, Weakness/syncope)
Observation
- Body condition may be poor with severe congestive heart failure due to loss of muscle mass
- Cachexia is more common with right-sided failure
- Small dogs with mitral valve disease are often overweight

Inspection
- Mucous membrane colour
  - Cyanosis (uncommon) – see Section 2
    - Assess cranial and caudal mucous membranes as differential cyanosis can occur. Uncommon
    - Pallor suggests poor peripheral circulation with vasoconstriction or reduced haemoglobin – check PCV to differentiate
- Capillary refill
- Jugular veins
  - Jugular distension is an indicator of right-heart failure: right atrial pressure is elevated and jugular veins can fill beyond their normal position
  - Hepatojugular reflux: apply firm pressure to the cranial abdomen for 1 minute, which will displace blood from congested liver into the caudal vena cava and cause jugular filling if the right atrium is unable to accommodate the increased venous return

Auscultation
- Ideally perform with animal standing
- Auscultate left and right sides over all valve areas (see Figure 1)

ORGAN SYSTEMS

ORGAN SYSTEMS

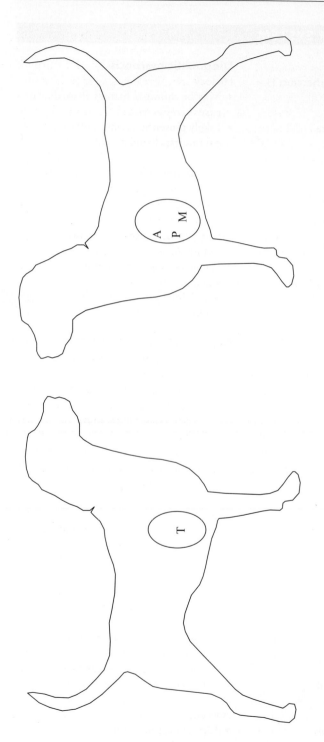

Figure 1   The approximate position of the heart valves. T=tricuspid valve, A=aortic valve, P=pulmonic valve, M=mitral valve.

- Normal heart sounds: only two are heard
  - S1 – 1st sound 'lub' – this is associated with closure of mitral/tricuspid valves, and is heard loudest over the apex
  - S2 – 2nd sound 'dup' – this is associated with closure of aortic/pulmonic valves, and is heard loudest over the heart base
- Audibility
  - Decreased by pleural effusion, mediastinal mass, pericardial effusion, obesity
  - Increased by cardiomegaly, anaemia, thin body condition, pneumothorax
  - Intrathoracic mass may displace sounds
- Heart rate
  - Decreased
    - Bradydysrhythmia
    - Increased vagal tone (CNS depression, GI disease)
    - Small brachycephalic dogs often have very slow heart rates
  - Increased
    - Cardiac failure
    - Fear, exercise, excitement, fever, pain
    - Tachyarrhythmia
- Rhythm: assess for regularity, equality with pulse and pattern of rhythm
  - Sinus arrhythmia = normal rhythm:
    - Regularly irregular, i.e. rhythm speeds up with inspiration and slows with expiration
  - Abnormal rhythms
    - Premature beats: isolated irregularities in rhythm can be supraventricular or ventricular in origin
    - Atrial fibrillation: chaotic, irregularly irregular rhythm, i.e. no consistency
  - Abnormal sounds
    - Usually indicate heart disease but not heart failure
    - Murmurs are vibrations due to turbulence of blood

- Friction sounds due to pericardial or pleural effusions
- False murmurs vary with stage of respiration, heart rate and day to day
- Gallop sounds often indicate cardiac failure
- Atrial overload: accentuates third (S3) and fourth (S4) heart sound
- Ventricular dilation or delayed closure of pulmonic or aortic valve causes duplication of second heart sound (S2)
- Abnormal respiratory noises: e.g. crackles with pulmonary oedema, decreased audibility with pleural effusion

Murmurs
- Intensity/grade
  - I   Soft murmur – not heard immediately on auscultation or in noisy surroundings
  - II Soft murmur but easily heard
  - III Moderate intensity murmur – prominent and immediately audible but not loud
  - IV Loud murmur, audible over large area and no precordial thrill
  - V   Loud murmur with a precordial thrill
  - VI Very loud, can be heard with the stethoscope off the chest wall, with a precordial thrill
- Phase of cardiac cycle
  - Murmurs are usually systolic created by high pressures, e.g. mitral and tricuspid regurgitation, aortic and pulmonic stenosis
  - Continuous murmurs – Patent ductus arteriosus (PDA), aortic-pulmonary window, aortic stenosis plus regurgitation
  - Diastolic are less common, usually found with systolic, e.g. endocarditis
- Pitch/frequency
  - Soft, blowing – mitral incompetence

- Harsh, crescendo-decrescendo – pulmonic stenosis
- Ejection – aortic stenosis
- Machinery – PDA
- Site
  - Identify the point of maximal intensity (PMI) of murmur (see Figure 1) as it may indicate origin/valve
  - Radiation
    - Widely radiating murmurs more often associated with clinically significant lesions than localised murmur
    - Depends on direction of flow of stenotic or regurgitant jet and the energy of the blood flow
    - Murmurs can radiate up the neck – auscultate this area

Palpation
- Abdomen
  - Ascites (if also jugular distension: suggests right-sided heart failure)
  - Hepatomegaly due to congestion
- Apex beat
  - Prominent in thin-skinned and narrow-chested dogs
  - Also more prominent with increased sympathetic tone: post exercise and in hyperkinetic conditions, e.g. anaemia
  - Less obvious in obese, barrel-chested animals or with pericardial or pleural effusions
  - Apex beat can be displaced to the right with ventricular enlargement or mediastinal pleural or pulmonary masses
- Extremities
  - Cold periphery suggests poor cardiac output and peripheral circulatory shut down
- Precordial thrill
  - Vibrations from blood turbulence can be felt; helps to identify point of maximal intensity of murmurs that radiate widely

- Pulse
  - Pulse quality affected by:
    - Difference between systolic and diastolic blood pressure, i.e. pulse pressure
    - Arterial pressure: dependent on myocardial contractility and blood viscosity
    - Peripheral vascular resistance: vasoconstriction or vasodilatation, AV shunts
    - Palpability: varies with conformation of hindlimbs and physical condition of dog
    - Palpate femoral pulse at same time as auscultation of the heart
    - Note pulse deficits, i.e. heart sounds but no pulse
  - Pulse character
    - Hypokinetic: reduced stroke volume (SV) and increased peripheral resistance, e.g. cardiac tamponade, DCM, hypoadrenocorticism, low output heart failure
    - Hyperkinetic: increased SV or reduced PR, e.g. PDA, aortic insufficiency, bradycardia (large SV), anaemia
    - Aortic insufficiency and PDA have been described to have 'water hammer' pulse with rapid rise and then rapid collapse in pressure
    - Variable: usually associated with dysrhythmias
    - Absent: iliac thrombosis, neoplasia, cardiac arrest/severe hypotension
    - *Pulsus paradoxus*: exaggerated fall in pressure associated with inspiration; can be found in pericardial effusions
    - *Pulsus alternans* can occur with severe myocardial failure: the pulse alternates in strength despite normal sinus rhythm, reflecting an

alternation in the strength of left ventricular contraction

- Pulse rate
  - Normal 70–140 beats per minute
  - Slow
    - Bradydysrhythmia
    - Increased vagal tone (brachycephaly, CNS depression, GI disease)
  - Rapid
    - Cardiac failure
    - Reflex tachycardia (exercise, shock, anaemia, fever, pain)
    - Tachyarrhythmia
  - Pulse deficit with dysrhythmias
    - Atrial fibrillation (AF)
    - Ventricular premature complexes (VPCs)
  - Pulse rhythm
    - Auscultation is more valuable

Percussion
- Abdominal percussion (ballottement) to detect fluid thrill with ascites
- Chest percussion may indicate cardiomegaly by enlarged area of dullness
- Horizontal line of dullness in the ventral thorax with pleural effusion

Laboratory analysis
- Generally mild changes

Haematology
- Mild anaemia and leukocytosis may be seen in CHF
- Neutrophilia and left shift may be found in endocarditis
- Polycythaemia in right to left shunts (adaptive)

Serum biochemistry
- Liver enzymes – slight elevation is common in congestive or right-sided heart failure
- Muscle enzymes (CPK, LDH) may increase in acute myocardial disease (not cardiac-specific)
- Plasma proteins tend to fall in CHF

- Urea – slight elevation is common in CHF (pre-renal azotaemia)

Imaging
Radiography
- Views
  - Lateral – usually right
  - Dorsoventral (DV) – better than VD for cardiac silhouette and pulmonary vessels
  - VD can be helpful to identify small amounts of pleural effusion
- Wide variation of 'normal' size
  - Upright in lateral, and smaller and rounder in DV in deep-chested dogs
  - More rounded right side with increased sternal contact and increased width in shallow, wide-chested breeds
  - Heart size varies with phase of contraction and phase of respiration
    - Inspiration: less sternal contact, caudal vena cava horizontal, minimal or no cardiophrenic contact
    - Expiration: increased sternal contact of heart, caudal vena cava is oblique, increased cardiophrenic contact
- Heart size (see Figures 2 and 3)
  - Evaluates volume load (e.g. CHF, hypovolaemia)
  - Normal heart size does not exclude cardiac disease
  - Increased heart size more likely to be significant if present in both lateral and DV radiograph (see Figures 2 and 3)
  - Vertebral heart scoring (VHS) system
    - Length of heart (L) is measured on lateral inspiratory radiograph and then measured against the number of vertebral bodies starting at the cranial edge of thoracic vertebra T4
    - Width of the heart (W) is measured from the same radiograph and then measured against the vertebrae, again starting at T4
    - The number of vertebral bodies equivalent to L is added to W

ORGAN SYSTEMS

- VHS = L+W
- Dog normal range 8.5–10.5
- Intercostal spaces
  - Lateral radiograph: canine heart is usually 2.5–3.5 intercostal spaces wide and occupies ¾ of the depth of the thorax
  - DV radiograph: heart should occupy less than 2/3 width thorax
- Position of anatomical structures of the heart on DV radiograph (clockwise) (see Figures 2b and 3b)
  - 11–1 o'clock – Aortic arch
  - 1–2 o'clock – Main pulmonary artery
  - 2–3 o'clock – Left auricular appendage
  - 2–6 o'clock – Left ventricle border – usually straight
  - 6–11 o'clock – Right ventricle border
- Left atrium is superimposed over caudal third of the silhouette
- Generalised cardiomegaly
  - Pericardial effusions
  - Peritoneo-pericardial diaphragmatic hernia
  - Some cases of DCM
- Individual chamber enlargement
  - Left atrium indicated by elevation of trachea, straightening of caudal border of heart, elevation of caudal vena cava, compression of the mainstem bronchi
  - Right-sided enlargement indicated by increased sternal contact
  - Ventricular enlargement can displace the apex either to left or right on DV and will appear as a more round outline in the relevant area
  - Left ventricular enlargement indicated by straight caudal border of heart on lateral, increased apico-basilar length of the heart
  - Left-sided congestive failure (CHF)
    - Generalised oedema (alveolar pattern): acute left CHF
    - Perihilar oedema (alveolar pattern): chronic left CHF

- Vascular congestion: distended vessels
- Right-sided congestive failure (CHF)
  - Ascites
  - Enlargement of caudal vena cava
  - Hepatomegaly
  - Pleural effusion
- Miscellaneous
  - Pulmonary hypovascularity ± microcardia with hypovolaemia with right to left shunts, haemorrhagic shock and hypoadrenocorticism

Echocardiography
- Useful information on structure and function of heart
- Aids the diagnosis of congenital abnormalities, myocardial failure, degenerative valvular disease, pericardial effusions, localise the source of a murmur, e.g. pulsed or continuous wave Doppler
- Bubble echocardiography provides contrast to track blood flow
- The reader is referred to specialist texts for full information

Special investigative techniques
- Angiography
  - Selective by cardiac catheterisation to identify intracardiac or vascular lesions
  - Non-selective via a catheter into jugular vein
  - Use iodine-based solutions
- Blood pressure measurement (should be routine part of cardiovascular investigation)
- Electrocardiography
  - Part of minimum database for suspected cardiac disease
  - Usually record in right lateral recumbency in dogs
  - Artefacts are common with gross movement, fine movement (muscle tremor), respiration, A/C interference, poor baseline definition, poor electrode contact

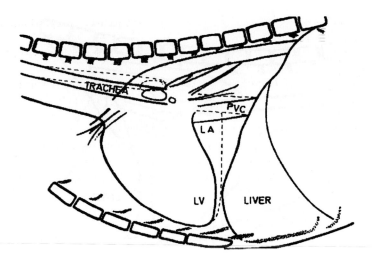

Figure 2(a)   Diagram of a lateral view of the thorax, showing changes found in left-sided cardiac failure. --- indicates displacement of structures. LA, left atrial enlargement; LV, left ventricle; PVC, posterior (caudal) vena cava.

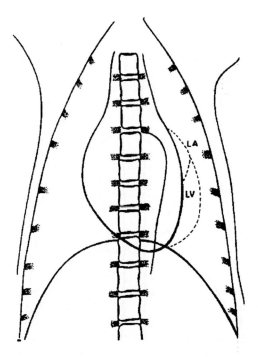

Figure 2(b)   Diagram of a dorsoventral view of the thorax, showing changes found in left-sided cardiac failure. --- indicates enlarged structures. LA, left atrial enlargement; LV, left ventricular enlargement.

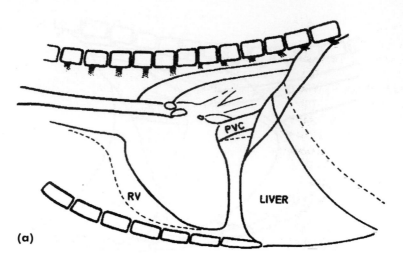

(a)

Figure 3(a) Diagram of a lateral view of the thorax, showing changes found in right-sided cardiac failure. --- indicates enlarged structures. RV, right ventricular enlargement; PVC, enlarging posterior (caudal) vena cava.

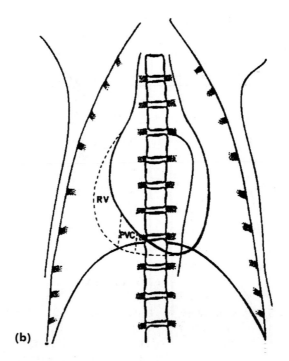

(b)

Figure 3(b) Diagram of a dorsoventral view of the thorax, showing changes found in right-sided cardiac failure. --- indicates enlarged structures. RV, right ventricular enlarge-ment; PVC, enlarging posterior (caudal) vena cava.

- Measures
  - Heart rate
  - Rhythm and impulse conduction
- May assess
  - Altered myocardial metabolism, e.g. electrolyte imbalance/hypoxia
  - Evidence of chamber enlargement/ hypertrophy but not very sensitive or specific
- Does not indicate cardiac output, e.g. ECG can be normal in an animal dying of cardiac failure
- For ECG measurement/inter- pretation, the reader is advised to refer to cardiology texts
- Real-time ECG monitoring
  - Event monitor
  - 24-hour Holter monitor
  - Telemetry
- Cardiac catheterisation
  - Assess central venous pressure in patients with suspected CHF
  - Measure chamber pressures
  - Obtain samples for blood gas analy- sis to help identify shunts
- Fluoroscopy
  - Can be useful in angiographic studies or to diagnose pericardial effusions or monitor drainage
- Phonocardiography
  - To record cardiac sound waves can be helpful to aid identification of timing of murmur in relation to the normal heart sounds, the duration, frequency and form of murmurs
- Plasma atrial natriuretic peptide meas- urement as an indicator of volume over- load

HEART FAILURE

Aetiology
- Deficiency of cardiac output sufficient to cause clinical signs, as an end result of:
  - Acquired heart disease

- Arrhythmias
- Congenital heart disease
- Pericardial disease
- Depending on the condition, there may be right- or left-sided failure, or com- plete congestive failure

LEFT HEART FAILURE
Major signs
- Exercise intolerance or lethargy
- Dyspnoea/tachypnoea/orthopnoea
- Coughing
  - Bronchial compression from LA en- largement
  - Pulmonary oedema rarely causes coughing
- Syncopal episodes (forward failure of cardiac output)
- Nocturnal restlessness
- Sudden death

Minor signs
- Anorexia
- Weight loss

Physical examination
- Abnormal cardiac rate and rhythm
- Changes in pulse quality
- Gallop rhythms and sounds
- Murmur
- Pale mucous membranes
- Prominent or displaced apex beat
- Pulmonary crackles (pulmonary oede- ma versus primary lung disease)

RIGHT HEART FAILURE
Major signs
- Ascites
- Dyspnoea (pleural effusion)
- Exercise intolerance
- Syncope

Minor signs
- Inappetence
- Subcutaneous oedema
- Weight loss

Physical examination

- Ascites
- Hepatojugular reflux
- Hepatomegaly
- Jugular venous distension ± jugular pulse
- Pleural effusion (dullness on percussion ventrally, reduced heart sounds)
- Subcutaneous oedema

Treatment of CHF

Diuresis

Indicated for the management of pulmonary oedema and right-sided CHF

Frusemide
- First-choice diuretic
- Potent loop diuretic
- Can cause hypotension and potassium depletion
- Ideal in emergency situation
  - 2–4 mg/kg every 1–2 hours, initially i/v
- Maintenance
  - 1–2 mg/kg PO BID or TID, and titrate to lowest effective dose

Spironolactone
- Potassium-sparing diuretic
- Competitive antagonist of aldosterone in the renal tubule
- Co-administration with loop diuretics may be beneficial in resistant fluid retention
- 2–4 mg/kg PO SID

Inotropic agents

Cardiac glycosides – Digoxin
- Indications
  - Positive inotrope – systolic failure, e.g. DCM
  - Negative chronotrope – management of supraventricular tachycardia (SVT)
- Contraindications
  - Bradydysrhythmias
  - Hypertrophic myocardial disease

- Side effects: depression, anorexia, vomiting, diarrhoea, bradycardia, arrhythmias
- Dose: 0.22 mg/m^2 PO BID
- Monitor therapeutic levels 10–14 days after starting/altering therapy and periodically if the dog is unstable
  - Serum sample 6–8 hours after last pill is assayed for digoxin levels

Pimobendan
- Phosphodiesterase III inhibitor and calcium sensitiser ('inodilator')
- Indications
  - Chronic degenerative mitral valve disease
  - DCM
- Contraindications
  - Not to be used in cases of hypertrophic cardiomyopathies or clinical conditions where augmenting cardiac output is not possible for functional or anatomical reasons, e.g. aortic stenosis
- Side effects
  - A moderate, dose-dependent, positive chronotropic effect
  - Vomiting may occur
- Dose 0.2–0.6 mg/kg/day given 1 hour before food, divided BID

Vasodilating agents
- Decrease myocardial workload.
- Arteriodilators may promote cardiac output by increasing the forward stroke volume, i.e. reduce the afterload
- Venodilators decrease ventricular diastolic pressures by increasing venous capacitance, i.e. reduce the preload

ACE inhibitors
- Inhibit angiotensin-converting enzyme (ACE), blocking angiotensin II production
- Arterial and venodilator
- Decrease salt and water retention

ORGAN SYSTEMS

- Indications
  - Mitral valve disease
  - Myocardial systolic failure
  - Volume overload
  - Hypertension
  - Reduction of renal proteinuria
- Dose examples
  - Enalapril 0.25–0.5 mg/kg PO SID or BID
  - Benazepril 0.25 mg/kg PO SID

Nitroprusside
- Balanced vasodilator
- Direct-acting, rapid onset of action, short half-life and potent vasodilator
- Indications
  - Acute, severe, life-threatening myocardial failure
  - Mitral or aortic regurgitation
  - Systemic hypertension
- 1–5 µg/kg/min i/v constant infusion initially and increase by 3–5 µg/kg/min increments
- Can cause severe hypotension: must be able to monitor blood pressure
- Discontinue drug gradually

Glyceryl trinitrate
- Venodilator applied transdermally
- Indications
  - To reduce congestion in combination with diuretics
- 2% gel [5–15 mg (0.5–5 cm)] every 6–8 hours transdermally
- Wear gloves when applying to dog

ACQUIRED HEART DISEASE

CHRONIC DEGENERATIVE VALVULAR DISEASE
Aetiology
- Endocardiosis, an age-related myxomatous changes in the valve, leads to deformation of leaflets
- Mitral valve primarily affected

- Incompetence of the valves leads to regurgitation and a murmur is produced
- Significant regurgitation eventually leads to heart failure
- Endocardiosis has been linked to macrothrombocytosis in the CKCS, but it is not clear whether this is cause or effect

Major signs
- Anorexia
- Coughing
- Dyspnoea
- Exercise intolerance
- Lethargy
- Nocturnal restlessness

Minor signs
- Syncope
- Weight loss

Potential sequelae
- Development of CHF
- Rupture of chordae tendineae can lead to acute decompensation
- Rupture of left atrium can result in sudden death

Predisposition
- Increased prevalence in small breed, male dogs: CKCS, Chihuahua, Miniature poodle, Miniature pinscher, Whippet
- Middle-old aged dogs
- Multifactorial, polygenic, threshold trait in CKCS; mitral valve prolapse as early as 1–2 years and predisposing to degenerative valvular disease

Historical clues
- In CKCS, murmur may be present by 1 year
- Loss of sinus arrhythmia and development of tachycardia indicate cardiac dysfunction

Physical examination
- Systolic murmur over left cardiac apex

ORGAN SYSTEMS

- Increased intensity, duration and radiation of the murmur as the disease progresses
- ± Precordial thrill in severe disease
- Signs of left-heart failure
  - Pulmonary crackles
  - Tachycardia

Imaging
Thoracic radiography
- Progressive left-sided (or global) cardiomegaly
- Pulmonary venous congestion
- Interstitial or alveolar pattern with left CHF

Echocardiography
- LA and LV enlargement in MVD
- Valvular endocardiosis lesions
- Myocardial failure can develop
- Colour-flow Doppler will identify a systolic regurgitant jet in the left atrium

Special investigations
- Cardiac catheterisation and angiography
  - Can be used to make a definitive diagnosis
  - Rarely required
- Electrocardiography in MVD
  - Wide P waves
  - Tall R waves
  - Arrhythmias in advanced cases – supraventricular usually

Treatment
- Weight loss if indicated
- Controlled exercise regime
- Management of left-sided CHF in MVD
  - Diuretics to control pulmonary oedema, e.g. frusemide
  - Anti-arrhythmic therapy based on ECG diagnosis and clinical signs
  - ACE inhibitor/Pimobendan

Monitoring
- Clinical response
- Imaging

Prognosis
- Guarded: the disease is progressive, but management for several years is possible

DILATED CARDIOMYOPATHY (DCM)
Aetiology
- Intrinsic failure of myocardium due to unknown causes
- In other species
  - Genetic defects
  - Viral infections
- As the myocardium fails, the heart dilates and AV valves become incompetent

Major signs
- Ascites
- Cough
- Dyspnoea/tachypnoea
- Lethargy/weakness
- Reduced exercise tolerance
- Syncope
- Weight loss

Potential sequelae
- Sudden death is possible in all cases
- Death from congestive heart failure (CHF)

Predisposition
- Young to middle-aged dogs (6 months to > 10 years)
- Predisposed breeds: Dobermann, Boxer, Cocker and Springer spaniels, Giant breeds (Irish wolfhound, St Bernard, Great Dane, Newfoundland)

Historical clues
- May be asymptomatic
- Arrhythmias
- Development of murmur in susceptible breed

Physical examination
- Soft systolic murmur secondary to valvular incompetence

- Arrhythmia – supraventricular and ventricular
- Gallop sounds may be detected on auscultation
- Hypokinetic pulse (poor stroke volume)
- Sluggish CRT
- Weight loss

Laboratory findings
- Pre-renal azotaemia

Imaging
Thoracic radiography
- Alveolar pattern (pulmonary oedema)
- Left-sided (or global) cardiomegaly
- Pleural effusion if concurrent right CHF
- Pulmonary venous congestion

Echocardiography
- Assess chamber size and global myocardial function
- Cardiac chamber dimensions > normal
- End-systolic diameter is increased due to reduced myocardial contractility
- Hypokinesis: left ventricular fractional shortening is decreased
- Doppler echocardiography used to assess valvular incompetence/regurgitation

Special investigations
Electrocardiography
- Wide P waves
- Tall R waves
- Arrhythmia – various ventricular and/or supraventricular: atrial fibrillation and VPCs are common

Holter monitor
- Identify paroxysmal arrhythmias in syncopal cases if not detected on routine ECG

Treatment
- Manage CHF
  - Diuretics

- ACE inhibitors
- Positive inotrope: digoxin (may not have inotropic action) or pimobendan
- Anti-arrhythmics – depends on the ECG diagnosis and clinical signs
- Severe crisis
  - Cage rest and oxygen
  - Intravenous frusemide
  - Vasodilators
  - Intravenous dobutamine infusion
  - Anti-arrhythmics
  - Monitor renal function and electrolytes

Monitor
- Echocardiography
- ECG

Prognosis
- Prognosis varies according to breed and severity of disease at presentation
  - Giant breeds identified because of arrhythmia may remain clinically silent for years
  - Cocker and Springer spaniels seem to have a long course of disease
  - Dobermanns have high incidence of sudden death with short clinical course
- Can survive several years with careful management in some breeds
- Outlook is poor when cardiac failure is associated: die or are euthanased within 6–12 months

ARRHYTHMIAS

Aetiology
- All cardiac tissue has intrinsic rhythmicity: the sinus node is the dominant pacemaker
- If there is no stimulus from the SA node, then other sites in the conduction tissue may act as substitute pacemakers; this is usually seen as bradycardia, with escape beats

ORGAN SYSTEMS

- Myocardial lesions can act as irritant foci creating ectopic pacemakers, which can precede the normal activation from the sinus node if they are premature

Major signs
- Asymptomatic, weakness, syncope or sudden death, depending on specific arrhythmia

Potential sequelae
- Cardiac arrest and death

Predisposition
- See specific arrhythmia

Historical clues
- Precipitating event may be noted

Physical examination
Auscultation
- Intensity of sounds
- Pattern of rhythm
  - Regular: sinus
  - Regularly irregular: sinus arrhythmia
  - Irregularly irregular: atrial fibrillation, ventricular arrhythmias
- Compare cardiac rhythm with pulse – any pulse deficit should be noted

Laboratory findings
- Electrolyte disturbances
- Often unremarkable, or reflecting underlying disease

Imaging
Radiography
- Altered heart size from under- or over-filling
- Signs of underlying disease

Echocardiography
- See specific arrhythmia

Special investigations
Electrocardiography
- Identify if sinus rhythm exists
- Identify arrhythmia
- If ectopics are they supraventricular or ventricular in origin?

Treatment
- See specific arrhythmia

Monitoring
- ECG

Prognosis
- See specific arrhythmia

NORMAL RHYTHMS
Sinus rhythm
- Normal regular activation of the atria and via the conduction system the ventricles by the pacemaker (sinus node) at a normal rate

Sinus arrhythmia
- Common in normal dogs: regular phasic acceleration and deceleration in heart rate, often synchronous with respiration
- P wave usually normal shape, but wandering pacemaker seen
- Accentuated in respiratory disease/airway obstruction
- Sign of a normal or a well-compensated diseased heart
- Lost with tachycardia

Sinus tachycardia
- Regular rhythm of sinus node origin at rates of 150–200 per minute
- Significance
  - Physiological: exercise, stress, fear, pyrexia, anaemia
  - Pathological: response to cardiac failure
  - P-QRS-T normal complexes but at faster rate
- Treatment is aimed at the primary cause

BRADYDYSRHYTHMIAS
Aetiology
- Excessive vagal tone, e.g. GI disease
- Myocardial lesions invading the conduction tissue, e.g. abscess, fibrosis, neoplasia
- Myocardial or pacemaker depression
  - Cardiac glycosides
  - Electrolyte disturbances
  - Toxaemia

Major signs
- Asymptomatic
- Syncope
- Weakness/collapse

Treatment
- Treat any underlying causes
- Parasympatholytic drugs can be helpful if vagally induced bradycardia
  - Atropine 0.02–0.04 mg/kg i/v, i/m, s/c
  - Glycopyrrolate 0.005–0.01 mg/kg i/v, i/m or 0.01–0.02 mg/kg s/c
- Side effects: miosis, vomiting, diarrhoea, tachycardia, reduced secretions
- Sympathomimetic drugs to increase ventricular escape rate
  - Temporary management in complete heart block
  - Isoproterenol 5 µg/kg i/v [0.05–1.0 µg/kg/min]
- Pacemaker implantation

Sinus arrest/pause
- Long pauses between groups of beats
- If prolonged can cause syncope
- Pause in pulse concurrently
- May be synchronised with respiration
- May be accentuated sinus arrhythmia
- Occasional ventricular escape beats can occur
  - Causes:
    - Common, normal variation in brachycephalics
    - Atrial pathology
    - Drugs

- Electrolyte imbalances (hyperkalaemia)
- Hypothyroidism
- Thoracic surgery
- ECG
  - Pause in rhythm with no QRS complex
  - If pause = 2 × RR interval, it is sinus block
  - If pause > 2 × RR interval, it suggests sinus arrest
  - Atropine may abolish disturbance if due to excessive vagal tone

Sinus bradycardia
- Heart rate < 60–70 beats per minute
- P-QRS-T have normal conformation but occur at a lower rate
- Causes
  - Normal in some fit dogs, giant breed dogs
  - Drugs, e.g. tranquillisers
  - Hyperkalaemia
  - Hypothermia
  - Hypothyroidism
  - Increased intracranial pressure
  - Systemic disease, e.g. uraemia
- Management
  - Treat the primary condition
  - Atropine response test to determine if vagally mediated: 20–40 µg/kg s/c and repeat ECG 30 minutes later. Increased rate suggests vagally mediated bradycardia
  - Usually no treatment as resolves with management of primary condition
  - Pacemaker would be effective if necessary

Bradycardia-tachycardia syndrome
- Sometimes misnamed 'Sick Sinus Syndrome'
- Alternating bradycardia-tachycardia rhythm
- Long periods of sinus arrest with a failure of escape beats to occur
- Clinical signs of syncope and weakness

- Reported most commonly in female, Miniature Schnauzers > 6 years old
- ? Idiopathic
- ECG
  - Persistent sinus bradycardia
  - Episodes of sinus arrest
  - May be atrial premature complexes or alternating bradycardia and tachycardia
- Treatment
  - Treatment of choice is pacemaker implantation

Atrial standstill
- Absence of any atrial activity
- Causes
  - Persistent atrial standstill in English Springer Spaniels
  - Temporary atrial standstill with hyperkalaemia and digoxin toxicity
- Clinical signs: asymptomatic weakness or syncope
- ECG
  - No P waves
  - Regular slow escape rhythm < 60 beats per minute
  - QRS complex often normal shape, but can be of prolonged duration
  - Sinus node still fires and impulses are conducted by internodal pathways to AV node but cause no atrial activity
- Treatment
  - Treat primary cause if identified
  - Persistent atrial standstill: pacemaker implantation not always successful

Atrioventricular block
- AV block is a failure to conduct impulses normally through the AV node

First-degree heart block
- P and QRS are normal in conformation but the PR interval is prolonged
- Causes
  - Normal at slow heart rates
  - Ageing changes in AV node
  - Drugs, e.g. digoxin, propranolol

- Hyperkalaemia
- Management aimed at underlying cause

Second-degree heart block
- P wave is normal, but there is an occasional or frequent failure of conduction through the AV node so there is an absence of the associated QRS complex
- Clinical signs – asymptomatic weakness or syncope
- Auscultation – occasional dropped beats
- Causes:
  - AV nodal fibrosis in older dogs
  - Drugs, e.g. digoxin
  - Hereditary in the Pug
  - High vagal tone, e.g. brachycephalics
  - Hyperkalaemia
  - Idiopathic
- Management aimed at the primary cause. Other treatments only if signs are severe
  - Some improvement may be seen with:
    - Parasympatholytic drugs (atropine, glycopyrrolate)
    - Sympathomimetic (isoprenaline or terbutaline)
  - Pacemaker implantation in cases unresponsive to medical therapy

Complete (third-degree) AV block
- Persistent failure of impulse conduction through AV node
- Pacemaker below the AV node discharges to control the ventricles with a rate of discharge slower than the AV node
  - Lower AV node/bundle branches = junctional escape rhythm 60–70 bpm with normal QRS
  - Purkinje cells = ventricular escape rhythm 30–40 bpm with abnormal QRS
- Associated with: cardiomyopathy, cardiac neoplasia, digoxin toxicity, AV

node fibrosis, endocarditis, electrolyte imbalance, hypothyroidism, Lyme disease
- Clinical signs
  - Weakness, lethargy, syncope, sudden death
  - Generalised cardiomegaly in chronic cases with slow ventricular rate and may develop CHF
  - Hyperdynamic femoral pulse
  - Regular but slow rhythm on auscultation
- ECG
  - Regular P waves at fast rate
  - QRS-T at regular slow rate
  - P and QRS-T are independent of each other
- Management
  - Most cases require pacemaker implantation if control of the primary disease cannot be achieved

TACHYARRHYTHMIAS
Aetiology
- Myocardial lesions acting as ectopic pacemakers, preceding the normal activation from the sinus node

Treatment
- Distinguish supraventricular or ventricular in origin
- Supraventricular
  - Attempt to slow AV nodal conduction
    - Beta-blockers, e.g. atenolol @ 0.5–2 mg/kg PO BID
    - Cardiac glycosides, e.g. digoxin @ 0.22 mg/m^2 PO BID
    - Calcium-channel blockers, e.g. diltiazem @ 1.5–2.5 mg/kg PO TID
- Ventricular
  - Reduce myocyte automaticity, decrease impulse conduction, prolong refractory period
  - Lignocaine (lidocaine)
    - @ 2–6 mg/kg i/v, then 25–80 µg/kg/min i/v
    - Not suitable for oral administration due to first-pass hepatic metabolism
  - Procainamide
    - @ 2 mg/kg i/v, then 25–40 µg/kg/min i/v, or 10–25 mg/kg PO or i/m QID, or sustained-release TID
  - Mexilitine
    - @ 4–8 mg/kg PO BID
  - Beta-blockers
    - Always start with a low dose and increase according to response
    - Atenolol as above
    - Propranolol @ 0.1 mg/kg i/v or 0.2–1.0 mg/kg PO TID
    - Sotalol @ 1–2 mg/kg PO BID

Supraventricular tachyarrhythmias
Premature complexes (SVPCs)
- Arise from an ectopic focus or foci above the ventricles
- Ventricles are depolarised normally: QRS shape is normal
- Auscultation – early beats interrupt normal rhythm (similar to VPC)

Supraventricular tachycardia (SVT)
- Often rapid rate with rapid onset and offset
- Pulse deficits can occur with SVPCs and weak pulse with SVT
- SVT may cause weakness, syncope, or CHF

Atrial premature complexes (APC)
- Arise in atria – produce 'ectopic' P wave – abnormal in shape, can be negative or positive or biphasic, PR interval is often prolonged
- No compensatory pause

Junctional premature complexes (JPCs)
- Arise in AV node or bundle of His
- Depolarisation wave spreads through ventricles normally but also retrograde through atria producing a P wave

ORGAN SYSTEMS

- abnormal in shape and usually negative in Lead II
- P wave can occur before, during or after the QRS complex
- If before the QRS the PR interval is usually shorter than normal and the SA node is reset
- Associated conditions with supraventricular tachyarrhythmias
  - Congenital/acquired AV valve disease
  - Congenital cardiac shunts
  - Digoxin toxicity
  - Right atrial haemangiosarcoma
  - Ventricular pre-excitation syndrome
- Management:
  - Single SVPCs usually do not require treatment
  - Management of the underlying cause often reduces SVT to acceptable rate
  - Vagal manoeuvre (ocular or carotid sinus massage) in paroxysmal or sustained SVT may terminate the rhythm
  - Symptomatic SVT: intravenous beta-blocker (e.g. esmolol) or calcium channel blocker
  - Oral therapy with calcium-channel blocker, beta-blocker or digoxin

Ventricular premature complexes (VPCs)

- Arise from an ectopic focus or foci within ventricular myocardium
- A run of three or more VPCs is called ventricular tachycardia (VT)
- VT usually occurs at rates > 100 per minute
- Clinical signs
  - None with single VPCs
  - Weakness, syncope and sudden death with VT (especially fast VT)
- Auscultation – normal rhythm is disrupted by premature beats followed by pause

- Pulse
  - Deficits are usually present
  - With VT, pulse can be very weak
- ECG
  - QRS complex is wide and bizarre
  - T wave is usually opposite in direction to the QRS and large
  - Occur prematurely (normal sinus complex hidden by VPC)
  - Compensatory pause as AV node is not stimulated again till next sinus beat
- Associated with:
  - Cardiac disease – CHF, cardiomyopathy (Dobermann, Boxer), myocarditis, endocarditis
  - Drugs, e.g. digoxin, anaesthetic agents
  - Systemic disease – hypoxia, acid-base disorders, uraemia, GDV, pyometra, pancreatitis, splenic disease
- Management
  - Treat underlying disease will often reduce the number of VPCs
  - If VT is considered life-threatening
    - i/v lignocaine bolus ± infusion
    - Oral therapy, e.g. mexiletine, procainamide

Fibrillation and flutter

- Fibrillation is rapid irregular small movements of fibres
- Flutter means to wave or flap regularly

Atrial fibrillation (AF)

- Random depolarisation waves throughout atria conducted to the AV nodes and ventricles at rate determined by AV node conduction velocity and refractory period
- Usually associated with dilation and stretching of the atria or with primary atrial pathology
- Common in medium-large breed dog with dilated cardiomyopathy

- Can occur without obvious atrial pathology in giant breeds at a low rate
- Effect on cardiac output depends on ventricular rate
- Often animal is in CHF
- Auscultation
  - cardiac rhythm is chaotic
  - marked pulse deficits
- ECG
- Irregular chaotic ventricular (QRS) rate and rhythm (irregular RR intervals)
- QRS varies in amplitude with no recognisable P waves preceding it, usually at a fast rate
- Rapid, irregular saw-tooth movement of baseline at 300–500 per minute (F waves)
- Management
  - Reduce ventricular response rate < 150–160 bpm
  - Digoxin is the drug of choice
  - Additional anti-arrhythmics if needed, e.g. beta-blocker or calcium-channel blocker

Ventricular fibrillation (VF)

- Random depolarisation throughout ventricles
- No co-ordinated contraction – very poor cardiac output
- Causes similar to VPCs and VT
- ECG
  - coarse or fine, rapid
  - irregular and bizarre movement with no recognisable waveforms or complexes
- Management
  - Treatment is the start of cardiopulmonary resuscitation (CPR)
- Grave prognosis; common cause of cardiac arrest and death

CONGENITAL HEART DISEASE

Aetiology

- Aortic stenosis: comprise 20–35% of reported canine congenital anomalies
- Mitral valve dysplasia
- PDA: comprise 20% of reported canine congenital anomalies
- Pulmonic stenosis
- Tetralogy of Fallot
- Ventricular septal defect (VSD)

AORTIC STENOSIS (AS) OR SUB-AORTIC STENOSIS (SAS)

Aetiology

- Congenital stenosis
  - Most commonly below the valvular ring, i.e. sub-aortic
- Occasionally causes LHF, especially if mitral regurgitation

Major signs

- Asymptomatic
- Exercise intolerance
- Syncope

Minor signs

- Hindlimb weakness

Potential sequelae

- Mild – moderate stenosis survival reported as 30–50 months
- Severe cases survive to < 3 years old
- Sudden death can occur due to arrhythmia development
- Bacterial endocarditis

Predisposition

- Breed predisposition: German Shepherd dog, Boxer, Golden retriever [Newfoundland, German short-haired pointer, Rottweiler, Samoyed, Great Dane, Bull terrier]

Historical clues

- May be asymptomatic for some time

ORGAN SYSTEMS

- Murmur should be detectable at vaccination

Physical examination
- Murmur
  - Crescendo-decrescendo murmur, radiates to thoracic inlet and right base
  - PMI is third-fourth intercostal space left-hand side near heart base
  - Murmur may also be auscultated in mitral valve region
- ± Precordial thrill
- Hypokinetic pulse
- Prominent apex beat

Laboratory findings
- Usually unremarkable

Imaging
Thoracic radiograph – right lateral and DV
- Usually normal unless LHF (uncommon)
- Left ventricular enlargement may be seen
- ± Post-stenotic dilation of ascending and descending aorta

Echocardiography
- 2D and M mode – may be no abnormalities in mild cases
- Concentric left ventricular hypertrophy
- Anatomic abnormalities of the left ventricular outflow tract and aortic valve
- Post-stenotic dilation of ascending aorta
- Doppler: normal maximal aortic velocity > 2 m/s = aortic stenosis measured from sub-costal view
  - Mild < 3.5 m/s
  - Moderate 3.5–4.5[5] m/s
  - Severe 4.5 –5 m/s
  - Turbulent high velocity aortic flow with Doppler but actual aortic insufficiency is often trivial

- May be evidence of mitral valve (MV) regurgitation
- MV dysplasia reported in combination with SAS in Golden retriever

Special investigations
Cardiac catheterisation
- Will demonstrate small left ventricular chamber, subvalvular obstruction and post-stenotic dilation

Electrocardiography
- May be unremarkable
- Tall R waves
- ± ST segment depression (hypoxic change)
- ± Notched QRS complex
- Ventricular ectopics due to myocardial hypoxia/ischaemia

Treatment
- Mild cases usually do not require treatment
- Severe cases
  - Avoid extreme exertion
  - Ventricular arrhythmias controlled with anti-arrhythmics
  - If concentric left ventricular hypertrophy use beta-blockers to improve diastolic filling and decrease myocardial oxygen consumption
  - Balloon valvuloplasty: 50% reduction in gradient but may attenuate over time and high-risk procedure
  - Surgical correction – requires bypass
  - Results of balloon and surgical valvuloplasty are disappointing

Monitoring
- Clinical signs
- Regular repeated ECG, echocardiography and radiographs

Prognosis
- Excellent for mild cases
- Poor for severe cases

MITRAL VALVE DYSPLASIA
Aetiology
- Congenital defect in mitral valve: absent, abnormal or fused valve leaflets
- Left-heart failure develops though mitral regurgitation

Major signs
- Coughing (LA enlargement and bronchial compression)
- Dyspnoea
- Exercise intolerance

Potential sequelae
- Development of left-sided CHF

Predisposition
- Predisposed breeds: Bull terrier, GSD and Springer spaniel

Historical clues
- Murmur detected at routine check, e.g. vaccination
- Gradual development of exercise intolerance

Physical examination
- Murmur over mitral valve (left, 5th intercostal space) area, holo- or pansystolic and loud
- Can radiate extensively and grade can be variable
- Murmur grade does not correlate with severity
- Arrhythmia may be auscultated/palpated – e.g. atrial fibrillation due to severe left atrial enlargement
- Adventitious lung sounds if in left-sided CHF

Laboratory findings
- Usually unremarkable

Imaging
Thoracic radiography
- LA and LV enlargement
- Pulmonary venous congestion and oedema if left-sided CHF

Echocardiography
- LA and LV enlargement (dilation)
- Dysplastic mitral valve
- ± Abnormal M-mode mitral valve motion
- Doppler
  - Increased mitral inflow velocity
  - Mitral regurgitation ± stenosis

Special investigations
Electrocardiography
- ± Wide P waves
- ± Tall R waves
- ± Arrhythmias

Treatment
- Medical management of left-sided CHF
  - Diuretics
  - ACE inhibitors
  - Pimobendan

Monitoring
- Clinical signs
- Echocardiography

Prognosis
- Guarded, depending on degree of mitral regurgitation

PATENT DUCTUS ARTERIOSUS (PDA)
Aetiology
- The ductus arteriosus is a foetal link between aorta and pulmonary artery which normally closes shortly after birth
- With a PDA this vessel remains patent
- Normally, PDAs shunt left to right; rarely right to left

Major signs
- Asymptomatic
- Left-sided heart failure

Minor signs
- Differential cyanosis (cyanotic caudally) with reverse PDA

Potential sequelae
- CHF
- Death

Predisposition
- Sex predisposition females: males = 3:1
- Autosomal dominant mode of inheritance?
- Predisposed breeds: GSD, Border collie (and crosses), CKCS

Historical clues
- May be asymptomatic for some time
- Murmur should be detectable at vaccination

Physical examination
- Murmur
  - Continuous murmur: 'machinery murmur'
  - Waxing in systole and waning through diastole
  - Loud murmur with precordial thrill
  - Can radiate widely to right base and thoracic inlet or can be very localised to high left base
  - Separate MV systolic murmur may be heard due to MV regurgitation
- Femoral pulse collapses rapidly (due to loss of volume through PDA): hyperkinetic 'water-hammer' pulse
- Left-sided CHF: dyspnoea and adventitious lung sounds
- Right to left shunting PDA (very rare) – differential cyanosis

Laboratory findings
- Usually unremarkable

Imaging
Thoracic radiography
- LA enlargement 2–3 o'clock on DV
- LV enlargement
- Dilated pulmonary trunk 1–2 o'clock on DV
- Dilated descending aorta 12–1 o'clock on DV
- Pulmonary over-circulation
- ± Pulmonary oedema

Echocardiography
- LA and LV enlargement (eccentric LV hypertrophy)
- Dilated main pulmonary trunk
- Hyperkinetic LV (progresses to myocardial failure with reduced fractional shortening)
- Ductus may be imaged between main pulmonary trunk and descending aorta (difficult)
- Doppler:
  - Turbulent flow in main pulmonary artery during diastole
  - Continuous turbulent flow at bifurcation of pulmonary trunk and in descending aorta
  - Ductus imaged with colour flow mapping
  - Mitral regurgitation is common

Special investigations
Cardiac catheterisation and angiography
- In suspected cases without a diagnosis after the above investigations

Electrocardiography
- Wide P waves (P mitrale)
- Tall R waves
- Various arrhythmias, particularly atrial fibrillation

Treatment
- If CHF is present, this should be treated before occlusion
- Management of CHF
  - ACE inhibitors
  - Diuretics
  - ? Digoxin if atrial fibrillation with high heart rate

- Occlusion of the PDA
  - Surgical double ligation
  - Transcatheter placement of intravascular coils

Monitoring
- Clinical signs

Prognosis
- Without intervention, 64% die by 1 year old
- Surgery in older dogs carries a higher risk as the ductus and dilated pulmonary arteries are friable
- Prognosis is good to excellent if diagnosed early before the development of myocardial failure

PULMONIC STENOSIS (PS)
Aetiology
- Congenital stenosis
- Development of right-sided CHF, e.g. ascites

Major signs
- Asymptomatic
- Syncope
- Exercise intolerance
- Stunted

Minor signs
- Dyspnoea
- Prominent jugular pulse
- Ascites

Potential sequelae
- Mild to moderate disease may have no effect on life expectancy
- Moderate to severe cases can develop exertional syncope, arrhythmias, tricuspid valve insufficiency, atrial fibrillation, CHF and sudden death

Predisposition
- Breed predisposition: Cocker spaniel, Miniature Schnauzer, Boxer

Historical clues
- May be asymptomatic for some time
- Murmur should be detectable at vaccination

Physical examination
- Murmur
  - Crescendo-decrescendo murmur
  - Left-sided, cranial (third intercostal space) and ventral
  - Mid-systolic ejection type
  - Radiates dorsally
- Precordial thrill and wide radiation in some high-grade stenoses
- Apex beat may be more prominent on right due to right ventricular hypertrophy
- Pulse quality good
- Signs of right CHF: jugular distension, hepatomegaly, ascites, hepatojugular reflux

Laboratory findings
- Usually unremarkable

Imaging
Thoracic radiography
- Normal if mild case
- Normal heart/hypoperfused pulmonary vasculature
- Right ventricular enlargement
- Post-stenotic dilation of pulmonary trunk

Echocardiography
- Abnormal pulmonic valve leaflets
- Interventricular septum flat or paradoxical motion
- Post-stenotic dilation of pulmonary trunk
- Right ventricular hypertrophy
- Doppler: high velocity and turbulent flow across the pulmonic valve
  - Normal transvalvular velocity < 2 m/s
  - Mild 2–3 m/s
  - Moderate 3–5 m/s

ORGAN SYSTEMS

- Severe > 100mmHg
- ± Tricuspid regurgitation

Special investigations
Cardiac catheterisation
- Angiography demonstrates narrowed pulmonic orifice, dysplastic valve leaflets, right ventricular hypertrophy, dynamic obstruction

Electrocardiography
- Deep S waves in leads I, II, III and aVF
- Right axis deviation
- ± Ventricular ectopics

Treatment
- Mild cases do not require treatment
- Moderate cases are best candidates for balloon valvuloplasty, but may need repeated treatments
- Surgery for those cases where balloon valvuloplasty has failed

Monitoring
- Clinical signs
- Regular repeated ECG, echocardiography and radiographs

Prognosis
- Mild to moderate disease may have no effect on life expectancy
- Moderate to severe cases can develop exertional syncope, arrhythmias, tricuspid valve insufficiency, atrial fibrillation, CHF and sudden death

TETRALOGY OF FALLOT
Aetiology
Combination of congenital defects:
- Over-riding aorta
- Pulmonic stenosis
- Right ventricular hypertrophy
- Ventricular septal defect

Major signs
- Cyanosis
- Severe exercise intolerance

- Syncope
- Stunting

Potential sequelae
- CHF rarely
- Right to left shunt with cyanosis
- Sudden death

Predisposition
- Predisposed breeds: Golden retriever, Wirehaired fox terrier, Labrador retriever, Siberian Husky, Toy poodle
- Keeshond has an autosomal dominant mode of inheritance with variable penetrance

Historical clues
- Ill-thrift from early age

Physical examination
- Mucous membranes are cyanosed
- Murmur
  - Left 3rd intercostal space and right 4th intercostal space
  - Radiates dorsally and to left apex
  - Mid- or holosystolic murmur, crescendo-decrescendo, ejection-type murmur
- Pulse quality usually normal

Laboratory findings
- Polycythaemia

Imaging
Thoracic radiography
- Right ventricular enlargement
- Hypovascular lung fields

Echocardiography
- RV hypertrophy
- Flat or paradoxical motion of interventricular septum
- VSD
- Over-riding aorta (overlying VSD)
- Hypoplastic pulmonary trunk
- Doppler
  - Pulmonic stenosis
  - VSD

Special investigations
- Bubble study to identify VSD
- Electrocardiography
  - Deep S waves in leads I, II, III and aVF
  - Right axis deviation

Treatment
- Conservative
- Closure of VSD and bypass the pulmonic stenosis
- Create AV shunt to increase pulmonary blood flow and oxygenation
- Phlebotomy to control polycythaemia
- Acute crisis – rest, oxygen, treat acidosis and viscosity

Prognosis
- Tolerate defect for some time if pulmonary blood flow is maintained and hyperviscosity controlled
- Sudden death is common
- If right to left shunt with cyanosis: usually die by 12–18 months

VENTRICULAR SEPTAL DEFECT (VSD)
Aetiology
- Congenital failure of closure of ventricular septum
- Left to right shunt more common
- Reversal of the shunt can occur (i.e. right to left) if pulmonary hypertension develops

Major signs
- Asymptomatic
- Exercise intolerance
- Coughing

Minor signs
- Cyanosis in right to left shunting VSD

Potential sequelae
- Partial/complete closure can occur with tricuspid adherence, right ventricular hypertrophy, aortic valve fibrosis

- Can develop *cor pulmonale* from pulmonary hypertension
- Left heart failure from high ventricular output

Predisposition
- Predisposed breeds: West Highland white terrier and Cocker spaniel
- Genetic base in Keeshond

Historical clues
- Asymptomatic: murmur identified at routine examination
- Exercise intolerance

Physical examination
- Holosystolic diagonal murmur – heard loudly on right craniosternal (2nd–4th intercostal spaces) area and left side more caudally (5th–6th intercostal spaces)
- Grade of murmur is inversely correlated with the size of the defect
- ± Precordial thrill
- A separate murmur of pulmonic stenosis (relative) may be heard due to increased blood flow across a normal valve

Laboratory findings
- Polycythaemia may be present if right to left shunting

Imaging
Thoracic radiography
- LV enlargement
- ± LA enlargement
- RV enlargement
- Pulmonary over-circulation if significant left to right shunting

Echocardiography
- LA enlargement
- LV enlargement (eccentric hypertrophy)
- RV dilation

- Hyperkinetic left ventricle
- VSD may be imaged in membranous part of septum below aortic valve and septal leaflet of tricuspid valve in long axis
- Doppler:
  - Turbulent high-velocity flow is identified
  - Measure pressure gradient across VSD
  - Mitral regurgitation is common

Special investigations
Bubble echocardiogram
- The reader is advised to consult cardiology texts for more information

Cardiac catheterisation
- Measure intracardiac pressures

Electrocardiography
- May be unremarkable
- Tall R waves
- ± wide P waves
- Deep Q waves in leads I, II, III and aVF ± right axis deviation

Treatment
- Management of left-sided heart failure
  - Restricted exercise
  - Diuretics
  - ACE inhibitors
- Phlebotomy if severely polycythaemic
- Pulmonary artery banding
  - Palliative to protect the pulmonary vascular bed, so not for mild to moderate cases

Monitoring
- Clinical signs
- Echocardiography

Prognosis
- High-velocity gradients but with small defects may be well tolerated with minimal signs
- Guarded with large VSD or if pulmonary hypertension develops

PERICARDIAL DISEASE

Aetiology
- Accumulation of fluid, usually blood in pericardium
- Pericardium is indistensible acutely, and the raised intra-pericardial pressure causes compression of right heart, i.e. tamponade
- Several conditions can lead to pericardial effusion
  - Common causes:
    - Idiopathic pericardial haemorrhage most common
    - Intrapericardial neoplasia – quite common cause
  - Uncommon causes
    - Congenital
    - Peritoneo-pericardial diaphragmatic hernia (PPDH)
    - Pericardial defect
    - Pericardial cyst
    - Constrictive pericardial disease
    - Unknown aetiology? subsequent to previous inflammation of the pericardium
    - Left atrial rupture
    - Pericardial transudate
    - Reported as an effect of right-heart failure, neoplasia and rarely renal failure
    - Purulent pericardial effusion/ pericarditis – very uncommon
    - Penetrating injury, foreign body or haematogenous spread

Major signs
- Ascites
- Dyspnoea (pleural effusion)
- Exercise intolerance/lethargy
- Inappetence
- Syncope
- Weight loss

Potential sequelae
- Right-heart failure – see below
- Death

Predisposition
Idiopathic pericardial haemorrhage
- Predisposed breeds: Golden retriever and St Bernard
- No age or sex predisposition

Intrapericardial neoplasia
Haemangiosarcoma
- Right atrium predilection site
- GSD and Golden retriever
- Older dogs more likely to be affected

Chemodectoma – heart base tumours
- Tend to occur in older, brachycephalic (or crossbred) dogs, e.g. Boxer

Left atrial rupture
- Small breed dogs with advanced mitral disease

Historical clues
- Sudden onset of clinical signs
- Recurrent haemorrhage is characteristic of tumours and idiopathic disease

Physical examination
- Apex beat less pronounced than normal
- Heart sounds muffled
- Weak pulse
- Pulsus paradoxicus (strength of pulse decreases with inspiration)
- Signs of right-heart failure
  - Ascites
  - Jugular venous distension
  - Hepatomegaly
  - Pleural effusion – reduced heart sounds, dullness on percussion
  - Subcutaneous oedema (uncommon)

Laboratory findings
- Clotting profile to ensure pericardial fluid is not secondary to a coagulopathy
- Pericardial fluid analysis
  - Culture: infectious pericardial disease may be currently under-diagnosed

- Cytology: difficult to interpret as reactive mesothelial cells behave in similar manner to neoplastic cells
- pH: inflammatory effusion pH < 6.5, neoplastic/non-inflammatory lesions pH > 7.5, not very discriminatory

Imaging
Thoracic radiography
- Large, round cardiac silhouette – depends on volume of effusion
- Cardiac outline is sharper than normal (not seen if pleural effusion is present)
- Pneumopericardiography (remove fluid, inject air or CO_2) to highlight masses (rarely used now)

Echocardiography
- Hypoechoic space between pericardium and heart
- Collapse of right atrium due to cardiac tamponade can be imaged
- Pendulum swinging of heart within pericardial sac
- Pericardial masses

Special investigations
Electrocardiography
- Electrical alternans: QRS complex voltages alter from beat to beat (reflects swinging heart within pericardium with a large effusion)
- QRS voltages may be small due to electrical dampening by fluid
- ST elevation common

Treatment
- Pericardiocentesis – diagnostic and therapeutic
- Diuretics must be used with care to reduce the ascites after drainage
- Prednisolone has been suggested at anti-inflammatory doses for cases of idiopathic pericardial haemorrhage; evidence is lacking
- Recurrent pericardial effusions – pericardial surgery

ORGAN SYSTEMS

- Pericardial strip at exploratory thoracotomy
- Pericardiectomy by thoracoscopy
- Balloon pericardiostomy for incurable neoplasia

Monitoring
- Clinical signs
- Echocardiography

Prognosis
- Idiopathic pericardial haemorrhage may require surgical pericardiectomy if recurrent disease; generally fair to good prognosis
- Neoplasia: poor prognosis, could consider aggressive surgical resection
- Left atrial rupture: very poor prognosis, usually rapidly fatal
- Pericarditis: prognosis depends on underlying cause, often require surgical pericardiectomy for effective treatment
- PPDH: good prognosis with surgical repair, often asymptomatic and diagnosed incidentally

ENDOCRINE SYSTEM

Problems
Presenting complaints (see Section 1)
- Alopecia
- Exercise intolerance
- Polyphagia
- PU/PD
- Seizures
- Weakness/lethargy
- Weight gain
- Weight loss

Physical abnormalities (see Section 2)
- Abdominal enlargement
- Bradycardia
- Hepatomegaly

Laboratory abnormalities (see Section 3)
- Calcium
- Glucose
- Lipids/cholesterol
- Liver enzymes
- Potassium/sodium
- Urea

Diagnostic approach
- Suspect endocrinopathy from problem list
- Screening by routine laboratory testing
- Perform specific endocrine tests

Diagnostic methods
History
- See individual diseases below

Physical examination
- See individual diseases below

Clinicopathological findings
- See individual diseases below

Imaging
Plain radiographs
- Altered fat distribution
- Hepatomegaly in diabetes mellitus (DM) and hyperadrenocorticism (HAC)
- Osteopenia in hyperparathyroidism and HAC
- Pulmonary calcification
- Soft tissue calcification

Ultrasound
- Endocrine organ enlargement

Special investigative techniques
- Specific hormone assays and dynamic function tests are used as indicated to confirm the diagnosis. See individual diseases below

DIABETES MELLITUS (DM)

- Insulin is normally secreted by the pancreas in response to hyperglycaemia
- It acts to lower blood glucose, promoting uptake of glucose by peripheral tissues

Aetiology
- Hyperglycaemia due to:
  - Absolute lack of insulin [Type I; insulin-dependent DM (IDDM)]
  - Insulin resistance [Type II; non-insulin-dependent DM (NIDDM)]
- IDDM is the more common
  - Idiopathic
  - End-stage chronic pancreatitis
- NIDDM is secondary
  - Acromegaly
  - HAC
  - Obesity
- Signs relate to:
  - Disturbance of intermediary metabolism
  - Osmotic diuresis

Major signs
Early
- Polyphagia
- PU/PD
- Weight loss

Advanced – suggests ketoacidosis
- Anorexia
- Collapsed
- Depressed
- Ketotic breath
- Vomiting

Minor signs
- Exercise intolerance/decreased activity
- Inappropriate urination
- Recurrent infections, e.g. urinary tract, conjunctivitis

Potential sequelae
- Acute renal failure in diabetic ketoacidosis (DKA)

- Cataracts
- Hepatic disease can occasionally complicate DM therapy
- Hepatocutaneous syndrome can be associated with DM
- Hypoglycaemia is a potential complication with insulin therapy
- Hyperosmolar DM, i.e. markedly elevated blood glucose without ketosis, develops occasionally
- Predisposition to infection
  - Conjunctivitis
  - Cystitis
  - Stomatitis
  - Urinary tract infection

Predisposition
- Breeds over-represented, e.g. cross-bred terriers, poodles, Schipperke, but variations in different geographical areas
- Breeds under-represented, e.g. GSD, Golden retriever
- Females may be at greater risk to develop diabetes than males, but this is age-associated, i.e. < 7 years equal risk for both sexes
- Entire females at 8–10 years are three times more likely to develop DM than neutered females of the same age
- Mammary tissue can cause progesterone-induced growth hormone (GH) secretion (powerful insulin antagonist)
- Neoplastic mammary tissue may induce greater levels of GH secretion
- Peak incidence > 7 years

Historical clues
- Initially well and polyphagic
- Owner notices extreme PU/PD and weight loss
- Later, DKA causes anorexia, depression and vomiting
- Sometimes cataracts are the first sign noted
- Long history of chronic GI signs suggests end-stage chronic pancreatitis

ORGAN SYSTEMS

Physical examination

- Cataracts
- Emphysematous cystitis – bladder 'crackles' on palpation
- Hepatocutaneous syndrome
  - Hyperkeratotic foot pads
  - Lameness because of foot pain
- Hepatomegaly
- Hyperosmolar
  - Extreme lethargy to comatose state
- Ketoacidosis
  - Depression
  - Dehydration
  - Ketotic breath
  - Tachypnoea
  - Vomiting
  - Weakness
- Obesity or weight loss (depends on severity/chronicity/type of disease)

Laboratory findings

Haematology

- Dehydration may lead to elevated haematocrit
- Infection may cause leukocytosis ± left shift
- Non-regenerative anaemia associated with chronic disease may be seen
- If severe hypophosphataemia (diabetic ketoacidosis), can develop haemolysis

Serum biochemistry

- Hyperglycaemia
- Hypercholesterolaemia
- Hypertriglyceridaemia
- Ketonaemia
  - Dipsticks are more sensitive to acetoacetate and acetone than to beta-hydroxybutyrate
  - Beta-hydroxybutyrate can be quantitatively assayed
- Lipaemic blood samples
- Increased liver enzymes (ALP and ALT) due to hepatic lipid storage ('hepatic lipidosis')
- DKA causes marked abnormalities of serum electrolytes, urea and creatinine, etc.

Urinalysis

- Glucosuria when blood glucose is greater than renal threshold of 10–12 mmol/L
- Ketonuria – usually worsens with effective therapy and then resolves [reflects shift from beta-hydroxybutyrate to acetoacetate production, which urine strips are more sensitive at detecting]
- Sediment suggestive of urinary tract infection: pyuria, haematuria, proteinuria, bacteriuria

Imaging

Plain radiographs

- Generally unremarkable except diffuse hepatomegaly
- Emphysematous cystitis occasionally seen
- Emphysematous cholecystitis seen rarely

Ultrasound

- Pancreas – try to identify pancreatitis as underlying disease

Special investigations

Arterial blood gas analysis

- Acid–base information in the ketoacidotic diabetic

Glucagon response test (rarely performed)

- Insulin concentration measured at 0, 5, 10, 15 and 30 minutes after injection of 1 mg glucagon
- This can provide information about the ability of the islet cells to produce insulin
- May identify dogs with insulin insensitivity as opposed to true deficiency

Glycosylated serum proteins

- Fructosamine
- Glycosylated haemoglobin

Intravenous glucose tolerance test
- Useful for evaluating diabetics where disease appears to have resolved. Not a useful test in general practice

Serum insulin concentrations
- Generally not helpful

TLI
- May be increased with pancreatitis
- Decreased with end-stage chronic pancreatitis causing DM and EPI

Treatment
Ketoacidotic diabetic (DKA)
It is beyond the scope of this book to detail management of the DKA; the reader is advised to refer to other texts.

1. Correct fluid/electrolyte losses

- 0.9% sodium chloride with potassium/phosphate supplementation as indicated by blood results
- Rate depends on degree of dehydration.
- Maintenance requirements, etc. – normally 1.5–2 × maintenance (= 3–4 ml/kg/hour)

2. Insulin

- Aim to normalise intermediary metabolism
  - Intermittent i/m regime – regular/soluble insulin
  - Constant low-dose insulin infusion technique – regular insulin
  - Intermittent high-dose i/m or s/c protocol – regular insulin
- Longer-acting insulin once dog is stable: dose similar to that of the regular insulin

3. Correct acidosis

4. Identify precipitating factors for the illness

5. Provide carbohydrate substrate when dictated by insulin therapy

6. Aim to return parameters to normal SLOWLY – too rapid correction can be harmful and can create osmotic and biochemical problems

Non-ketotic diabetic
Stabilisation period
Diet
- Daily regime constant in composition, volume and timing of meals
- High levels of complex carbohydrates including fibre to slow digestion and absorption giving smoother glycaemic curves

Exercise
- Regular plan during stabilisation
- Avoid exercising at times of expected low blood glucoses, e.g. 6–8 hours after lente insulin

Insulin
- Preparation
  - Intermediate-acting, e.g. lente
  - Starting dose of 0.5 i.u./kg
- Frequency
  - Twice-daily injections generally recommended over once-daily
- Feeding
  - Once-daily lente insulin with 75% food and 25% food fed 6–8 hours later at predicted peak of lente activity
- Monitoring
  - Daily urine glucose or blood glucose
- Adjustment doses
  - Usually takes 1–3 days to obtain a consistent response to a specific dose of insulin
- Most dogs stabilise at 1–1.5 IU/kg of lente insulin daily
- 24-hour blood glucose curve after the initial stabilisation period to assess duration of action of insulin and stability and help to determine ideal meal times

- Often need to consider twice-daily injections of the same insulin or once-daily injections of a longer-acting preparation.

Maintenance therapy
Insulin
- Adjust based on occasional or serial nadir blood glucose concentrations – initially weekly, then every 2 weeks, then once a month

Monitoring
- Routine clinical examination
- Occasional minimum database including urinalysis to identify problems early
- Occasional or serial nadir blood glucose concentrations

Fructosamine
- Measure plasma proteins which have undergone non-enzymatic glycation
- This relates to the mean blood glucose in the lifetime of those proteins, i.e. usually 1–3 weeks
- Can be assessed at any time of day
- > 400 μmol/L suggests poor control

Glycated haemoglobin
- Reflects control over the preceding 1–3 months
- Useful for animals that are not rechecked frequently
- Problems with valid assays being available

Prognosis
- Survival times are likely to be decreased compared to the unaffected dog population
- DM can be very difficult at time of dioestrus to control if bitch is not spayed
- Hepatocutaneous syndrome is difficult to manage

- Hyperosmolar DM has very poor prognosis
- Underlying diseases, e.g. HAC, can make diabetes more difficult to manage. The investigations should aim to identify concurrent disease and to try to manage it.

DIABETES INSIPIDUS (DI)

- Antidiuretic hormone (ADH) is produced by the pituitary in response to increases in plasma osmolality
- ADH increases water reabsorption by the renal tubules

Aetiology
- Lack of ADH or failure of renal collecting ducts to respond
- Can be partial or complete

Central DI (CDI)
- Absolute or relative deficiency of ADH
- Idiopathic
- Congenital (rare)
- Acquired
- Secondary to head trauma or large pituitary or hypothalamic tumour

Nephrogenic DI (NDI)
- Results from a defect in renal tubular receptor that leads to an insensitivity to ADH
- Congenital (rare)
- Secondary to renal, metabolic and electrolyte disorders
  - CRF
  - Hepatic failure
  - HAC
  - Hypercalcaemia
  - Hypokalaemia
  - Pyelonephritis
  - Pyometra

Major signs
- PU/PD

Minor signs
- CNS signs if chronic hypernatraemia due to gradual water restriction
  - Aimless wandering
  - Incoordination
  - Seizures
  - Visual deficits
- Dehydration (mild)
- NDI – signs referable to inciting disease may be present
- Nocturia
- Restlessness and weight loss secondary to severe PD
- Urinary incontinence

Potential sequelae
- CNS signs from large expanding tumour of pituitary or hypothalamus
- Gradual deterioration as dog perpetually craves water

Predisposition
- Congenital CDI recognised
- No age, sex or breed predisposition for CDI

Historical clues
- Onset of profound PU/PD
- No other major signs in CDI

Physical examination
- Often unremarkable
- With secondary NDI there may be clinical findings referable to the underlying disease (see earlier list)

Laboratory findings
Haematology and serum biochemistry
- To rule out other causes of PU/PD
- Slight increases in PCV, total proteins and plasma osmolality may be seen secondary to mild dehydration with DI
- If total water depleted, urea, creatinine, sodium and chloride may be increased
- Further assessment of hepatic function or pituitary-adrenal axis may be indicated

Urinalysis
- Hyposthenuria – urine SG 1.001–1.007
- Urine osmolality 40–200 mOsm/kg

Imaging
Thoracic and abdominal radiographs
- Performed to assess for other disease causing PU/PD
- In many cases a large bladder will be observed due to overstretching from the severe PU

Special investigations
Hickey-Hare test
- Aims to assess the ability of the hypothalamic-pituitary-renal axis to decrease urine volume in response to increasing plasma osmolality
- This test is rarely indicated

Water deprivation test
- Should *never* be performed in azotaemic or hypercalcaemic animals
- Aims to establish if ADH is released in response to dehydration
- Before performing a water deprivation test it is essential, in the authors' view, to rule out HAC conclusively by means of ACTH stimulation and LDDS (see HAC, pp. 233–7)
- Animals with HAC will not fully concentrate urine in response to water deprivation and this may lead to a misdiagnosis of partial DI
- ADH response test is commonly performed after the water deprivation test to classify whether the dog has CDI or NDI

Absolute water deprivation test
- This test acutely restricts water intake and assesses any increase in urine SG
- Failure to concentrate the urine may indicate
  - CDI
  - NDI

ORGAN SYSTEMS

- Medullary washout – prolonged polyuria depletes the renal medulla of sodium, so that urine concentrating ability is decreased

Modified water deprivation test

- Medullary washout is a controversial concept, but the modified test is designed to prevent it
- The modified test restricts water intake for several days before the test to rule out medullary wash-out as an explanation for failure to concentrate urine on water restriction

Day 1 – weigh dog and allow 120 ml water/kg body weight (BWT) given as small amounts during 24-hour period
Day 2 – weigh dog and allow 90 ml water/kg BWT as above
Day 3 – weigh dog and allow 60 ml water/kg BWT as above
Day 4 – remove all water and perform water deprivation test as below

Monitor hydration and urine specific gravity on a daily basis.

Protocol for water deprivation test (absolute or modified)

- The dog receives no food or water for the duration of the test.
- An indwelling urinary catheter is preferred over repeated catheterisations.
- It is preferable to measure urine osmolality and plasma osmolality during this protocol if the equipment is available.
1   Empty the bladder and collect urine sample, weigh dog.
2   The bladder is emptied every hour, the urine SG measured and the dog weighed. The urine SG is checked every hour.
- Record body weight, urine SG

3   The test is stopped when:
- 5% of initial body weight has been lost (usually within 3–8 hours for DI cases)
or
- Urine SG >1.030 indicates normal concentrating ability
- Dog shows CNS signs: depression, stupor, seizures
4   ADH response test is commonly performed immediately after the water deprivation test.

Interpretation

- Urine SG after water deprivation
  - < 1.010 – highly suggestive of CDI or NDI
  - 1.020–1.030 is equivocal may be seen with partial ADH deficiency or medullary washout (or HAC)
  - > 1.030 is normal

ADH response test

Indicated for dogs failing to concentrate urine adequately in response to dehydration at end of water deprivation test.

1   Catheterise and empty bladder
2   Check urine SG (and preferably osmolalities as above)
3   Desmopressin (DDAVP – synthetic ADH) administered 1–4 µg i/v or i/m
4   Empty bladder every 15–30 minutes for 2 hours
5   Collect urine for SG and osmolality check every 15–30 minutes
6   Collect plasma samples for osmolality concurrently
7   Check hydration and CNS status

Interpretation

- Failure to increase urine SG above 1.030 after DDAVP highly suggestive of NDI
- Increase of urine SG > 1.030 indicative of CDI

At end of test
- Introduce small amounts of water every 30 minutes for 2 hours
- Monitor for vomiting and CNS signs
- Return to *ad libitum* water after 2 hours if dog is well

Treatment
CDI or partial NDI
- DDAVP subcutaneously 0.5–2 µg once or twice daily
- DDAVP intranasal drops (via conjunctival sac) – 1 to 4 drops once or twice daily
- DDAVP tablets @ 10 µg/kg given before food twice daily has been used successfully in one dog
- Duration of action is variable (8–24 hours) and usually has maximal effect between 6–10 hours
- Side effects uncommon
- Thiazide diuretics may decrease water intake by 50% (see NDI), but often unavailable

NDI
- Treat underlying disease
- Thiazide diuretics, e.g. chlorothiazide or hydrochlorothiazide, but often unavailable
- Reduce water intake by 30–50% in some cases
- Mechanism
  - Thiazide reduces total body sodium by inhibiting reabsorption in the ascending loop of Henle
  - Decreased sodium and plasma osmolality inhibits the thirst centre and reduces water consumption
  - This results in decreased GFR, increased proximal tubular reabsorption of sodium and water and decreased delivery of sodium to distal tubule and net reduction in urine volume

- Hydrochlorothiazide @ 2.5–5 mg/kg twice daily
- Chlorothiazide @ 10–20 mg/kg twice daily
- Salt intake should be restricted

Monitoring
- Water intake

Prognosis
- Water intake can be reduced by more than 50% in some cases
- CNS signs may develop in some cases of CDI secondary to tumour growth

HYPERADRENOCORTICISM (HAC)

- Cortisol, the main glucocorticoid, is produced by the adrenal cortex
- Its secretion is controlled by ACTH from the pituitary
- It has a negative feedback on ACTH release

Aetiology
- Excessive production of endogenous glucocorticoids
  - Adrenal tumour (ADH)
  - Pituitary-dependent (PDH)
- Excessive administration of exogenous glucocorticoids
  - Iatrogenic

Major signs
- Abdominal distension ('pot-belly')
- Hepatomegaly
- Lethargy/exercise intolerance
- Muscle weakness/wasting
- Panting
- Polydipsia – (>100 ml/kg/day)/polyuria – (>50 ml/kg/day) (PU/PD) causing nocturia/incontinence/inappropriate urination
- Polyphagia
- Skin changes/alopecia

ORGAN SYSTEMS

Minor signs
- Calcinosis cutis (white/cream plaques, surrounded by erythema, develop cracks and secondary infection)
- Myotonia
- Neurological signs (due to expansion of pituitary macroadenoma)
- Reproductive failure
- Slow wound healing

Potential sequelae
- Progression of major signs
- DM from insulin resistance
- Immunosuppression
- Neurological signs due to expansile pituitary mass (Nelson's syndrome)
  - Gradual alteration in level of consciousness
  - Acute blindness
  - Seizures
- Pancreatitis?
- Pulmonary thromboembolism (PTE)
- Secondary infections
  - Pyoderma
  - Urinary tract infection
- Sudden death

Predisposition
- < 20% of cases develop ADH
- > 80% of cases develop PDH
- ADH
  - Females more likely to develop than males
  - More frequently in large breed dogs (50% weigh > 20 kg)
  - Tend to be older than PDH – (median 11–12 years)
- PDH
  - Dachshunds, Poodles, small terriers at increased risk
  - No sex predisposition
  - Usually mid- or old-aged dogs (median 7–9 years)

Historical clues
Owner feels dog is generally well:
- Eating

- Gaining weight

but is concerned by:

- Exercise intolerance/lethargy
- Hair loss
- Panting
- Polyphagia
- PU/PD
- Poor wound healing

Dogs that are anorexic, unwell, or losing weight do not normally have HAC as the primary cause of their problem

Physical examination
- Alopecia – usually bilaterally symmetrical, affects flank, ventral abdomen and thorax, perineum and neck
- Calcinosis cutis occasionally: predilection sites – ventrum, neck, inguinal, axilla
- Comedones frequently
- Decreased muscle mass especially on limbs, spine and temporal region
- Excessive surface scale
- Myotonia rarely – stiff, stilted hindlimb gait
- Pot-bellied appearance
- Thin, inelastic skin over ventrum
- Bruising after blood sampling

Laboratory findings
Haematology
- Stress leukogram
  - Eosinopenia
  - Lymphopenia
  - Neutrophilia
  - Monocytosis
- RBC – normal or mildly increased numbers
- Platelets – mild elevation increased nRBCs

Serum biochemistry
- Alkaline phosphatase (ALP) ↑ in > 90% cases

- 5× to 40× upper end of reference range
- Induction of hepatic isoenzyme of ALP (steroid-induced)
- Alanine aminotransferase (ALT)
  - Mild increase, ?secondary to glycogen accumulation in hepatocytes
- Bile acids
  - Mild/moderate elevations
- Cholesterol and triglycerides
  - due to increased lipolysis
- Glucose
  - Usually high normal
  - Diabetes mellitus develops in 10% cases due to insulin antagonism by cortisol
- Urea and creatinine
  - Low-normal due to increased urinary loss

Urinalysis
- Specific gravity < 1.015 (often < 1.008)
- Glucosuria in cases with overt DM
- Urinary tract infection
  - Present in 50% cases
  - Sediment may appear inactive due to immunosuppression

Imaging
Thoracic radiographs
- Tracheal/bronchial wall/pulmonary mineralisation
- Pulmonary metastasis from adrenocortical carcinoma
- PTE (rarely positive findings on X-ray)
- CHF (rare)

Abdominal radiographs
- Hepatomegaly
- Good contrast (++ fat in abdomen)
- Pot-bellied appearance
- Large/distended bladder (secondary to PU/PD)
- Adrenal enlargement/mineralisation
- General poor bone density = osteoporosis (lumbar vertebral bodies good place to assess)

- Soft tissue mineralisation
  - Aorta
  - Calcinosis cutis
  - Kidneys

Ultrasonography
Adrenal ultrasound
- Normal
- Bilateral enlargement = hyperplasia
- Unilateral enlargement = tumour?

Liver
- To assess hepatomegaly and if adrenal tumour to check for visible metastasis

Special investigations
Test protocols
ACTH stimulation test (ACTH stim)
1 Collect 3 ml plasma or serum for basal cortisol concentration.
2 Inject 0.25 mg synthetic ACTH i/v (slowly) to dogs > 5 kg (0.125 mg to dogs < 5 kg).
3 Collect a second sample for cortisol concentration 30–90 minutes after i/v ACTH (the author is routinely using 60 minutes).
4 Recent administration of glucocorticoids will affect results.

Low-dose dexamethasone suppression test (LDDS)
1 Collect 3 ml plasma or serum for basal cortisol concentration.
2 Inject 0.01 mg/kg dexamethasone i/v (it is a very small volume, so either place an i/v catheter to ensure complete administration, or dilute 1 in 10 with water for injection of a larger volume).
3 Collect further samples for cortisol determination at 3 and 8 hours after dexamethasone administration.
4 The dog should be kept quiet and unstressed during the test period.
5 This test can be modified to be performed at home, using oral dexamethasone, collecting urine samples

to measure urinary cortisol. It is not routinely performed in the UK.

Urine cortisol: creatinine ratio (UCCR)
- A 5 ml sample of morning urine is collected, urine cortisol and creatinine are measured, and a ratio is obtained.

High-dose dexamethasone suppression test (HDDS)
- As for LDDS, but 0.1 mg/kg dexamethasone is injected i/v

High-high-dose dexamethasone suppression test (HHDDS)
- As for LDDS, but 1.0 mg/kg dexamethasone is injected i/v

Plasma endogenous ACTH concentration
1 Collect 5 ml blood into cooled plastic EDTA tube and centrifuge immediately @ 4°C.
2 Separate plasma and freeze at < –20°C in a plastic tube.
3 Transport to the laboratory in a frozen state.

Screening tests
ACTH stim
- Identify > 50% cases with ADH and > 85% cases with PDH

LDDS
- Diagnostic in all cases ADH (do not suppress at all) and 90–95% cases PDH (suppress at 3 hours and escape at 8 hours)

UCCR
- Healthy dogs < 10×10^{-6}
- > 10×10^{-6} – could be HAC or non-adrenal illness

Discriminatory tests
HDDS
- Use 0.1 mg/kg dexamethasone
- Differentiate between PDH and ADH
- Suppression @ 8 hours with PDH

- 20–30% of PDH cases will not suppress at 0.1 mg/kg dexamethasone
- No suppression with ADH

HDDDS
- Use 1.0 mg/kg dexamethasone
- Differentiate between PDH and ADH
- Suppression @ 8 hours with PDH
  - Much higher percentage of PDH cases will suppress than with HDDS
- No suppression with ADH

Endogenous ACTH
- Normal dogs: 20–80 pg/ml
- PDH > 45 pg/ml
- ADH < 10 pg/ml

CT/MRI
- To assess adrenal disease/pituitary tumours

Treatment
Medical
Trilostane
- Competitive enzyme inhibitor in the steroid synthesis pathway
- Only licensed product in UK (Vetoryl)
- Body weight 5–20 kg, give 60 mg PO SID
- Body weight 20–40 kg, give 120 mg PO SID
- Body weight > 40 kg, give 120 mg PO SID
- Licensed for once-daily usage, but some dogs require twice-daily dosing
- If overdose, withdrawal of the drug should reverse signs within 24–48 hours

Mitotane (o,p'-DDD)
- Selective destruction of zona fasciculata and reticularis of adrenal cortex
- Induction: orally @ 50 mg/kg/daily with food (fatty meal aids absorption)
- Then dose @ 50 mg/kg/week with food as maintenance when:
  - Water intake reduces to < 60 ml/kg/day

- Reduced appetite (takes longer to eat food)
- Vomiting/diarrhoea
- Lethargy/depression develop
- Lymphocyte count $> 1 \times 10^9/L$ or eosinopenia abolished (but unreliable markers)
  - Post-ACTH stimulation serum cortisol between 20–120 nmol/L
- Average 6–14 days for dogs to respond to induction
- Adjust dosage based on results ACTH stimulation testing
- If relapse – short re-induction course or increase maintenance dose
- Higher doses required for adrenal tumours
- Side effects:
  - Overdose can lead to hypoadrenocorticism (5–17% cases)
  - Stop maintenance therapy and treat with replacement glucocorticoid and mineralocorticoid

NB – Complete chemical adrenalectomy with high daily doses, until dog has hypoadrenocorticism; this reduces the chance of relapse, but is potentially fatal.

L-Deprenyl (selegiline hydrochloride)
- Monoamine oxidase inhibitor
- Inhibits ACTH secretion via alteration of hypothalamic/pituitary axis
- Dose: 1 mg/kg daily increased to 2 mg/kg/day if inadequate response after 2 months
- At least 50% of dogs do not respond

Ketoconazole
- Imidazole antifungal drug that suppresses steroidogenesis
- Dose: 5 mg/kg BID for 7 days to assess drug tolerance, then 10 mg/kg BID for 14 days
- Monitor with ACTH stimulation test and increase dose by 5-mg increments if not effective
- 25% of dogs do not respond

- Side effect: can cause hepatopathy

Cyproheptadine
- May reduce ACTH concentrations via anti-serotonin activity
- Low success rates

Pituitary irradiation
- If showing neurological signs

Surgical
Hypophysectomy
- High morbidity and mortality

Bilateral adrenalectomy for PDH
- Treat as hypoadrenocorticism for life
- Glucocorticoid and mineralocorticoid supplementation peri- and post-operatively

Unilateral adrenalectomy for ADH
- Glucocorticoid (and mineralocorticoid) supplementation peri- and immediately post-operatively
- If successful, all steroid replacement therapy can be gradually withdrawn

Monitoring
- ACTH stimulation
- Clinical signs

Prognosis
- Improvement in appetite and drinking seen soon after effective treatment commenced
- Minimum of 6–8 weeks on treatment before marked improvement will be seen in dermatological signs and hepatomegaly/pot belly
- Treatment may unmask steroid-responsive disease, e.g. flea bite hypersensitivity, osteoarthritis
- Mean survival time reported for mitotane-treated dogs 30 months (range: days to 7 years)
- Anecdotal reports of sudden death after initiation of trilostane

ORGAN SYSTEMS

ORGAN SYSTEMS

- Highest mortality in first 16 weeks of treatment with mitotane
- Prognosis with ADH depends on the ability to remove tumour surgically and the extent of metastases

HYPOADRENOCORTICISM (ADDISON'S DISEASE)

The adrenal gland produces:
- Glucocorticoid
  - Cortisol is major hormone
  - Controlled by ACTH secretion from pituitary
- Mineralocorticoid
  - Aldosterone
  - Part of renin-angiotensin-aldosterone system (RAAS) stimulated in response to sodium delivery to the juxta-glomerular apparatus
- Sex hormones

Aetiology
- Adrenocortical insufficiency – lack of cortisol and aldosterone
- Clinical signs are only evident when 90% of the adrenal cortex is non-functional

Primary
- Destruction of the adrenal cortices
  - Idiopathic/immune-mediated
    - Typical = lack of glucocorticoid and mineralocorticoid production
    - Atypical Addison's = hypocortisolaemia without mineralocorticoid deficiency and electrolyte changes (rare)
- Infectious/infiltrative/bleeding diseases – rare cause of disease

Secondary
- Deficient ACTH secretion by the pituitary
  - Destructive lesion in pituitary or hypothalamus, e.g. neoplasia/ inflammation/trauma

- Iatrogenic secondary to long-term glucocorticoid therapy causing suppression of the normal adrenal axis – effect can last for weeks to months after cessation of therapy
- Only glucocorticoid production affected, as RAAS intact

Major signs
- Anorexia
- Collapse – hypovolaemic shock
- Diarrhoea
- Lethargy
- PU/PD
- Vomiting
- Weight loss

Minor signs
- Melaena/haematochezia
- Shaking/shivering

Potential sequelae
- Hypovolaemic shock
- ARF
- Death

Predisposition
- Average age 2–7 years (range: 2 months to 14 years)
- Female dogs reportedly more commonly affected than males
- Higher incidence in castrated males than intact males
- Genetic predisposition suggested in some breeds by a familial occurrence, e.g. Standard Poodle, Leonberger, Nova Scotia duck tolling retriever
- Increased risk suggested in other breeds, e.g. Great Dane, Saint Bernard, Springer spaniel, WHWT and others

Historical clues
- Vague/non-specific signs
- Clinical signs compatible with many other diseases, e.g. primary gastrointestinal/ renal or neuromuscular disease
- Waxing-waning course of disease probably due to progressive destruction of

the adrenal cortex which cannot cope with 'stress'
- Temporary improvement with intravenous fluid therapy or glucocorticoids
- Eventual crisis with profound collapse

Physical examination
- Abdominal pain
- Bradycardia in < 30% of cases
- Collapse
- Depression
- Hypothermia
- Weak peripheral pulse
- Weakness

Laboratory findings
Haematology
- Mild to severe normochromic, normocytic anaemia in 20–30% cases
  - Non-regenerative anaemia of chronic disease
  - GI blood loss, which can be severe
- Hypovolaemia may mask anaemia due to haemoconcentration – recheck after rehydration
- Reverse stress leukogram would be expected – only seen in < 20% of cases
- However, in a dog with severe illness the presence of normal lymphocyte and eosinophil counts (instead of decreased) should alert the clinician to the possibility of hypoadrenocorticism

Serum biochemistry
- Hyperkalaemia: 90% of cases
- Hyponatraemia: 83% of cases
- Hypochloraemia: 46% of cases
- Decreased sodium: potassium ratio: 92% of cases [normal > 27:1, hypoadrenocorticism < 23:1]
- Pre-renal azotaemia: 60–80% of cases
- Inorganic phosphate increased: 66% of cases
- Hypoglycaemia: 20% of cases; rarely of clinical significance

- Hypercalcaemia: 30% of cases; correlates with hyperkalaemia and severity of disease
- Hypoalbuminaemia: < 40% of cases – various mechanisms
- Mild to moderate increases in ALT and ALP: 30–50% of cases; could be secondary to poor tissue perfusion or may reflect primary hepatic disease

Urinalysis
- Urine SG should be > 1.030 as azotaemia is pre-renal in origin
- Often, SG < 1.030 due to impaired concentrating ability as a result of chronic sodium loss reducing the renal medullary concentrating gradient
- Ultimately, ARF may occur due to renal ischaemia, and urine may be isosthenuric

Imaging
Thoracic radiography
- Changes reflect hypovolaemia and decreased tissue perfusion, or muscle weakness, i.e. not specific for hypoadrenocorticism
  - Hypoperfusion of the lung fields
  - Megaoesophagus is present in < 1% of cases
  - Microcardia
  - Narrowed caudal vena cava and descending aorta

Abdominal radiography
- Liver and kidneys may appear slightly small due to hypovolaemia

Ultrasonography
- Significant decrease in the length and width of the adrenal glands

Special investigations
Blood pressure
- 90% humans with hypoadrenocorticism are hypotensive; likely to occur, but insufficient evidence in dogs

ORGAN SYSTEMS

- Arterial blood gas analysis
  - Mild to moderate acidosis common
  - Total carbon dioxide and serum bicarbonate values reduced

ECG
- Classical ECG changes reportedly due to hyperkalaemia, but also depend on acid–base and other electrolyte changes
- The ECG changes occur as listed below – the higher the potassium, the more changes are evident
1   Peaking of T wave
2   Shortening of QT interval
3   Increased QRS duration
4   Decreased P-wave amplitude
5   Prolonged PR interval
6   Absence of the P wave (sinoatrial standstill)
7   Severe bradycardia

Hormone assays
ACTH stimulation test
- Follow the protocol of the laboratory analysing samples
- Cross-reactivity of dexamethasone with cortisol in the assay is negligible compared with other glucocorticoid preparations
- Perform after i/v fluid replacement, before glucocorticoids are administered
- Diagnosis of hypoadrenocorticism – low basal cortisol and lack of response/ stimulation to exogenous ACTH
- Does not differentiate between primary and secondary disease

Aldosterone assay
- Concentration should be normal after ACTH stimulation with secondary hypoadrenocorticism and decreased in cases of primary hypoadrenocorticism.
- Can be used in cases with an ACTH stimulation suggestive of hypoadrenocorticism, but with normal serum electrolytes.

Endogenous ACTH
- Useful in dogs with abnormal ACTH stimulation and normal electrolytes. Cases of primary hypoadrenocorticism should have markedly elevated levels of plasma ACTH (> 90% of cases) and low or non-measurable levels of plasma ACTH in secondary hypoadrenocorticism. Follow laboratory directions for handling of the sample.

Treatment
Acute crisis
- Hypovolaemia and shock is life-threatening

Fluid therapy
- 0.9% normal saline is fluid of choice
- Initial rate 20–80 ml/kg/hour for 1–2 hours, depending on severity
- 1.5 to 2× maintenance (3–4 ml/kg/ hour) once hypovolaemia is corrected
- Monitor urine output
- Fluid therapy is gradually reduced and stopped when hydration, urine output, serum electrolytes and serum creatinine concentrations are normal

Glucocorticoid therapy (one of drugs below)
- Hydrocortisone @ 5–10 mg/kg i/v and repeated every 6 hours, has glucocorticoid and mineralocorticoid effects
- Methyl prednisolone sodium succinate @ 1–2 mg/kg i/v
- Dexamethasone @ 0.5–2 mg/kg i/v single dose
- Methyl prednisolone and dexamethasone can be repeated 2–6 hours later according to response

Mineralocorticoid therapy
- Hydrocortisone i/v provides some mineralocorticoid action
- Oral administration of fludrocortisone
- Desoxycorticosterone acetate (DOCA), a short-acting injectable mineralocorti-

coid preparation, is currently unavailable in the UK

Management of hyperkalaemia
- Usually resolves with aggressive fluid therapy
- If the hyperkalaemia does not respond to fluid therapy or there are severe bradydysrhythmias, then specific therapy may be indicated (e.g. insulin/dextrose, bicarbonate)
- The ability to measure potassium levels and acid–base is important for safe correction of the hyperkalaemia
- Refer to specialist endocrinology or critical care manuals for management of hyperkalaemia

Maintenance therapy
Mineralocorticoids
Fludrocortisone acetate
- @ 0.015–0.02 mg/kg daily (once-daily or divided twice-daily)
- Adjust dose by 0.05–0.1 mg/day
- Re-check electrolytes 1–2 weeks after discharge, and repeat at this frequency until electrolytes are stable
- Once stable, electrolytes should be checked two to three times yearly
- Required dose usually increases during first 6–18 months of therapy
- Side effects PU/PD, polyphagia and hair loss

Desoxycorticosterone pivilate (DOCP)
- Longer-acting depot mineralocorticoid preparation
- Dose @ 2.2 mg/kg every 25 days s/c or i/m
- Adjust dose based on serum electrolyte concentrations
- Unfortunately, this drug is not available in the UK

Glucocorticoids
- Use in all cases in the early stages of stabilisation

- Approximately 50% of cases on maintenance mineralocorticoid therapy require glucocorticoid supplementation long-term

Prednisolone
- Dose @ 0.2 mg/kg/day

Hydrocortisone
- Dose @ 500 µg/kg twice daily: benefit of mineralocorticoid action which may help to reduce the requirements for fludrocortisone
- All owners should have a small supply for 'at home' use during stressful episodes, e.g. exertion, trauma, surgery, illness
- During stressful periods, increase the dose 2- to 10-fold

Salt
- Mild and persistent hyponatraemia can be corrected by adding salt to the diet
- Do not use LOSALT, as this is potassium chloride not sodium chloride
- Dose @ 0.1 mg/kg/day

Secondary hypoadrenocorticism
- Only glucocorticoid supplementation required

Monitoring
- Clinical signs
- Creatinine and urea initially
- Sodium/potassium

Prognosis
- Excellent once therapy has been started
- Owner education is important with regard to the necessity for daily therapy and the risk factors and signs of destabilisation
- Acute addisonian crisis can result in intrinsic renal damage if hypovolaemia is not rapidly addressed: this alters the prognosis for full recovery

ORGAN SYSTEMS

ORGAN SYSTEMS

- It is important to consider hypoadrenocorticism in animals that appear to have ARF, as the prognoses for these two conditions are very different

HYPOTHYROIDISM

- Thyroid hormone secretion is regulated by the circulating concentration of thyroid-stimulating hormone (TSH) produced by the pituitary gland.
- Thyroxine (T4) and tri-iodothyronine (T3) are highly protein bound, and only the free hormone is active.
- Thyroid hormones have an effect on most metabolic reactions.

Aetiology
- Decreased production of T4 and T3 by the thyroid gland
- Primary hypothyroidism (95% cases)
  - Idiopathic thyroid atrophy
  - Lymphocytic thyroiditis (at least 50% cases)
    - Believed to have an immune-mediated basis: anti-thyroglobulin antibody present
- Secondary hypothyroidism due to inadequate pituitary TSH secretion is rare
- Tertiary hypothyroidism due to decreased hypothalamic secretion of thyroid-releasing hormone (TRH) is very rare

Major signs
- Alopecia
- Cold intolerance
- Exercise intolerance
- Lethargy
- Pyoderma
- Seborrhoea
- Weight gain/obesity

Minor signs
- Disproportionate dwarfism (congenital hypothyroidism)

- Female infertility
- Myxoedema – thickened, oedematous dermis
- Neurological dysfunction – possible association, but cause-and-effect rarely shown
  - Peripheral neuropathy
  - Megaoesophagus
  - Vestibular disease
- Ocular disorders
  - Corneal lipodystrophy

Potential sequelae
- Myxoedema coma is rare, but is associated with a poor prognosis

Predisposition
- Castrated males and neutered females may be at greater risk
- Decreased risk in greyhounds
- High incidence in Doberman pinscher and Golden Retriever
- Lymphocytic thyroiditis inherited in laboratory Beagles and a family of Borzois
- Middle-aged (mean 7 years), pure-bred dogs are over-represented

Historical clues
- Weight gain
- Lethargy
- Bilaterally symmetrical alopecia
- 'Heat-seeking'
- Response to empirical therapy is an unreliable diagnostic criterion

Physical examination
Dermatological
- Alopecia
- Change in haircoat colour/quality
- Comedones
- Dry/scaly skin
- Hyperkeratosis
- Hyperpigmentation
- Myxoedema – classically facial – 'tragic face'
- Otitis externa
- Poor wound healing/increased bruising

- Seborrhoea
- Superficial pyoderma

Cardiovascular
- Bradycardia
- Muffled heart sounds
- Pallor and slow CRT
- Poor peripheral pulse volume
- Weak apex beat

Neurological
- Central nervous disease
- Peripheral neuropathy – either local (e.g. vestibular disease, facial paralysis) or generalised

Ocular
- Corneal lipid dystrophy
- Other lesions secondary to hyperlipidaemia, e.g. retinopathy

Laboratory findings
Haematology
- Mild non-regenerative normocytic, normochromic anaemia
- Mild increase in platelet count and decrease in platelet size
- No evidence of bleeding abnormalities (e.g. von Willebrand's factor) as was previously thought

Serum biochemistry
- Hypercholesterolaemia – in 75% of cases, it is often > 10 mmol/L
- Hypertriglyceridaemia is also common
- Mild elevations of creatine kinase can be seen due to myopathy or reduced clearance
- Serum ALP is often mildly elevated

Imaging
- Likely to be unremarkable apart from increased subcutaneous and intracavitary fat

Special investigations
Hormone assays
Basal thyroid hormone concentrations
- Total T3
  - Less accurate than total T4 (TT4)
- Total T4
  - More reliable than total T3
  - If well within normal range – likely to be euthyroid (unless rare cases of cross reaction of antithyroid antibodies)
  - Decreased TT4 does not give a diagnosis of hypothyroidism as non-thyroidal disease/drugs can cause this (sick euthyroid syndrome)
  - Greyhounds and Scottish deerhounds have lower TT4 compared with other breeds
  - Small breeds – higher T4 than medium/large breeds
- Free (unbound) T4 (fT4)
  - Active hormone – therefore more representative of true thyroid function
  - Only useful if equilibrium dialysis method is used, but this is time-consuming and expensive
  - Other methods underestimate fT4 level and so have no benefit over TT4
- Problems of test interpretation:
  - Drugs, e.g. prednisolone, phenobarbitone, trimethoprim sulphonamides, etc. can alter thyroid hormone concentration
  - Any drug that may decrease thyroid hormone levels should be stopped (if possible) before investigating hypothyroidism
  - Dogs with non-thyroidal illness may have decreased TT4 levels – investigation of thyroid disease should be postponed to allow recovery from the illness or, if that is not possible, stabilisation of the pre-existing disease

ORGAN SYSTEMS

Endogenous TSH (cTSH)
- Elevated cTSH with decreased TT4 or fT4 is specific for hypothyroidism
- Elevated cTSH with normal TT4 – may be early hypothyroidism with TT4 maintained in normal range by increased cTSH
- Elevated cTSH with normal TT4 could reflect drug therapy or recovery from non-thyroidal illness
- Up to 38% of hypothyroid dogs will have normal cTSH level

TSH response/stimulation test
- Considered the 'gold standard' of diagnosis for a long time
- TSH is expensive and difficult to obtain
- Measure TT4 before starting the test, and then again 6 hours after i/v or i/m administration of 0.1 IU/kg bovine TSH (maximum 5 units)
- Anaphylaxis has been reported after i/v TSH, and i/m injection is painful
- Minimum response expected is a two-fold increase and TT4 > 30 nmol/L post-TSH
- If dog is receiving L-thyroxine supplementation, this must be stopped for 6–8 weeks before TSH stimulation is performed

TRH response test
- Follow the laboratory's protocol
- TRH stimulates release of TSH and thus TT4
- The change in TT4 after administration of TRH is much smaller in dogs than with TSH stimulation
- cTSH also increases after TRH administration – again, this is a smaller response
- Interpretation of TRH response test is more difficult than the TSH stimulation test due to smaller magnitudes of change

Other tests
Antibodies
- Anti-thyroglobulin and anti-thyroid hormone antibodies can be measured
- Detect immune-mediated thyroid damage, but do not predict hypothyroidism
- Clinical use is limited

Thyroid biopsy
- Rarely indicated clinically

Scintigraphy
- Limited studies available

Treatment
L-Thyroxine
- Treatment of choice because it results in normalisation of T4 and T3
- Bioavailability can vary with products – use licensed product
- Consider twice-daily administration because half-life of T4 is 9–15 hours
- L-Thyroxine dose: 11–22 µg/kg twice daily
- If concurrent disease, e.g. diabetes mellitus, hypoadrenocorticism, CHF, start at 25% of dose and increase by 25% every 2 weeks until full dose is achieved at 6 weeks

Response to treatment
- Increased activity/improved attitude within 1 week
- Weight loss within 2–4 weeks
- Dermatological changes will take months
- Improved cardiovascular function by 8 weeks
- Peripheral neuropathies should improve in 8–12 weeks

Monitoring
- Collect blood samples for therapeutic monitoring 4–8 weeks after starting therapy
- TT4 should be within reference range immediately before pill and at high end/

above reference range for 4–6 hours after administration
- Check TT4 every 6–8 weeks for first 6–8 months, as metabolism of T4 will alter as the metabolic rate stabilises
- Once stable, check TT4 levels once or twice yearly

Prognosis
- Oral therapy is effective in most cases
- Resolution of clinical signs in puppies with congenital disease depends on early recognition and treatment

HAEMOPOIETIC SYSTEM

Problems
Clinical presentations (see Section 1)
- Anorexia
- Bleeding
- Dyspnoea
- Exercise intolerance
- Haematemesis
- Haematochezia
- Haematuria and discoloured urine
- Haemoptysis
- Melaena
- Nasal discharge
- Stiffness and joint swelling
- Weakness-lethargy-collapse/syncope
- Weight loss

Physical abnormalities (see Section 2)
- Anaemia
- Hepatomegaly
- Icterus/jaundice
- Pulmonary alveolar pattern
- Splenomegaly
- Tachycardia

Laboratory abnormalities (see Section 3)
- Anaemia, see Section 2, p. 89
- Bilirubin
- Liver enzyme alterations
- Pancytopenia
- Polycythaemia
- Leukocytosis
- Leukopenia

Diagnostic approach
- For anaemia, see Section 2
- For bleeding, see Section 4, Haemostatic system
- For leukocytosis, see Section 3
- For leukopenia, see Section 3
- For WBC neoplasia, see Section 4, Immune system
- For pancytopenia, see Section 3
- For bleeding disorders, see Section 4, Haemostastic system

Diagnostic methods
History
- See individual diseases below

Physical examination
- See individual diseases below

Laboratory findings
- See individual diseases below

Imaging
- See individual diseases below

Special investigative techniques
- Bone marrow aspirate and core biopsy
- Serum iron and total iron-binding capacity

ORGAN SYSTEMS

ANAEMIA OF CHRONIC RENAL DISEASE

Aetiology
- The hormonal stimulus for RBC production, erythropoietin (EPO), is normally synthesised by the kidney, so that in CRF, the production of EPO declines, leading to a non-regenerative anaemia.
- Secondary hyperparathyroidism associated with renal disease can lead to myelofibrosis and may have direct inhibitory effect on erythropoiesis.

Major signs
- Anorexia
- Lethargy
- Pallor
- PU/PD
- Tachycardia
- Tachypnoea
- Weakness

Predisposition/patient details
- Middle- to older-aged patients with CRF
- Younger patients with familial/congenital nephropathies
- GI bleeding in uraemic dogs can contribute to development of anaemia

Potential sequelae
- Anaemia can be profound
- Death from uraemia is usual end result

Physical examination
- Typical signs of anaemia as above
- May be signs of uraemia; see Section 4, Urogenital system
- Systolic heart murmur if severe anaemia

Laboratory findings
Haematology
- Assess degree of anaemia and type (usually normocytic-normochromic) and non-regenerative (check reticulocyte count)

NB – Often the dog is dehydrated and this may mask the anaemia; therefore re-evaluate after rehydration.

Serum biochemistry (see Section 4, Urogenital system)
- Azotaemia expected if renal disease advanced enough to cause anaemia
- If urea is disproportionately increased compared to creatinine, this suggests GI blood loss
- Hypoalbuminaemia may suggest blood loss

Urinalysis
- Urine SG is likely to be submaximally concentrated in an azotaemic animal, suggesting loss of concentrating ability
- Urine SG in advanced renal disease is usually isosthenuric

Imaging
Radiography
- Small kidneys associated with chronic renal disease
- Osteopenia occasionally
- Renal calcification sometimes
- Ultrasonography of the kidneys and urinary tract is indicated

Special investigations
Blood pressure assessment
- Arterial hypertension is reported in up to 69% of dogs with chronic renal disease
- Retinal examination for evidence of hypertension – see pp. 130–31, 312

ACTH stimulation test
- Hypoadrenocorticism can also present with azotaemia, isosthenuria and anaemia

PTH concentration
- May be helpful for identifying secondary hyperparathyroidism

NB – Special collection and transport of this sample to the laboratory is required.

Serum erythropoietin (EPO) concentration
• If EPO level is increased, a further investigation for a cause of the anaemia other than renal disease should be carried out

Treatment
• Treat renal disease – see pp. 318–19

Gastrointestinal and other blood loss
• Reduce gastric ulceration with gastric protectants, etc.
• If iron-deficient: supplement with oral ferrous sulphate, e.g. 100–300 mg/day per dog

Blood transfusion
• Whole blood or packed RBCs
  • Useful for acute cases requiring rapid improvement
  • Difficult to restore PCV to normal in these dogs
  • Repeated transfusions are usually required and even with cross-matching, incompatibility can occur
  • Availability of donors often limits the number of transfusions that can be given

Recombinant human erythropoietin
• PCV usually increases by 0.5–1% per day, with red cell mass restored in 1 month
• Improves appetite, physical activity and general well-being
• Used in patients with moderate to severe anaemia due to EPO deficiency
• In the long term, dogs can develop anti-EPO antibodies which reduce the benefit of therapy. Recombinant canine EPO is not yet available commercially

Monitor
• PCV

• Progression of renal disease – see Section 4, Urogenital system

Prognosis
• Poor to guarded as the renal disease is usually advanced and will progress regardless of the management of the anaemia

IMMUNE-MEDIATED HAEMOLYTIC ANAEMIA (IMHA)

Aetiology
• Primary, autoimmune (AIHA)
• Secondary IMHA: sometimes a precipitating event can be identified
  • Drugs, e.g. cephalosporins, penicillins, trimethoprim sulphonamides
  • Infectious/parasitic, e.g. *Babesia*, *Dirofilaria*, *Ehrlichia*, *Leishmania*, *Haemobartonella*
  • Immunological, e.g. transfusion reaction, post vaccine
  • Neoplastic, e.g. lymphoma, leukaemia

Major signs
• Bounding pulse
• Lethargy
• Pale mucous membranes
• Tachycardia
• Tachypnoea
• Weakness

Minor signs
• Collapse (acute onset, severe cases)
• Dyspnoea
• Haemic heart murmur
• Lymphadenopathy
• Pyrexia

Potential sequelae
• Failure to respond to therapy with immunosuppressive drugs or recurrence once treatment stops should prompt a thorough search for possible underly-

ORGAN SYSTEMS

ing disease and an assessment of the adequacy of immunosuppression
- Pulmonary thromboembolism (PTE)
- DIC and death

Predisposition/patient details
- Young adult to middle-aged dogs
- Common in some breeds, e.g. Cocker Spaniel, English Springer spaniel, Poodles, Old English Sheepdog, Collies
- May be more common in females

Historical clues
- One report of increased incidence of IMHA following vaccination

Physical examination
- Bounding pulse
- Heart murmur
- Hepatosplenomegaly
- Jaundice and discoloured urine
- Lymphadenopathy
- Pallor
- Pyrexia
- Tachycardia
- Tachypnoea

Imaging
- Radiographs and ultrasound will demonstrate hepatosplenomegaly
- Screening radiographs and abdominal ultrasound are indicated to search for underlying disease

Minimum database
Haematology
- Moderate to severe anaemia which is usually regenerative
  - Anisocytosis
  - Polychromasia
  - High corrected reticulocyte count
  - Increased numbers of nucleated red blood cells

NB – It can take 3–5 days from onset for marrow regeneration to be evident.

- Spherocytosis (rounded RBCs) and agglutination are consistent with diagnosis of IMHA
- Neutrophilic leukocytosis, as haemolysis is 'inflammatory'
- Platelets are usually normal unless concurrent ITP (Evans syndrome): see Section 4, Haemostatic system

Serum biochemistry
- Mild to moderate increase in liver enzymes secondary to hepatic hypoxia
- Hyperglobulinaemia, usually normal albumin
- Mild to moderate hyperbilirubinaemia is usually transient; it is seen with severe and acute anaemia, until the liver adjusts to the increased bilirubin turnover
- Haemoglobinaemia with intravascular haemolysis

Urinalysis
- Bilirubinuria
- Haemoglobinuria with intravascular haemolysis

Special tests/investigations
- Slide agglutination test to differentiate agglutination and rouleaux: if positive, it is highly suggestive of IMHA
- Immunological testing
  - Positive Coombs' test confirms IMHA, but not AIHA
  - Negative Coombs' test is sometimes reported with IMHA
- Lymph node cytology/biopsy to try and identify underlying disease
- Bone marrow analysis
  - Non-regenerative form of IMHA
  - Pure red cell aplasia
  - Myelodysplasia or bone marrow neoplasia

Treatment
- Manage underlying/predisposing disease, e.g. treat infectious disease, lymphoma, etc.

Immunosuppressive therapy
- Prednisolone @ 2 mg/kg/day PO (given once or split twice daily)
  - Initially may want to use intravenous preparation, e.g. dexamethasone @ 0.1–0.2 mg/kg
  - Should see response with increased PCV by 3–7 days
  - Tailor therapy according to response, gradually decreasing to alternate-day therapy
  - Treatment should not stop until the patient becomes Coombs' test negative
- Other immunosuppressants are used if inadequate response to prednisolone alone.
  - Lag period before they are effective, so some clinicians start them immediately
  - Azathioprine 2 mg/kg/day PO reducing after 1 week to 2 mg/kg every other day
  - Cyclophosphamide 50 mg/m² for 4 days of each week

Supportive therapy
- Cage rest to reduce oxygen demand
- Oxygen supplementation for very severe cases
- Fluid therapy to maintain urine output

NB – These patients are normovolaemic, so do not give too much fluid.

- Prophylactic treatment of DIC and PTE with heparin @ 75–100 IU/kg s/c three to four times daily is advised by some clinicians

Blood transfusion
- Indicated in patients with severe, acute-onset anaemia who are showing clinical signs of compromise or with PCV < 10%
- Transfused cells have a short life in dogs with IMHA and potentially can increase the rate of haemolysis, but they can be life-saving in critical situations
- Packed red cells are preferable to whole blood as these patients are normovolaemic
- Cross-matching should be performed, particularly if multiple transfusions are anticipated
- Oxyglobin might be an alternative to blood transfusions as it provides means for oxygen transport to the tissues

Alternatives for refractory cases
- Cyclosporin A has been used successfully to treat some cases of refractory IMHA
- Danazol reported to be useful in chronic poorly responding cases
- Splenectomy: the spleen is the major site of red cell destruction and an important site of antibody production

Newer therapies
- High-dose human intravenous gamma globulin
- Plasmapheresis

Monitor
- Monitor PCV daily until > 20%, then monitor weekly
- If using cyclophosphamide, monitor for development of sterile haemorrhagic cystitis and myelosuppression
- If using azathioprine, monitor for development of myelosuppression
- Tailor therapy according to response
- Treatment can be stopped once the patient is Coombs' negative and the anaemia has been in remission for 3–6 months
- PCV should be monitored after stopping therapy

- Some dogs remain Coombs' positive for a very long period of time, possibly indefinitely
- Dogs with bone marrow immune-mediated disease, e.g. pure red cell aplasia (PRCA), may require transfusion and up to 3 months before improvement is seen in the PCV

Prognosis

- Negative prognostic indicators include profound jaundice, haemoglobinaemia, haemoglobinuria, poor regenerative response and positive slide agglutination
- Mortality rates are high: 33–50% of all presented cases die or are euthanased because of severe anaemia or PTE during the acute crisis, or recurrent/persistent disease, or unacceptable drug side effects
- High-risk for developing PTE: if an anaemic patient develops severe and persistent dyspnoea consider a PTE. The prognosis is grave
- Can develop DIC: grave prognosis

IRON-DEFICIENCY ANAEMIA

Aetiology

- Insufficient intake of iron, e.g. newborn puppies
- Chronic blood loss
  - External parasites, e.g. severe flea infestation
  - Internal parasites, e.g. *Ancylostoma* hookworm
  - Chronic GI bleeding, e.g. neoplasia, ulcer
  - Excessive bleeding of blood donors
- Rapid erythropoiesis
  - EPO therapy in anaemia (increased demand for iron)

Major signs

- Evidence of bleeding, e.g. melaena, haematemesis, etc.
- Lethargy
- Pallor
- Weakness

Predisposition

- Chronic NSAID therapy
- Parasitism

Potential sequelae

- Severe anaemia

Historical clues

- Melaena
- NSAID administration

Physical examination

- Depends on underlying cause – may be normal
- Abdominal mass may be palpable with bleeding intestinal neoplasms
- Evidence of external parasitism, e.g. parasite, flea dirt

Laboratory findings

- Microcytic hypochromic anaemia
- Thrombocytosis
- Biochemical abnormalities may be present relating to the underlying disease, e.g. GI blood loss is often associated with hypoalbuminaemia
- Look for hookworm ova

Imaging

- Radiographs may demonstrate the cause
  - Intestinal mass
  - GI ulcer
- Ultrasonography is indicated for a thorough abdominal evaluation for evidence of GI disease, particularly localised tumours

Special investigations
- Serum iron concentration is low
  - Also seen with acute/chronic inflammatory reactions, hypothyroidism
- Total iron-binding capacity (TIBC) can be within normal range or higher than normal
- % saturation (serum iron/TIBC %) is low
- Serum ferritin concentrations are decreased
- Bone marrow iron stores depleted/absent
- Endoscopy/surgery to look for source of bleeding and to obtain biopsies

Treatment
- Treat underlying cause
  - Gastric protectants, etc. if gastric ulceration
  - Resection of localised neoplasm
  - Treat for internal and external parasites
- Iron supplementation @ 2–10 mg/kg/day based on iron content of preparation
  - Ferrous sulphate is recommended
- Food reduces iron absorption, therefore give on an empty stomach
- If dog has malabsorption or does not tolerate oral medication, inject with iron dextran

Monitor
- PCV should increase within 4–7 days and should be normal within 4 weeks
- If inadequate response, reassess diagnosis
- Supplementation is recommended for 4–9 months to allow replacement of body stores and not just correction of PCV

Prognosis
- If underlying disease is appropriately managed and iron is supplemented, the prognosis can be good

LEUKAEMIA

LYMPHOID LEUKAEMIA
Aetiology
- Arises in bone marrow, is manifested in blood, and spreads, e.g. to liver, spleen, lymph nodes (LNs)

Acute lymphoblastic leukaemias (ALL)
- Acute malignant disease characterised by immature lymphoid cells (lymphoblasts) present in large quantities in circulating blood, lymphoid tissue and bone marrow

Chronic lymphocytic leukaemia (CLL)
- Neoplastic proliferation of small lymphocytes, usually of B-cell origin, in the peripheral blood and haemopoietic tissues

Intermediate grade leukaemia
- Circulating cells are less mature than in CLL, but marrow infiltration and haematological changes are less marked than in ALL. Probably should be treated as ALL

Major signs
Clinical signs with ALL are acute/severe, but with CLL are often vague:
- Anorexia
- Dyspnoea
- Lameness
- Lethargy
- PU/PD
- Vomiting and diarrhoea
- Weight loss

Predisposition
- ALL has a wide age range; mean age at presentation is 6 years, and is more commonly reported in large breed dogs
- CLL more common in middle-aged and older dogs

ORGAN SYSTEMS

Historical clues
- CLL can often be an incidental finding on a blood screen

Physical examination
- May be normal
- Hepatosplenomegaly
- Mild lymphadenopathy
- Neurological abnormalities
- Pallor
- Pyrexia

Laboratory findings
ALL
- Leukocytosis due to circulating blasts
- Usually, there is accompanying thrombocytopenia and neutropenia due to myelophthisis (marrow 'crowding') and variable degrees of anaemia
- Increased liver enzyme activity, mild azotaemia and hypercalcaemia can be found
- ALL is differentiated from lymphoma on the basis of severe marrow infiltration, lack of markedly enlarged lymph nodes and acute clinical progression
- Differentiation of lymphoblast and myeloblasts can be difficult and (immuno)cytochemistry may be necessary to differentiate the cells

CLL
- Moderate to marked peripheral lymphocytosis with small, mature lymphocytes
- Marrow infiltration and splenic, hepatic and lymph node enlargement
- If high tumour burden in marrow – thrombocytopenia and anaemia (usually normocytic, normochromic) can also be present
- Occasionally there is hyperglobulinaemia which can be due to a monoclonal spike

Imaging
- Hepatosplenomegaly sometimes found

Special investigations
- Bone marrow aspirate and core biopsy

Treatment
- ALL is treated with various chemotherapy protocols: the reader is advised to refer to current texts for the current treatment recommendations
- Treatment of CLL is controversial. Chemotherapy is used, but it is suggested that only symptomatic or cytopenic dogs should be treated

Monitor
- Haematology

Prognosis
- Poor for ALL – survival times of 4–6 weeks are average with therapy
- CLL much better than ALL, usually 1–2 years, regardless of treatment

OTHER HAEMOPOIETIC NEOPLASMS
Aetiology
Acute myeloid leukaemia (AML)
- Accumulation of blast cells (myeloblasts, monoblasts, megakaryoblasts) in the circulation and extramedullary tissues.

Chronic myeloid/granulocytic leukaemia (CML/CGL)
- Rare neoplasm of granulocytes

Chronic eosinophilic leukaemia
- Malignant cells of eosinophilic origin in bone marrow and peripheral blood
- May be organ infiltration, e.g. liver, spleen, intestines, mesenteric lymph nodes with mature and immature eosinophils

- Distinguished from hypereosinophilic syndrome where the infiltrating cells are mature

Myelodysplastic syndrome (MDS)
- Characterised by abnormal maturation of cells and production resulting in anaemia, thrombocytopenia, neutropenia or pancytopenia.

Major signs
- Anorexia
- Lameness
- Lethargy
- PU/PD
- Vomiting and diarrhoea
- Weight loss

Potential sequelae
- Clinical course in MDS can be prolonged for months
- Death

Predisposition
- No specific predisposition noted

Historical clues
- None

Physical examination
- May be normal
- Hepatosplenomegaly
- Mild lymphadenopathy
- Pallor
- Pyrexia

Laboratory findings
- AML: peripheral leukocytosis, anaemia and thrombocytopenia
- CML/CGL: marked neutrophilia with left shift
- Chronic eosinophilic leukaemia: marked peripheral eosinophilia with immature forms in peripheral blood and cytopenia of other cell lines

Imaging
- Hepatosplenomegaly in some cases

Special investigations
- Bone marrow examination
  - Classes of AML are based on the percentage of each type of blast cell in the marrow
    - Blast cells are identified with cytochemical stains for specific diagnosis
  - Bone marrow shows granulocytic hyperplasia and erythroid hypoplasia ± disordered maturation in CML/CGL
- Biopsy of infiltrated organs: liver, spleen, LN

Treatment
- Chemotherapy; consult specialist text for latest advice

Prognosis
- Guarded to poor

LEUKOPENIA

For causes of leukopenia and an approach to investigation, see Section 3.

Treatment of neutropenia
- Manage underlying disease
- Isolation if high risk of acquiring infection from other animals – generally dogs are better at home, as in hospital situation they risk nosocomial infections with potentially resistant organisms
- Consider antibiotic therapy: prophylactic antibiotics against intestinal flora if neutrophil count $< 0.5 \times 10^9/L$
- Recombinant haemopoietic factors to stimulate neutrophil production, e.g. recombinant granulocyte-colony stimulating factor (G-CSF) @ 5 µg/kg/day s/c for 5–20 days

ORGAN SYSTEMS

ORGAN SYSTEMS

THROMBOSIS

Aetiology
- Thrombi (fibrin-platelet masses) form at sites of endothelial damage, abnormal blood flow, and in hypercoagulable states
- Thrombosis is the ischaemic condition caused by intravascular deposition of a thrombus
- Fragmentation of a thrombus produces emboli that may cause ischaemia at remote sites

Major signs
- Depend upon site, i.e. which organs involved and to what extent
- Pulmonary thromboembolism (PTE)
  - Acute respiratory distress
  - Dyspnoea, haemoptysis, tachycardia, tachypnoea, pyrexia
- Renal thrombosis
  - Haematuria, flank pain
- Aortic thrombus
  - Painful, cool, paretic, pulseless, pale hindlegs

Minor signs
- Visceral arterial thrombosis
  - Abdominal pain, vomiting
- Neural thrombosis
  - Neurological signs dependent upon site of thrombosis

Potential sequelae
- Thrombosis of other organ systems
  - Pulmonary hypertension ± tricuspid regurgitation
- Worsening signs and death

Predisposition
- Dislodged catheter tips
- DM
- HAC
- IMHA ± corticosteroids
- Neoplasia

- Nephrotic syndrome causing antithrombin III (ATIII) deficiency
  - Amyloidosis, glomerulonephritis
  - Protein-losing enteropathy (PLE)
- Vascular endothelial damage
  - Bacterial endocarditis, Dirofilaria, immune complex vascular disease

Physical examination
- See Major signs above

Laboratory findings
- Haematology and biochemistry to assess for co-existent disease, e.g. hypoalbuminaemia, thrombocytopenia
- Screening coagulation tests are usually normal, but may be slightly shortened and fibrin degradation products (FDPs) and D-dimer increased

Imaging
- Thoracic radiographs in case of PTE may be normal or may show acute truncation of the pulmonary vessels or increased lung density

Special investigations
- Angiography or Doppler echography of the affected area
  - High-velocity pulmonic and/or tricuspid regurgitation
- Arterial blood gas analysis
- ATIII measurement: reduced in 50–70% cases of nephrotic syndrome
- Nuclear imaging (scintigraphic) scan [perfusion scan]
- Platelet aggregation

Treatment
- Correct underlying predisposing factors/diseases
- Limit further thrombus formation
  - Heparin, warfarin, aspirin
- Direct thrombolytic therapy
  - Urokinase, streptokinase and tissue plasminogen activator
- Supportive therapy
  - Oxygen, fluids, etc.

Monitor

- Perfusion and function of affected organ

Prognosis

- Prognosis is guarded but depends upon location, severity and underlying cause
- Unless the underlying cause can be managed, the prognosis is poor

HAEMOSTATIC SYSTEM

Haemostasis is the maintenance of vascular integrity and blood fluidity that is necessary for the normal function of blood.

There are three stages of repairing a vascular injury:

- Primary haemostasis = formation of a platelet plug at the injury site.
- Secondary haemostasis = stabilisation of the plug with mesh of fibrin formed via the coagulation cascade.
- Fibrinolysis = balance between clot formation and clot dissolution.

Dysfunction of one or more of these stages may lead to prolonged bleeding.

Problems

Clinical presentations (see Section 1)
- Abdominal discomfort/pain
- Anorexia
- Bleeding
- Cough
- Dyspnoea
- Exercise intolerance
- Haematemesis
- Haematochezia
- Haematuria and discoloured urine
- Haemoptysis
- Melaena
- Nasal discharge
- Stiffness and joint swelling
- Weakness-lethargy-collapse/syncope

Physical abnormalities (see Section 2)
- Abdominal enlargement
- Anaemia
- Pleural effusion
- Pulmonary alveolar pattern
- Splenomegaly
- Tachycardia

Laboratory abnormalities (see Section 3)
- Anaemia (see Section 2)
- Hypoproteinaemia (hypoalbuminaemia)
- Pancytopenia
- Leukopenia

Diagnostic approach

1   Determine whether bleeding is localised or generalised.
2   Differentiate platelet problems from coagulopathy by type of bleeding.
3   Assess platelet function and numbers and clotting times as appropriate.

Diagnostic methods

For history, physical examination, laboratory findings and imaging, see Section 1, Bleeding.

Tests of primary haemostasis
Buccal mucosal bleeding time (BMBT)
- Time taken for bleeding to stop from a standardised superficial incision
- Reflect upper lip (hold in place with gauze bandage)
- Make an incision in mucosa with spring-loaded cutting device (template) or no. 11 scalpel blade
- Use filter paper to absorb blood (do not touch incision, dab below)
- Time for bleeding to stop is recorded
- 1.7–4.2 minutes is normal

ORGAN SYSTEMS

- Prolonged times with vWD, thrombocytopenia and qualitative platelet defects

Platelet number and morphology
- Automated platelet counts
  - Use veterinary laboratories with validated machine

NB – CKCSs have macrothrombocytes which are excluded from the automated count.

- Manual platelet count
  - Lyse RBCs and then manual count using haemocytometer chamber
- Smear evaluation
  - One platelet in an oil immersion field (×1000 total magnification) approximates to 15×10^9/L platelets
  - Normal 11–25 platelets per oil immersion field ($\cong 165 \times 10^9$/L platelets)
- Platelet morphology should be assessed from smear by an experienced haematologist

Platelet function
- Clot retraction is a crude method of assessing platelet function when numbers are normal

Platelet aggregation tests
- Assess ability to aggregate and release granule contents by adding reagents to induce these responses in healthy patients – specialist assay

von Willebrand factor (vWF) antigen
- Assayed by electroimmunoassay or ELISA
- vWF levels can be increased by exercise, liver disease, etc., so do not sample within 2 weeks of any systemic illness/stress or from females during oestrus or pregnancy

- vWF antigen levels are low in patients with bleeding disorders caused by vWF deficiency

Tests of secondary haemostasis
Activated clotting time (ACT)
- Time taken for whole blood to clot in the presence of a substance (diatomaceous earth) that initiates contact activation of coagulation
  - Pre-warm ACT tube to 37°C, minimise tissue factor collection when taking blood sample, i.e. discard first 0.5 ml of blood
  - Add 2 ml blood to ACT tube – start timing as soon as blood enters tube
  - Mix sample by inversion and place in 37°C water bath
  - Tilt sample every 10 seconds until first clot is observed
  - Normal dogs = 60–110 seconds
- Prolongation suggests abnormalities of intrinsic and common clotting pathways
- Also prolonged in severe thrombocytopenia and hypofibrinogenaemia

Whole blood clotting time
- Use glass tubes instead of ACT tubes: add 1 ml blood to each of two glass tubes and tilt every 30 seconds until blood has coagulated. Do not use plastic tubes
- Normal = 6–7 minutes
- Prolonged for same reasons as ACT

Clotting tests
- Collect sample into sodium citrate anticoagulant, separate plasma and freeze at −20°C if not to be assayed immediately
- One-stage prothrombin time (OSPT)
  - Coagulation disorders of extrinsic (Factor VII) and common pathways (Factors II, V and X) identified
  - Prolongation relative to laboratory reference indicates a significant deficiency of factors (< 30% normal levels)

- Prolonged in acquired vitamin K deficiency, liver disease, specific factor deficiencies, DIC
- Activated partial thromboplastin time (aPTT)
  - Coagulation disorders of intrinsic (Factors VIII, IX, XI, XII) and common pathways identified
  - Variation with different reagents so need to establish ranges in each laboratory
  - Prolongation relative to laboratory reference indicates a significant deficiency of factors (< 30% normal levels)
  - Not useful to detect carriers of haemophilia with 40–60% or higher levels of normal Factor VIII or IX activity

Tests of fibrinolysis
Fibrinogen
- Fibrinogen concentration ranges from 1.5–3.0 g/L in normal dogs
- Hypofibrinogenaemia with increased consumption in DIC or from advanced liver disease

D-dimer
- Assay for cross-linked fibrin degradation products, indicating clot formation and dissolution is occurring
- DIC is main cause of increased fibrinolysis

Fibrin degradation products (FDPs)
- Healthy dogs FDP levels < 10 µg/ml
- FDP > 40 µg/ml indicates increased fibrinolysis
- DIC is main cause of increased fibrinolysis
- FDPs increased with coagulopathy secondary to vitamin K antagonism, hepatic disease and thrombotic disease

Thrombin clot time (TCT)
- Time taken for citrated plasma to clot when exogenous thrombin and calcium are added

- Assesses only ability of thrombin to convert fibrinogen to fibrin
- TCT is prolonged with hypofibrinogenaemia or dysfibrinogenaemia or via inhibition of thrombin, e.g. by heparin, FDPs, abnormal serum proteins

Antithrombin III (ATIII)
- Circulating natural anticoagulant, main inhibitor of thrombin
- DIC causes decreased ATIII compared to normal pooled plasma
- ATIII decreases in hepatic disease due to reduced synthesis
- ATIII decreases in protein losing conditions (PLE, PLN) due to similarity in size to albumin, i.e. is lost with albumin

Specific factor assays
- Contact specialist laboratory

ANTICOAGULANT RODENTICIDES

Aetiology
- Vitamin K is a fat soluble vitamin absorbed in the gut and stored in the liver. Vitamin K is recycled to ensure sufficient is available for haemostasis.
- Factors II, VII, IX and X are produced in the liver in an inactive form; they become active in the presence of vitamin K.
- Functional deficiency of any of the coagulation factors leads to severe impairment of secondary haemostasis.
- Anticoagulant rodenticides inhibit the enzymatic process that regenerates vitamin K.
- Fat maldigestion/malabsorption can also cause vitamin K deficiency, e.g. lymphangiectasia, EPI, extrahepatic bile duct obstruction.

Rodenticides
First generation (e.g. warfarin)
- Single ingestion of massive dose or, more commonly, repeated ingestions of small doses
- Clinical signs usually develop after 4–5 days unless massive exposure
- Warfarin half-life ≈ 12 hours, once exposure is discontinued, toxicity unlikely to persist over 1 week
- Indanediones half-life 4–5 days, so toxicity can persist for over 1 month

Second generation (e.g. brodifacoum)
- Highly potent compared with warfarin
- Clinical signs within 24 hours of ingestion
- Toxicity can persist for > 1 month
- Secondary poisoning from ingestion of poisoned rodents is possible

Major signs
- Spontaneous bleeding
- Major episodes of acute haemorrhage into body cavity, e.g. pleura, mediastinum, pericardium, abdomen, joints
- Cutaneous ecchymoses
- Ocular haemorrhage – hyphaema, conjunctival/scleral bruising
- Development of large subcutaneous/ intramuscular haematomas at injection sites
- Oral bleeding, epistaxis, haemoptysis, haematemesis, melaena, vaginal/ preputial bleeding, haematuria

Minor signs
- Acute severe dyspnoea
- Cough (pulmonary/mediastinal/tracheal/laryngeal bleeding)
- Hypovolaemic shock, i.e. pallor, collapse, poor pulse volume, tachycardia
- Lame (muscular or joint bleeds)
- Neurological signs (bleeds into CNS)

Potential sequelae
- Death

Predisposition
- Farm dogs/country dogs

Historical clues
- Access to rodenticide
- Some baits contain dyes that colour faeces if ingested

Physical examination
- Usually no petechial haemorrhages as primary haemostasis should be intact
- Dyspnoea
- Pallor, hypovolaemia (poor peripheral pulse, tachycardia, slow CRT)
- Ocular haemorrhage, e.g. hyphaema

Laboratory findings
Haematology and serum biochemistry
- Anaemia and hypoproteinaemia
  - May take 24 hours for PCV to reduce with acute blood loss
  - Anaemia becomes regenerative within 5 days
- Liver function tests to ensure no biliary obstruction with secondary vitamin K deficiency or severe hepatic failure with failure to produce coagulation factors
- Assess for SI malabsorption
- Thrombocytopenia can be seen with rodenticide toxicity

Coagulation screen
- ACT
- APTT
- PT
- All the above tests will be affected by rodenticide anticoagulants. Factor VII has the shortest half-life and is a component of the extrinsic clotting pathway, thus theoretically the PT will be prolonged before the aPTT and ACT

Imaging
Thoracic radiographs
- Pleural effusion due to haemothorax
- Increased mediastinal density due to haemomediastinum

- Generalised mixed alveolar/interstitial opacities due to pulmonary haemorrhage and intra-airway bleeding

Abdominal radiographs
- Abdominal distension and loss of detail – haemoperitoneum

Ultrasonography
- Thorax, heart, abdomen to identify or locate internal bleeding or assess for concurrent disease

Special investigations
- Joint tap/thoracocentesis/abdominocentesis/pericardiocentesis or aspiration of haematomas to identify the nature of the fluid/swelling
- PIVKAs (protein induced by vitamin K absence or antagonism): non-functional factors which cannot be activated due to lack of vitamin K, spill over into blood and can be detected via the TCT test
- Toxicology to detect presence of anticoagulants in stomach contents, unclotted blood, urine, liver or kidney

Treatment
Vitamin K
- Use vitamin K_1, as K_3 is very much less effective
- Do not give i/v as this can cause anaphylaxis
- i/m administration is possible, but is associated with increased risk of haematoma formation
- Parenteral (s/c) treatment initially, then orally
- Treat for the duration the toxin will remain in body
  - Second generation > 1 month
  - Warfarin – treat for up to 1 week
- Vitamin K is better absorbed orally if given with a fatty meal

Dose
- First generation

- 5 mg/kg s/c in multiple sites
- 2.5 mg/kg s/c or orally 12 hours later and repeated every 12 hours for 1 week
- Second generation
  - Can follow above regime, but continue maintenance for at least 2–3 weeks
  - In view of the high incidence of treatment failures, it has been suggested to use 'double dose' maintenance therapy, i.e. 5 mg/kg divided twice daily for maintenance phase.

Blood transfusion
- Even with prompt vitamin K therapy it takes 1–2 days for the generation of functional clotting factors
- If the dog is severely dyspnoeic, etc., provision of functional clotting factors must be provided by transfusion
- Whole blood, or any fresh plasma product, is suitable

Symptomatic therapy for toxic incidents
- Gastric emesis/lavage with recent suspected/confirmed ingestion
- Strict cage rest
- Minimise injections/bleeding/surgery until haemostatic defect is corrected
- Treat shock with appropriate fluid therapy
- Dyspnoeic animals are likely to benefit from oxygen
- Therapeutic centesis, e.g. of thorax or pericardium, is only indicated if situation is life-threatening

Monitoring
- Coagulation parameters return to normal within 1–2 days of appropriate therapy
- Monitor PT time again 2 days after cessation of therapy; if it is prolonged, then maintenance therapy is continued for a further 2 weeks and the process repeated
- If using ACT to monitor progress – this should be assessed 4 days after stopping

therapy since the ACT is less sensitive than the PT in detecting early haemostatic abnormalities

Sequelae
- If recognised and adequate course treatment is administered, the prognosis is good
- Mortality estimated at 10–20% due to failure of prompt diagnosis or inadequate duration and/or dosage of vitamin K

DISSEMINATED INTRAVASCULAR COAGULATION (DIC)

Aetiology
DIC occurs when there is:
- Procoagulant activation
- Fibrinolytic activation
- Inhibitor consumption
- Microvascular thrombosis
- End organ failure

Numerous factors produce an overwhelming thrombotic process, depleting clotting factors and hence promoting bleeding elsewhere and organ failure:

- Endotoxin
- Exogenous toxins
- Hypoxia
- Pyrexia
- Sepsis
- Tissue necrosis
- Vascular stasis

Major signs
- Relate to haemorrhage or thrombosis

Acute
- Severe fulminant DIC – generalised bleeding from body orifices, mucosal petechiation or ecchymoses, haematuria
- Acute organ failure (due to microcirculatory obstruction with thrombi), e.g. acute

oliguric renal failure, dyspnoea, haemorrhagic vomiting and diarrhoea, coma
- Often, bleeding occurs late in the course of disease

Chronic
- Minimal clinical signs
- Low-grade consumption of platelets and clotting factors can lead to unexpected bleeding after surgery

Potential sequelae
- End-organ failure
- Uncontrollable haemorrhage
- Death

Predisposition
- Associated with many diseases of varying severity:
  - Immune-mediated disease, e.g. IMHA
  - Infectious disease, e.g. heartworm, bacterial sepsis, rickettsial diseases
  - Inflammatory disease, e.g. pancreatitis
  - Neoplasia, e.g. haemangiosarcoma
  - Miscellaneous, e.g. snake bites, severe trauma

Physical examination
- Dyspnoea
- Ecchymoses
- External bleeding, e.g. epistaxis, haematuria, melaena
- Petechiae

Laboratory findings
Haematology
- Moderate to severe thrombocytopenia $< 100 \times 10^9/L$
- Red blood cell morphology
  - Fragmented red cells – schistocytes

Serum biochemistry
- Organ function, e.g. liver, kidneys

Coagulation screen
- aPTT and PT prolonged by > 25% pooled plasma
- ATIII < 60% of normal levels
- Increased FDPs to greater than 1:10 dilution
- Increased D-dimer
- Hypofibrinogenaemia

Imaging
- Thoracic and abdominal radiographs to identify evidence of underlying disease

Special investigations
- Histological evidence of microthrombi

Treatment
- Remove/inhibit underlying disease
- Control hypovolaemia, hypoxia, endotoxaemia, acidosis
- Factor replacement
  - Transfusion whole blood or plasma
  - Can pre-incubate transfusion with heparin
- Heparin – to reduce the process of intravascular coagulation
  - Low-dose heparin @ 50–150 IU/kg s/c TID
  - Requires adequate ATIII concentrations to be effective

Monitor
- Clinical signs
- Coagulation screen, especially D-dimer, FDPs, platelets, OSPT and aPTT

Prognosis
- Often, high mortality which may be associated with poor control of underlying disease or insufficiently prompt therapy

FACTOR VIII DEFICIENCY (HAEMOPHILIA A)

Aetiology
- Haemophilia is an inherited deficiency of a specific coagulation protein
  - Haemophilia A is a deficiency of Factor VIII
- Severity of signs in any haemophiliac depends on which factor and degree of deficiency
  - Factor VIII deficiency can cause fatal haemorrhage

Major signs
Severe disease
- Persistent navel bleeding at birth
- Haematoma formation in puppies once they interact with littermates
- Gingival haemorrhage when teeth are shed
- Shifting/recurrent lameness due to haemarthroses, muscle haematomas
- Subcutaneous bleeds
- Mediastinal haemorrhage, haemothorax and retroperitoneal bleeds are common causes of death

Moderate disease
- Bleeding tendency after trauma
- Recurrent lameness
- Prolonged bleeding during OHE of carrier females

Potential sequelae
- Recurrent bleeding episodes in less severely affected patients
- Degenerative osteoarthroses following haemarthrosis
- Death before adulthood in severe cases

Predisposition
- Commonest inherited coagulopathy
- Sex linked – affected males and female carriers

ORGAN SYSTEMS

- Self limiting – affected males rarely survive to adulthood and reproductive capacity
- GSD – moderately severe form occurs and affected males may survive until adulthood and become stud dogs

Historical clues
- Recurrent episodes of bleeding with no history of access to anticoagulants

Physical examination
- Haematomas
- Joint effusions
- Pleural effusion, etc.
- Prolonged bleeding from wounds/ surgery sites

Laboratory findings
Haematology
- Normal platelet numbers
- Normal red cell parameters unless recent haemorrhage

Coagulation screen
- Prolonged clotting times that assess the intrinsic system – increased aPTT
- PT normal
- Buccal mucosal bleeding time (BMBT) normal

Imaging
- Thorax and abdomen to investigate intracavitary bleeds
- Joints to assess for effusion ± degenerative changes

Special investigations
- Measure Factor VIII activity levels: less than normal plasma pool in affected animals – < 20% in affected animals; 40–60% in carrier females
- Factor VIII-related antigen (vWF antigen) is normal or increased in affected animals
- Pedigree analysis to try and identify female carriers

Treatment
- Gene therapy – has been used successfully, but only short-term expression of the gene (1–2 weeks) due to development of antibodies
- Tranexamic acid (non-licensed) – inhibitor of fibrinolysis has been used to control bleeding episodes in haemophiliac patients @ 15–20 mg/kg orally, two to four times daily

Transfusion
- Fresh or fresh-frozen plasma @ 6– 10 ml/kg three times daily for 3–5 days or until bleeding stops
- Cryoprecipitate
  - Higher levels of Factor VIII – less incidence of side effects
  - Commercial Factor VIII concentrates from humans and pigs are effective, but increase risk of antibody formation and subsequent anaphylaxis
  - Give twice daily until the bleeding has stopped

Monitor
- Clinical signs

Prognosis
- Guarded to grave, depending on the severity of the deficiency

IMMUNE-MEDIATED THROMBOCYTOPENIA (ITP)

Aetiology
- Auto-immune
- Secondary – see Section 3 for causes

Major signs
- Ecchymotic haemorrhages
- Epistaxis, haematemesis, haematochezia and melaena
- Haematuria

- Petechial haemorrhages – examine oral, penile or vulval mucous membranes and the skin

Minor signs
- Anorexia
- Concurrent anaemia
  - Blood loss
  - IMHA (Evans's syndrome)
- Lethargy
- Weakness

Potential sequelae
- Recovery
- Recurrence
- Persistent haemorrhage
- Death
  - Blood loss
  - CNS haemorrhage

Predisposition
- Commonly middle-aged dogs for primary IMT
- Female predisposition for immune-mediated disease
- Breed association: Cocker spaniel, Miniature and Toy Poodle and Old English Sheepdog

Historical clues
- Recent drug therapy or vaccination
- Presence of petechiation is cardinal sign of thrombocytopenia

Physical examination
- Ecchymoses
- External blood loss, e.g. epistaxis, etc.
- Hyphaema
- Mucous membrane pallor
- Petechiae
- Pyrexia
- Retinal haemorrhages

Laboratory findings
Haematology
- Low platelet count; commonly < 10 000/mm^3
- If significant blood loss – regenerative anaemia may be seen – responsive to bleeding due to thrombocytopenia or part of immune-mediated process
- Microplatelets –? suggest primary IMTP
- Pancytopenia may be seen with hypoplasia/aplasia bone marrow
- Schistocytes and thrombocytopenia could suggest DIC
- Spontaneous bleeding is not usually seen until platelet count < 50 000/mm^3

Serum biochemistry
- Evidence of concurrent disease

Urinalysis
- Evidence of haematuria

Imaging
- Blood loss into body cavities
- Radiographic evidence of neoplasia
- Splenomegaly often seen with immune-mediated disorders

Special investigations
- aPTT normal to slightly increased
- BMBT increased
- Fibrin degradation products normal unless DIC
- OSPT normal
- Platelet count – decreased
- Bone marrow biopsy
  - If immune-mediated/infectious basis cannot be identified as the cause of the thrombocytopenia
- PF$_3$ release test
  - Detects anti-platelet antibody, but not reliable
- Platelet antibody tests
  - Determine platelet-bound immunoglobulin (IgG) and serum platelet-binding IgG

- Not readily available
- Not specific for primary immune-mediated thrombocytopenia; also false positives and negatives
- Anti-megakaryocytes antibodies tests are available at some institutions
- Coombs' test, antinuclear antibody to evaluate for immune-mediated disease
- Blood cultures, fungal titres, rickettsial disease serology

Treatment
- Identify underlying/concurrent disease and manage that specifically
- Withdraw any drug therapy which may have induced thrombocytopenia
- Severe bleeding may require transfusion of fresh-frozen plasma/fresh whole blood or platelet rich plasma
- Immunosuppressive therapy – suppress phagocytic activity of reticuloendothelial system
  - Prednisolone @ 2 mg/kg daily, tapering once platelet count returns to normal
- Other immunosuppressive therapy
- Other agents are usually used when prednisolone is not effective alone
  - Vincristine – increase platelet production
  - Cyclophosphamide 50 mg/m² four days a week
  - Azathioprine @ 2 mg/kg daily
  - Regular haematology – these drugs are myelosuppressive
- Danazol @ 5mg/kg PO BID is recommended by some authors for IMT
  - 3–6 weeks delay before therapeutic benefit
- Splenectomy has been advocated when medical therapy fails or has unacceptable side effects or with recurrent disease
- OHE in entire females as oestrogen exacerbates platelet destruction

Monitor
- Clinical signs
- Haematology, including platelet count

Prognosis
- Less than 30% of cases with IMT die or are euthanased during the initial episode or during recurrence
- More than 70% of dogs with primary IMT ± concurrent IMHA will have a platelet count > 100×10^9/L after initial therapy with immunosuppressive agents
- Approximately 40% of cases have recurrent disease
- Remaining cases are cured or lost to follow-up
- The prognosis when with IMHA is worse than with IMT alone

VON WILLEBRAND DISEASE

Aetiology
- von Willebrand factor (vWF, Factor VIII-related antigen) is an endothelial factor required for the binding of platelets
- von Willebrand disease is inherited as an autosomal trait
- vWF deficiency can cause generalised bleeding
- Range of severity is dependent upon the vWF concentration and the type of multimer deficient (more severe if lacking high molecular-weight multimer)
- Concurrent disease can accentuate signs, e.g. hepatic disease, renal disease,? hypothyroidism

Major signs
Excessive bleeding from mucosal surfaces
- Haematuria
- Epistaxis
- Melaena
- Uterine or gingival haemorrhage

Excessive bleeding after surgery or trauma

Minor signs
- Lameness
- Intracranial haemorrhage – neurological signs
- Poor wound healing

Potential sequelae
- Depends on severity
  - Asymptomatic
  - Only bleeds after trauma
  - Spontaneous bleeding
  - Death

Predisposition
- No sex predisposition
- Prevalent in Dobermann, Irish Wolfhound and GSD in the UK

Historical clues
- Episodes of bleeding following previous traumatic events

Physical examination
- Signs as for bleeding, e.g. haematomas, haemarthroses

Laboratory findings
- Platelet count normal

Coagulation screen
- Coagulation times normal
- BMBT
  - Useful as a presurgical assessment in susceptible breeds of unknown vWF status
  - Mild decreases in vWF:Ag concentration may have normal BMBT
  - Moderate/severe decreases in vWF:Ag concentration prolong BMBT

Imaging
- Normal unless intracavitary bleed, etc.

Special tests
- vWF:Ag testing quantifies plasma vWF, but not its function
- Genetic testing
  - Gene defects identified in certain breeds, e.g. Dobermann, Manchester terrier, Pembroke Welsh Corgi, Poodle, Shetland Sheepdog, Dutch Kooiker, Scottish terrier
  - No studies showing link between genetic defect and clinical disease, therefore check vWF:Ag levels also

Treatment
- Increase vWF:Ag concentration to a level to stop or prevent haemorrhage
  - Infusion of cryoprecipitate or fresh-frozen plasma
    - Avoid whole blood as risk of sensitising to further transfusions; use only if severe anaemia
  - Desmopressin (DDAVP)
    - Increases plasma vWF:Ag and Factor VIII levels by inducing release of vWF from endothelial cells
    - Only effective in dogs with Type I vWD who have endothelial stores
    - Repeat injections have reducing benefit due to depletion of stores
    - Can be used for pre-surgical treatment of 'at-risk' Dobermanns, or for donor dogs before transfusion is collected
    - Response is unpredictable
    - 1 µg/kg diluted to 1 ml with sterile saline injected s/c 30 minutes before surgery (intranasal preparation) – may shorten BMBT for up to 4 hours

Monitor
- Clinical signs

Prognosis
- Good to grave, depending on severity

ORGAN SYSTEMS

IMMUNE SYSTEM

Components of the immune system
These comprise:
- Accumulations of lymphocytes
  - Lymph nodes
  - Thymus
  - Within tissues
- Circulating WBCs
- Reticuloendothelial cells within tissues

Diseases of the immune system
These can be categorised as:
- Immune-mediated diseases of other organ systems
  - DM
  - Eosinophilic respiratory disease
  - Glomerulonephritis
  - Hypoadrenocorticism
  - IBD
  - IMHA
  - ITP
  - Lymphocytic thyroiditis
  - Myasthenia gravis
  - Polyarthritis
  - SRMA
  - Temporal myositis

Specific diseases of the immune system
  - Immunodeficiencies – rare
  - Lymphadenitis – rare
  - Myeloproliferative disorders – rare
  - Neoplasia of immune cells – common
    - Histiocytic diseases
    - Leukaemias
    - Lymphosarcoma – most common
    - Multiple myeloma
    - Mast cell tumours
  - SLE – uncommon

As the immune system is not confined to one organ system, many problems can be manifested (see Sections 1, 2 and 3). Hence, a complete list of their details, together with diagnostic approaches and methods, is beyond the limits of this book.

LYMPHOSARCOMA

Aetiology
- Spontaneous neoplasm of a single lymphocyte clone – B or T cells
  - T-cell lymphomas have been associated with development of hypercalcaemia
- Lymphosarcoma may be confined to:
  - Lymph nodes
  - Solid organs
    - CNS
    - GI tract
    - Kidneys
    - Liver
    - Lungs
    - Prostate
    - Skin (epitheliotropic)
    - Spleen
  - Bone marrow
- Multicentric lymphosarcoma involves more than one site, and is staged:
  - Stage 1 – limited to single LN or lymphoid tissue of single organ
  - Stage 2 – two or more LNs in same region
  - Stage 3 – multiple LNs (generalised)
  - Stage 4 – involvement of liver and/or spleen
  - Stage 5 – any of the above and including bone marrow and blood
  - Subclassify each stage as (a) without systemic signs or (b) with systemic signs

Major signs
Lymphosarcoma manifests in different ways:
- Anorexia
- Dull, depressed
- Weight loss
- Signs dependent on site and consequent local effects:
  - Bone marrow – pancytopenia: infection, bleeding

ORGAN SYSTEMS

- CNS – neurological signs
- GI – vomiting, diarrhoea, malabsorption, PLE
- Liver – icterus
- LNs – lymphadenopathy
- Lung – coughing, dyspnoea, tachypnoea
- Skin – alopecia, crusting
- Signs dependent on paraneoplastic effects:
  - PU/PD through hypercalcaemia caused by secretion of a PTH-related peptide (PTHrp)
  - Secondary IMHA
  - Secondary ITP

Potential sequelae
- Renal failure from hypercalcaemia
- Death

Predisposition
- None; can occur in young and old dogs

Historical clues
- Gradual or acute onset
- Signs may respond temporarily to steroid administration

Physical examination
- Hepatosplenomegaly
- Pale mucous membranes
- Peripheral lymphadenopathy

Laboratory findings
Haematology
- Anaemia
  - Often mild non-regenerative, but can be due to blood loss, immune-mediated or microangiopathic
- ITP
- Leukocytosis
- Leukopenia
- Pancytopenia
- Neoplastic cells may be identified in the circulation; usually lymphoblasts (immature cells) are seen. But < 60% affected dogs have circulating lymphoblasts, and the diagnosis must be confirmed by examination of tissue and not on blood smear examination alone

Serum biochemistry
- Azotaemia
- Hypercalcaemia – associated with PTHrp production by T-cell lymphosarcoma
- Hypoproteinaemia
- Jaundice
- Raised liver enzymes

Imaging
Plain radiographs
- Anterior mediastinal mass
- Enlargement of LNs
  - Bronchial
  - Mesenteric
  - Sternal
  - Sublumbar
- Hepatosplenomegaly
- Lung infiltrate – interstitial and/or alveolar
- Renomegaly

Ultrasound
- Enlargement of LNs
- Enlargement and altered echogenicity of LNs

Special investigations
- Bone marrow aspirate
- Fine-needle aspirate (FNA)
- LN and solid organ biopsy
- Immunophenotyping
  - Immunohistochemistry
  - Flow cytometry
- Serum PTHrp

Treatment
- Prednisolone
  - Used alone it induces partial remission, but barely prolongs median survival time
  - Induces resistance to other chemotherapy agents

- Combination chemotherapy
  - Various agents used in a variety of protocols, e.g. prednisolone, cyclophosphamide, vincristine, doxorubicin, methotrexate, L-asparaginase, chlorambucil
  - Given for an:
    - Intensive induction phase
    - Maintenance phase when in remission
    - Rescue protocol when relapse, but next remission shorter
  - Median survival time prolonged up to 10–12 months depending on protocol used

Monitoring
- Haematology
- LN size
- Renal function

Prognosis
- Grave with no treatment; median survival 6 weeks
- Significant improvement of multicentric form with combination chemotherapy, but nearly all cases will relapse and ultimately die
- Morphological appearance does not necessarily reflect biological behaviour
- Worse prognosis if:
  - Stage V – bone marrow involvement
  - Hypercalcaemia
  - Previous corticosteroid therapy inducing multi-drug resistance
  - T-cell origin

MAST CELL TUMOUR (MCT)

Aetiology
- Spontaneous tumour of mast cells
- Distribution
  - Cutaneous – most common
  - Occasionally in solid organs, e.g. liver, spleen, intestine

- Rarely systemic mastocytosis
- Malignant potential
  - Histological grading of MCT predicts biological behaviour
  - MCTs on limb extremities and in groin tend to be more malignant, i.e. local and metastatic invasion
- Histamine release may stimulate excess gastric acid secretion leading to gastric ulceration

Major signs
- Pruritus

Minor signs
- Lesions associated with self-trauma
  - Alopecia
  - Bleeding
  - Erythema
  - Scaling

Potential sequelae
- Gastric perforation and peritonitis
- Regrowth after removal
- Local LN metastasis
- Systemic metastasis

Predisposition
- Boxer dog

Historical clues
- Pruritic skin lesion

Physical examination
- Hairless, erythematous cutaneous mass

Laboratory findings
Haematology
- Anaemia if severe gastric bleeding
- Occasionally eosinophilia
- Rarely circulating mast cells
- Usually unremarkable

Serum biochemistry
- Raised urea if GI bleeding
- Usually unremarkable

Imaging
Plain radiographs
- Metastatic disease
  - Metastasis to lungs is uncommon

Ultrasound
- Hepatic and splenic metastasis

Special investigations
- FNA – mast cells and eosinophils
- Biopsy

Treatment
- Surgical excision
- Chemotherapy for high-grade tumours: many protocols tried:
  - Prednisolone
  - Vinblastine
- Acid blockers, e.g. H_2 antagonists, PPIs

Monitoring
- Tumour recurrence
- FNA of draining LN

Prognosis
- Excellent for low grade
- Guarded for high grade

MULTIPLE MYELOMA

Aetiology
- Spontaneous neoplasm of plasma cells within bone marrow
- Isolated extramedullary plasmacytomas occur rarely

Major signs
- Anorexia
- Pain
- Pyrexia
- Shifting lameness

Minor signs
- Lethargy/weakness
- Spontaneous haemorrhage

- Epistaxis
- Retinal haemorrhage

Potential sequelae
- Hyperviscosity syndrome
  - Cerebral dysfunction
  - Ocular changes and sudden blindness
  - CHF
- Death

Predisposition
- None

Historical clues
- Gradual onset of ill-thrift
- Shifting lameness

Physical examination
- Bone pain
- Hepatosplenomegaly
- Mild lymphadenopathy
- Poor condition
- Pyrexia

Laboratory findings
Haematology
- Anaemia
- Leukopenia
- Thrombocytopenia
- Pancytopenia

Serum biochemistry
- Hyperglobulinaemia

Urinalysis
- Para-proteins may be present, e.g. Bence-Jones proteins

Imaging
Plain radiographs
- Multiple lytic bone lesions

Special investigations
- Bone marrow aspirate
- Serum protein electrophoresis
- Urine protein electrophoresis

ORGAN SYSTEMS

Treatment

- Melphalan @ 2 mg/m^2 PO SID for 7–14 days induction then:
- Prednisolone @ 40 mg/m^2 PO for 7–14 days induction, then 20 mg/m^2 every other day
- Alternative protocols use cyclophosphamide, vincristine, chlorambucil

Monitoring

- Haematology
- Serum proteins

Prognosis

- Guarded
- Prolonged remission of several years is sometimes achieved

SYSTEMIC LUPUS ERYTHEMATOSUS (SLE)

Aetiology

- Autoimmune disease directed at more than one organ system
  - Bullous disease of mucocutaneous junctions – mouth, anus, prepuce, vulva, digits
  - Glomerulonephritis
  - IMHA
  - ITP
  - Meningitis
  - Polyarthritis
- The diagnosis of SLE is made on finding multi-organ system involvement and a positive ANA

Major signs

- Bleeding
- Pyrexia
- Shifting lameness

Minor signs

- Dull, depressed

Potential sequelae

- Nephrotic syndrome
- Severe lameness
- Fatal haemorrhage

Predisposition

- Middle-aged females

Historical clues

- Waxing-waning signs with pyrexia

Physical examination

- Ulcerative lesions at mucocutaneous junctions (intact bullae rarely found)
- Swollen joints

Laboratory findings

Haematology
- Anaemia
- Inflammatory leukogram
- Thrombocytopenia

Serum biochemistry
- Azotaemia
- Hypoalbuminaemia

Urinalysis
- Proteinuria

Imaging

Plain radiographs
- Polyarthritis

Special investigations

- ANA
- Coombs' test

Treatment

- Immunosuppression
  - Prednisolone and azathioprine

Monitoring

- Clinical response

LIVER AND BILIARY TREE

Problems

Clinical presentations (see Section 1)
- Abdominal discomfort/pain
- Altered consciousness
- Anorexia
- Bleeding
- Diarrhoea
- Haematemesis
- Haematochezia
- Haematuria and discoloured urine
- Melaena
- Polyuria/polydipsia
- Seizures
- Vomiting
- Weakness-lethargy-collapse/syncope
- Weight loss

Physical abnormalities (see Section 2)
- Abdominal enlargement
- Anaemia
- Ascites
- Hepatomegaly
- Icterus/jaundice
- Microhepatica
- Pleural effusion

Laboratory abnormalities (see Section 3)
- Anaemia – see above
- Bile acids
- Bilirubin – see Icterus above
- Hypoglycaemia
- Hypocholesterolaemia
- Potassium
- Hypoproteinaemia (hypoalbuminaemia)
- Hyperglobulinaemia
- Liver enzyme alterations
- Urea
- Leukocytosis

Diagnostic approach
- Identify potential hepatic disease from clinical signs and liver enzymes
- Check if primary hepatopathy by liver function test
- Evaluate by imaging technique
- Liver biopsy

Diagnostic methods

History

Signs may be acute, but may reflect either acute disease or end stage of chronic process.

A detailed history usually reveals signs of ill thrift for some time in chronic cases.
- Drug administration – barbiturates
- Environment – access to toxins
- Vaccination status – ICH, leptospirosis

Age
- Young
  - Congenital portosystemic shunt
  - Infections
  - Canine viral hepatitis
  - Canine herpes virus (neonates)
  - Juvenile hepatic fibrosis
- Older
  - Chronic hepatitis
  - Cirrhosis

Breed-associations
- See specific conditions below

Specific clinical signs
- Jaundice – not invariably present in severe liver disease
- Acholic (pale) faeces – indicates biliary obstruction or rupture
- Ascites if portal hypertension and/or hypoalbuminaemic
- Poor growth/stunting – especially with congenital PSS
- Hepatoencephalopathy (bizarre neurological signs)
  - Pacing, restlessness, intermittent blindness, head pressing, stupor, seizures, coma
  - Exacerbation by dehydration, azotaemia, GI bleeding, constipation and sometimes dietary protein intake

ORGAN SYSTEMS

Non-specific clinical signs
- Loss of appetite
- Weight loss
- Fever
- PU/PD
- Bleeding diatheses especially GI bleeding (haematemesis, melaena), DIC

Physical examination
Observation
- General body condition
- Icteric mucous membrane
- Neurological signs suggestive of hepatoencephalopathy
- Weight loss/stunting

Palpation
- Abdominal enlargement
- Ascites
- Hepatomegaly
- Cranial abdominal pain in acute disease
- Haemorrhage or petechiation
- Renomegaly in PSS

Laboratory findings
All dogs suspected of having hepatic disease should undergo laboratory investigation

Haematology
- Anaemia of chronic disease
- Microcytosis, especially in PSS
- Target cells and poikilocytosis
- Leukocytosis if infectious/inflammatory disease

Serum biochemistry
- Markers of liver damage
  - Liver enzymes
- Crude markers of chronic liver function
  - Hypoalbuminaemia
  - Hyperglobulinaemia
  - Hypoglycaemia
  - Low urea
  - Hypo- or hypercholesterolaemia
- Liver function tests

- Bile acids
- Ammonia
- Bilirubin
  - Van den Bergh test for the significance of conjugated and unconjugated bilirubin can be misleading

Urinalysis
- Bilirubinuria (small amount is normal in dog)
- Urate crystalluria
- Absence of urobilinogen in biliary obstruction

Imaging
Radiographs
Plain
- Liver size
  - Large hepatic masses
  - Microhepatica
- Liver size related to gastric axis: normally parallel to ribs
  - Microhepatica pushes axis cranially
  - Hepatomegaly pushes axis caudally
- Gallstones
- Emphysematous cholecystitis

Portovenography
- Single congenital shunts
- Multiple secondary (acquired) shunts

Ultrasound
- Liver size
- Hepatic architecture – masses, nodules, altered/disturbed echogenicity
- Gall bladder wall and contents
- Portal and hepatic veins
- PSS

Special investigative techniques
- Coagulation times are mandatory before liver biopsy
- Abdominocentesis
  - Transudate if pre-hepatic portal hypertension
  - Modified transudate if hepatic or post-hepatic portal hypertension

- Bile from bile duct or gall bladder rupture
- Liver biopsy + culture (tissue, bile)
  - FNA
  - Tru-cut
  - Laparoscopic
  - Surgical

Treatments
- Antibiotics
  - Bacterial cholangiohepatitis
  - *Leptospirosis*
- Anti-inflammatory
  - Prednisolone
- Immunosuppressive
  - Prednisolone
  - Azathioprine
- Anti-fibrotic
  - Prednisolone
  - Colchicine
- Choleretic
  - Ursodeoxycholic acid (UDCA)
- Decoppering
  - D-penicillamine
  - Trientine
  - Zinc
- Antioxidants
  - S-Adenosyl methionine (SAM)
  - Vitamin E
- Control hepatoencephalopathy
  - Lactulose
  - Moderate protein restriction
  - Neomycin, ampicillin or metronidazole

CHRONIC HEPATITIS/ CIRRHOSIS

Aetiology
- Chronic inflammatory disease of the liver, usually characterised by a lymphoplasmacytic infiltrate, with progression to bridging fibrosis and ultimately cirrhosis.

- Histological classification suggests several forms, but uniform classification not agreed
  - Chronic active hepatitis
  - Chronic persistent hepatitis
  - Lobular dissecting hepatitis
- Many cases are idiopathic, but a variety of potential causes have been identified
  - Bacterial cholangiohepatitis?
  - Copper accumulation
  - Drugs
  - ICH
  - Infection
  - Mebendazole
  - Metabolic defects
    - Alpha$_1$-antitrypsin abnormality?
  - Phenobarbitone
  - Primidone

Major signs
- Signs may wax and wane:
  - PU/PD
  - Icterus
  - Ascites
  - Hepatic encephalopathy
  - Bleeding diatheses

Minor signs
- Variable appetite – anorexia
- Weight loss
- Hepatocutaneous syndrome

Sequelae
- Cirrhosis
- End-stage liver failure and death

Predisposition/patient details
- Alpha$_1$-antitrypsin abnormality: Cocker spaniel
- Chronic active hepatitis: female Dobermann, Labradors
- Copper accumulation: Bedlington and Skye terrier, Doberman and WHWT
- Lobular dissecting hepatitis in young dogs: GSD, Standard poodle

ORGAN SYSTEMS

ORGAN SYSTEMS

Historical clues
- May be asymptomatic and be detected on routine blood testing
- Episodes of vague illness before presentation in acute crisis

Physical examination
- Signs of chronic liver disease – see above

Laboratory findings
- Anaemia of chronic disease
- Abnormal liver function tests
- Hyperbilirubinaemia
- Hypoalbuminaemia
- Persistently raised liver enzymes – can be mild at end-stage
- Terminal hypoglycaemia

Imaging
- Small irregular liver
- Ascites
- Altered/disturbed echogenicity on ultrasound

Special investigations
- Abdominocentesis
  - Modified transudate
- Liver biopsy
  - Special stains for collagen, copper

Treatment
The most effective treatment is unknown due to lack of controlled studies:
- Control hepatoencephalopathy
- Prednisolone?
- Azathioprine?
- UDCA
- Colchicine?
- Anti-oxidants?

Monitor
- Clinical signs
- Liver enzymes
- Albumin

NB – Bile acids cannot be used as an indicator of changes in hepatic function.

Prognosis
- Ultimately grave, but treatment may prolong life

CONGENITAL VASCULAR ANOMALIES (PSS)

Aetiology
- Congenital abnormalities of the portal circulation (portosystemic shunts; PSS) leading to by-pass of the liver
- The liver fails to grow because of lack of nutrients and trophic factors
- Delivery of ammonia and other toxins from the GI tract to the systemic circulation causes hepatoencephalopathy
- Signs of PSS are related largely to hepatoencephalopathy, and eventually to hepatic failure
- Congenital anomalies comprise
  - Intrahepatic microvascular dysplasia
    - Dysplasia is sometimes seen in association with a single PSS, but may occur alone and be asymptomatic
  - Single PSS, which may be:
    - Intrahepatic
    - Extrahepatic

Major signs
- Hepatic encephalopathy
- PU/PD
- Stunting

Minor signs
- Vomiting and diarrhoea
- Haematuria from renal and/or cystic urate calculi
- Recurrent pyrexia from repeated bacteraemia

NB – Ascites is rare, and icterus is *not* a feature

Potential sequelae
- Ascites due to severe hypoalbuminaemia
- Rarely, spondylitis following bacteraemia
- Hepatic coma
- Death

Predisposition
- Young dogs, usually less than 1 year
- Microvascular dysplasia in terrier breeds
- Extrahepatic shunts in small breeds
  - Portocaval
    - Terrier breeds
    - Yorkshire, WHWT, Norfolk/Norwich, JRT, Cairn
    - Lhasa Apso, Shih Tzu, Border collie
  - Porto-azygous
    - Irish setter
- Intrahepatic shunts in large/giant breeds
  - Irish wolfhound, Golden retriever

Historical clues
- Recurrent illnesses since early life
- Failure to thrive
- Intermittent neurological signs

Physical examination
- Often unremarkable except for body size, unless showing hepatoencephalopathy
- Renomegaly – reflects increased GFR
- Association with cryptorchidism
- Flow murmur due to volume overload

Laboratory findings
Haematology
- Microcytic anaemia

Serum biochemistry
- Abnormal liver function
  - Post-prandial bile acids is as sensitive as ammonia and less prone to laboratory artefact
- Hypocholesterolaemia
- Liver enzymes generally only mildly increased, but age-related increase in ALP anyway
- Low urea

Urinalysis
- Urate crystalluria

Imaging
Radiography
- Microhepatica
- Compensatory renomegaly
- Single shunt demonstrated by porto-venography

Ultrasound
- Single shunt may be demonstrated

Special investigations
- Liver biopsy if no macroscopic shunt identified

Treatment
- Surgical ligation (complete/partial)
- Ameroid constrictor
- Control hepatoencephalopathy medically if ligation not possible

Prognosis
- Guarded
- Surgical correction offers best prognosis
- Medical management may prolong life for years (see p. 273)

COPPER-ASSOCIATED CHRONIC HEPATITIS

Aetiology
- Accumulation of copper in the liver is potentially hepatotoxic
- In some breeds the failure to excrete copper is the primary event
- In other breeds, copper accumulation is believed to follow chronic cholestasis, and help perpetuate chronic hepatitis

Major signs
- Anorexia
- Icterus
- PU/PD
- Weight loss

Minor signs
- Acute haemolytic crisis

Predisposition/patient details
- Increasing incidence with age due to progressive copper accumulation
- Primary copper accumulation in Bedlington (and Skye terrier?)
- Probably secondary accumulation in Dobermann and WHWT

Potential sequelae
- Chronic hepatitis
- Cirrhosis
- Death

Historical clues
- May be asymptomatic and be detected on routine blood testing
- Episodes of vague illness before presentation in acute crisis

Physical examination
- Asymptomatic or signs of chronic hepatitis

Clinicopathological findings
- As for chronic hepatitis
- There are no characteristic changes in blood copper or caeruloplasmin concentrations

Imaging
- As for chronic hepatitis

Special investigations
- Liver biopsy
  - Quantitative copper analysis
  - Staining for copper with rhodanine or rubeanic acid

Treatment
- As for chronic hepatitis
- Low copper/high zinc diet
- Oral zinc acetate or gluconate
- D-penicillamine or 2,2,2-tetramine (Trientine)

EXTRAHEPATIC BILE DUCT OBSTRUCTION (EHBDO)

Aetiology
- Obstruction of the extrahepatic biliary tree results in post-hepatic jaundice
- Rupture of gall bladder or cystic or common bile ducts causes similar clinical signs initially, but bile peritonitis develops gradually

Common causes
- Acute pancreatitis
- Pancreatic carcinoma
- Traumatic rupture of gall bladder or cystic or common bile duct by RTA

Uncommon causes
- Chronic fibrosing pancreatitis
- Bile duct carcinoma
- Cholelithiasis
- Liver fluke (not in UK)
- Aberrant *Toxocara* migration
- Perforation of duodenum near major papilla
- Obstruction of duodenal papilla by foreign body

Major signs
- Jaundice
- Vomiting
- Ascites develops gradually if ruptured biliary tree

Minor signs
- Anorexia
- Weight loss

Sequelae
- Death if untreated

Predisposition
- Pancreatitis – obese, sedentary middle-aged bitches
- Pancreatic carcinoma in old dogs

Historical clues
- History of trauma for ruptured biliary tree

Physical examination
- Ascites
- Icterus
- Palpable pancreatic mass

Laboratory findings
- Hyperbilirubinaemia
- Increased ALP and GGT >> ALT and AST
- Hypercholesterolaemia

Imaging
Radiograph
- Cranial abdominal mass
- Loss of peritoneal detail
- Radiodense choleliths

Ultrasound
- Dilated gall bladder and common bile duct
- Choleliths
- Pancreatic changes
- Free abdominal fluid

Special investigations
- Abdominocentesis – bile-stained fluid if bile peritonitis
- Exploratory laparotomy

Treatment
- Surgery: repair, cholecystectomy, cholecystoduodenostomy
- Euthanasia

Monitor
- Clinical signs
- Bilirubin

Prognosis
- Guarded

HEPATIC LIPIDOSIS/ REACTIVE HEPATOPATHY

Aetiology
- Fat accumulation and a vacuolar hepatopathy is a common reactive change to metabolic diseases
- Causes:
  - DM
  - Drugs
  - Hypothyroidism
  - Hypoxia
  - Inflammatory disease elsewhere
  - Malnutrition
  - Over-nutrition
  - Phenobarbitone

Major and minor signs
- The signs reflect the primary disease

Predisposition
- None

Historical clues
- Depends on primary disease

Physical examination
- Depends on primary disease

Clinicopathological findings
- Changes related to primary disease, e.g. hyperglycaemia in diabetes mellitus
- Secondary increase in liver enzymes
- No or mild changes in liver function tests

Imaging
- Normal or increased liver size
- Diffuse or patchy changes in echogenicity

Special investigations
- Look for underlying disease

ORGAN SYSTEMS

Treatment
- Treat primary disease

Monitor
- Signs of underlying disease

Prognosis
- Good if underlying disease can be treated

HEPATIC NEOPLASIA

Aetiology
- Primary neoplasia of the liver is uncommon, but because of its highly vascular nature, it is a common site of metastatic disease and the third most common site of origin for haemangiosarcoma.
- Hepatic tumours may be:
  - Primary
    - Hepatocellular carcinoma
    - Biliary carcinoma
  - Infiltrative
    - Histiocytic
    - Lymphosarcoma
    - Mast cell
  - Secondary
    - Haemangiosarcoma
  - Metastatic
    - Carcinoma of pancreas, ovary, prostate, intestine, insulinoma, seminoma, or osteosarcoma

Major signs
- Non-specific signs of liver dysfunction
- Hepatomegaly
- Primary signs of primary organ if metastatic disease
- Intra-abdominal haemorrhage in haemangiosarcoma

Minor signs
- Anorexia
- Weight loss

Predisposition
- Older dogs

Historical clues
- Often asymptomatic until advanced disease

Physical examination
- Hepatomegaly
- Primary tumour may be palpable

Laboratory findings
Haematology
- Anaemia of chronic disease or haemorrhage

Serum biochemistry
- Raised liver enzymes
  - Hepatocellular carcinoma: ALT
  - Biliary carcinoma: ALP
- Liver function tests often normal

Imaging
Radiographs
- Hepatomegaly
- Irregular outline/masses
- Chest radiographs for metastatic disease

Ultrasound
- Nodules/masses of altered echogenicity

Special investigations
- Liver biopsy

Treatment
- Combination chemotherapy for lymphosarcoma
- Surgical lobectomy if tumour localised
- Euthanasia

Monitor
- Liver size and function

Prognosis
- Usually grave

INFECTIOUS HEPATITIS

Aetiology
- Infectious hepatitis became uncommon because of vaccination
- Emergence of new *Leptospira* serovars has caused a moderate resurgence
- Bacterial cholangitis and cholangiohepatitis is being recognised more frequently, and may be a previously unsuspected cause of some cases of chronic hepatitis

Causes
- Leptospirosis
- Canine herpes virus
- Infectious canine hepatitis (ICH, Rubarths, canine adenovirus)
- Ascending bacterial cholangiohepatitis

Major signs
- Pyrexia
- Jaundice
- Cranial abdominal discomfort

Minor signs
- Anorexia
- Vomiting and diarrhoea
- Petechiation

Potential sequelae
- Recovery
- Chronic hepatitis
- Death

Predisposition
- Young unvaccinated dogs
- Leptospirosis in dogs that hunt rats
- Canine herpes only significant as perinatal infection from bitch

Historical clues
- Contact with infected rodent or dog

Physical examination
- Pyrexia
- Icterus
- Cranial abdominal discomfort

Laboratory findings
- Inflammatory leukogram
- Raised liver enzymes

Imaging
- Swollen liver, but may be unhelpful

Special investigations
- Dark-field evaluation for leptospires
- Paired serology for ICH and leptospirosis
- Intranuclear inclusions in ICH
- Culture of liver and bile for bacterial cholangiohepatitis

Treatment
- Penicillins for leptospirosis
- Amoxycillin + metronidazole for ascending biliary infection
- Supportive care for viral hepatitis

Monitor
- Clinical signs
- Bilirubin
- Liver enzymes

Prognosis
- Guarded, but full recovery possible

JUVENILE HEPATIC FIBROSIS

Aetiology
- Development of hepatic fibrosis in the absence of an inflammatory response seen in young dogs
- Signs are related to hepatic function impairment and portal hypertension

Major signs
- Ascites
- Hepatoencephalopathy
- Late-onset icterus

ORGAN SYSTEMS

- Stunting
- Weight loss

Minor signs
- Loss of appetite
- Diarrhoea

Potential sequelae
- Ascites and secondary shunts from portal hypertension
- Death

Predisposition
- Young pure-bred dogs under 1 year of age
- GSD, Rottweiler

Historical clues
- Signs consistent with PSS

Physical examination
- Ascites
- Icterus
- Neurological signs
- Undersized/underweight

Laboratory findings
- Raised liver enzymes
- Abnormal function tests – ammonia, bile acids
- Hypoalbuminaemia, but insufficient to cause ascites alone
- Microcytic anaemia
- Prolonged PT and PTT
- Ascitic fluid is modified transudate

Imaging
- Ascites
- Microhepatica
- Increased echogenicity
- Multiple secondary PSSs

Special investigations
- Liver biopsy
- Special stain for collagen

Treatment
- Supportive
  - Moderate protein restriction
  - Vitamin E and antioxidants
- Prednisolone
- Colchicine
- Diuretics

Monitor
- Clinical signs
- Serum albumin

NODULAR HYPERPLASIA

Aetiology
- A benign, age-related change in the liver
- Its only significance is that it may misleadingly suggest HAC

Major signs
- Hepatomegaly if multiple nodules

Minor signs
- None

Predisposition/patient details
- Older dogs aged > 8 years

Historical clues
- Asymptomatic

Physical examination
- Palpable hepatomegaly occasionally

Laboratory findings
- Increased ALP
- Other liver enzymes and function tests unremarkable

Imaging
Radiographs
- Hepatomegaly may be noted

Ultrasound
- Nodules may or may not be apparent

Special investigations
- Liver biopsy

Treatment
- None

Monitor
- Not required

Prognosis
- Excellent

STEROID HEPATOPATHY

Aetiology
- The canine liver can be exquisitely sensitive to the effects of glucocorticoids, which cause accumulation of glycogen
- However, individual dogs vary in their response to specific dosages, and there is a suggestion that repeated exposure is more likely to cause changes

Causes
- HAC
- Exogenous glucocorticoids – parenteral, oral and topical

Major and minor signs
- The signs of steroid hepatopathy are the same as for HAC (see pp. 233–4)
- The enlargement of the liver and signs of PU/PD may misleadingly suggest a primary hepatopathy

Predisposition
- Same as for hyperadrenocorticism

- Dogs on chronic steroid therapy, e.g. atopics

Potential sequelae
- Progressive enlargement of liver

Historical clues
- Known administration of steroids

Physical examination
- Hepatomegaly
- Signs of HAC

Clinicopathological findings
- Marked increase in ALP, out of proportion to any rise in ALT
- Mild increase in bile acids (usually < 50 µmol/L)

Imaging
- Hepatomegaly
- Variable, diffuse alteration in echogenicity

Special investigations
- Dynamic cortisol testing for HAC
- Steroid-induced ALP isoenzyme – unreliable

Treatment
- As for HAC
- Withdrawal of exogenous steroids

Monitor
- Liver size
- ALP

Prognosis
- Excellent, completely reversible

ORGAN SYSTEMS

NEUROLOGICAL SYSTEM

ORGAN SYSTEMS

CENTRAL AND PERIPHERAL NERVOUS SYSTEMS (CNS AND PNS)
Problems
Presenting complaints (see Section 1)
- Altered consciousness
- Anorexia
- Ataxia
- Dysphagia
- Head posture abnormalities
- Seizures
- Tremors
- Weakness-lethargy-collapse/syncope

Physical abnormalities (see Section 2)
- Bradycardia

Laboratory abnormalities (see Section 3)
- Usually unremarkable if primary neurological disease
- Leukocytosis

Diagnostic approach
- Rule out metabolic and toxic causes of neurological signs
- Full neurological examination
- CSF tap
- Plain radiographs to rule out metastatic disease
- CT or MRI

Diagnostic methods
History
- Onset and time course of disease
- Initial clinical signs: progression of these signs and any new signs
- Character of disease: intensity, severity and exacerbating factors
- Response to previous treatment
- Specific questioning as to neurological functions, e.g. vision, gait

Clinical signs
Clinical signs associated with neurological

disease by anatomic location are detailed in Table 5.

Physical examination
- General physical examination
- Ophthalmological examination, especially retina
- Neurological examination
  - Observe
    - Behaviour, consciousness, alertness
    - Gait
    - Cranial nerve examination
    - Attitude and postural examination
    - Spinal reflexes (See Table 6)
    - Sensory evaluation
  - Interpret!
    - Is it neurological disease?
    - Is the disease above or below the foramen magnum?
    - Is it CNS or PNS?
    - Isolated cranial nerve deficits with no other signs = probably PNS lesion
    - Cranial nerve and limb deficits = probably CNS lesion
    - Disease is below foramen magnum with UMN reflex changes (CNS lesion)
    - All spinal reflexes are LMN = lesion is PNS
    - Try to localise disease – is it focal, multi-focal or diffuse?

Laboratory findings
- Often unremarkable in CNS and PNS disease
- Normal results help rule out metabolic disease

Imaging
- Plain spinal radiographs ± myelogram
- MRI/CT for central neurological or spinal lesions

Cerebrum and diencephalon	Cerebellum	Brainstem (midbrain, pons, medulla)	Vestibular system	Spinal cord injury	Peripheral spinal nerve injury	Peripheral cranial nerve injury
Mentation changes		Depressed mental state		Pain	Pain	
Visual deficits – normal pupils	Pathological nystagmus	Pathologic nystagmus	Pathological nystagmus and positional strabismus	Horner's syndrome (rarely)		
Circling	Head tilt ±	Head tilt and circling	Head tilt and circling			
Weakness – hemi- or tetraparesis	Normal strength	Weakness	Abnormal muscle tone	Weakness	Weakness and hypotonia	
Seizures	Intention tremors	Vestibular signs	Falling or rolling			
Delayed postural reactions	Ataxic postural reactions	Delayed postural reactions	Ataxic postural reactions	Delayed postural reactions	Delayed postural reactions	
	(Menace deficit)	Cranial nerve deficits		Abnormal spinal reflexes – depend on location of injury	Absent spinal reflexes	Loss of affected cranial nerve function
	(Torticollis)	Cardiac arrhythmias		± Urinary and faecal incontinence	Muscle atrophy	
	Ataxia	Ataxia	Ataxia	Ataxia		
		Respiratory depression		Respiratory distress (rarely)	Analgesia	

ORGAN SYSTEMS

Table 6

	Reflexes	Muscle tone	Gait
Upper motor neurone (UMN)	Normal/exaggerated	Increased	Paresis
Lower motor neurone (LMN)	Decreased	Decreased	Paresis

Special investigations
- Electromyography/nerve conduction velocity
  - If suspect PNS or neuromuscular lesion
- Electroencephalography (EEG)
  - To assess electrical brain activity
- Brainstem auditory-evoked potentials (BAER)

IDIOPATHIC EPILEPSY

See Section 1, Seizures for predisposition, approach to investigation, etc.

Aetiology
- Idiopathic epilepsy is any non-progressive intracranial disorder that induces recurrent seizure activity
- Status epilepticus is a state of continual seizure, which may cause permanent neurological damage or death

Major signs
- Seizures
- Normal neurological examination between seizures

Potential sequelae
- Treatment is generally not indicated for the first few seizures
- Some dogs have infrequent seizures and do not require therapy
- Majority require therapy to achieve reduction in seizure frequency/duration

- aim for 50% reduction in seizure frequency
- Some dogs are refractory to conventional therapy, and alternatives should be considered
- Some are refractory to all treatment and necessitate euthanasia
- Prolonged/untreated seizures or status epilepticus can result in hypoxic damage to the CNS and other tissues, with resultant clinical signs

Predisposition
- Idiopathic epilepsy can occur in any breed/mixed breed
  - Inheritance proven in Beagle
  - Suggested genetic determinance in Belgian Shepherd dog, GSD, Keeshond, Collie dogs
  - High incidence reported in Golden retriever, Irish setter, Saint Bernard, GSD, American Cocker spaniel
  - Higher incidence reported in male GSDs in UK, and Keeshond
- First seizure generally between 6 months and 5 years of age
- Increased frequency seizures in female dogs during oestrus or pregnancy

Historical clues
- Normal between episodes
- Seizure activity – see Section 1, Seizures

Physical examination
- General physical examination is normal, unless concurrent disease

- Neurological examination is normal (unless seizure occurred in past few hours to days)
- Ophthalmological examination is normal

Laboratory findings
- Usually unremarkable
- Hypoglycaemia can result from continued seizure activity
- Seizure activity may lead to short-term abnormalities in bile acids

Imaging
- Radiographs of thorax, abdomen and skull should be unremarkable

Special investigations
- *Toxoplasma/Neospora* serology negative
- Distemper CSF titre negative
- CSF analysis should be unremarkable
- MRI/CT should be normal
- EEG – may demonstrate abnormal electrical activity even in the interictal period

Treatment
Intermittent seizures
- Start therapy if more than one seizure in 6–8 weeks, or prolonged seizures
- Ideally, do not treat after first seizure to allow assessment of the natural seizure interval (unless cluster seizures or status epilepticus occur)
- Goal is to eradicate seizures; rarely happens so aim for reduction in frequency, severity and duration of seizures
- Phenobarbitone
  - Drug of choice for maintenance therapy
  - Dosage 2–8 (usually 2–3) mg/kg PO BID
  - 10–15 days for steady state to be reached, so need to wait this long before checking therapeutic levels
- Serum trough therapeutic range 20–40 μg/ml (ideally 30–35 μg/ml)
- Chronic use leads to increases in hepatic enzymes
- Sedation is a main side effect
- If inadequate seizure control despite serum phenobarbitone concentrations of 30–40 μg/ml for 1–2 months, consider adjunctive therapy
- Potassium bromide
  - Variable oral bioavailability
  - Long elimination half-life
  - Formulated as 250 mg/ml solution, or tablets now available
  - Dosage 22–30 mg/kg/day PO (SID or divided BID)
  - Loading doses can be used @ 400 mg/kg of KBr PO in divided doses over 24 hours
  - Side effects: ataxia, polydipsia, polyuria, polyphagia, sedation
  - Therapeutic range 1–3 mg/ml
  - Assess serum bromide levels at 1 and 4–6 months after starting therapy
  - If added to phenobarbitone, gradual reduction of the dose of phenobarbitone can be attempted once seizures are controlled
- Other therapies
  - Primidone
    - Metabolised to phenobarbitone, but has more severe side effects
  - Mephenytoin
    - Achieved seizure control in a limited number of dogs
    - Can be used as a sole agent or in combination with phenobarbitone and KBr

Status epilepticus
- Life-threatening cerebral event, so requires aggressive therapy
- Ensure patent airway
- Maintain cardiorespiratory function and adequate tissue oxygenation/perfusion
- Maintain normothermia

- Check for metabolic disorder
- Maintain fluid, electrolyte and acid–base balance

Anticonvulsant therapy
- Intravenous diazepam 0.5–1.0 mg/kg i/v
  - Onset of action 2–3 minutes
  - Repeat two to three times over several minutes to try and achieve control
  - Maintains therapeutic levels for about 20 minutes
  - Continuous intravenous infusion can be used if the drug is effective; infuse @ 1–2 mg/kg/hour for dogs
- Phenobarbitone 2–4 mg/kg i/v, repeated i/v or i/m at 20- to 30-minute intervals until a cumulative dose of 20 mg/kg has been given
  - Maintenance dose of 2–4 mg/kg i/v or i/m can be given every 4–6 hours for 24–48 hours before starting oral therapy
- Pentobarbitone
  - Use if no response to diazepam or phenobarbitone administration
  - Dosage @ 3–15 mg/kg i/v
  - Marked respiratory depression, so may require intubation and ventilation
- Propofol
  - Constant i/v infusion @ 0.1–0.6 mg/kg/minute, or bolus as required

Monitor
- Biochemical profile, haematology and phenobarbitone levels every 6 months
- Serum phenobarbitone trough therapeutic range 20–40 µg/ml (ideally 30–35 µg/ml)

Prognosis
- Guarded for good control
- Poorer if dog has clusters of seizures or presents in status epilepticus

VESTIBULAR DISEASE

VESTIBULAR SYSTEM
Anatomy
- Inner ear
- Peripheral cranial nerve VIII
- Brainstem vestibular nuclei
- Cerebellar nuclei that co-ordinate vestibular motor responses

Functions
- Maintains posture
- Regulates muscle tone
- Corrects for changes in body posture
- Controls involuntary eye movement
- Controls eye movements to correct for changes in head position

Aetiology
- Cranial nerve VIII injury
- Idiopathic vestibular disease: most common
- Inflammatory disease
- Inner ear infection
- Metabolic disease
- Neoplasia
- Trauma
- Vascular disease

Major signs
- Loss of balance
- Circling (tight circles generally towards side of lesion)
- Head tilt (usually affected side held lower)
- Rolling/falling – usually falls to the affected side
- Disorientated/confused/excited or restless
- Decreased extensor muscle tone on the affected side – leans/appears weak on that side
- Pathological nystagmus

Predisposition
- Idiopathic vestibular syndrome: mid- to old-aged dogs, seasonal incidence?

- Neoplasia: usually affects mid- to old-aged dogs

Potential sequelae
- Recovery
  - Often within days with idiopathic vestibular syndrome
- Partial deficits may persist
- Progressive leading to death if neoplasia

Physical examination
Details of physical examination for vestibular conditions are listed in Table 7.

Laboratory findings
- Usually unremarkable
- Assess for evidence of endocrine disease, e.g. hypothyroidism or bleeding disorders

Imaging
- Skull radiographs particularly of the tympanic bullae
- Chest radiographs for metastatic disease

Special investigations
- Otoscopy
- Endocrine assays, e.g. total T4 and TSH assay
- Blood pressure for hypertension
- CSF tap for cytology, culture, serology
- *Toxoplasma/Neospora* serology
- CT/MRI to localise lesion, e.g. petrous bone tumour, central lesions

Treatment
Cranial nerve VIII injury
- No specific treatment

Idiopathic vestibular disease
- Some suggest protracted course of antibiotics, e.g. cephalexin for clinically undiagnosed inner-ear infection
- Some suggest benefit of corticosteroids
- Probably no effective treatment as self-limiting disease, and likely that improvement with therapy is coincidental

Inflammatory disease
- Antibiotics if culture/CSF positive
- Corticosteroids

Inner-ear infection
- Systemic antibiotics
- Surgical drainage if poor response

Metabolic disease
- Treat the underlying disease, e.g. hypothyroidism, hyperadrenocorticism, etc.

Neoplasia
- Surgery ± radiation therapy, or palliative corticosteroids

Trauma
- Supportive care ± sedation to prevent self-injury

Vascular disease
- Corticosteroids for inflammation and oedema, treat any underlying disease

Monitor
- Clinical signs

Prognosis
- Inner-ear infection: fair prognosis if treated early, but head tilt and dry eye may remain
- Idiopathic vestibular syndrome: good prognosis and self-limiting disease, head tilt may remain
- Neoplasia: poor prognosis
- Metabolic disease: variable recovery
- Cerebellar disease
  - Depends on aetiology
  - Inflammatory: usually guarded prognosis
  - Neoplasia: grave prognosis
- Vascular disease: fair to good prognosis if idiopathic, otherwise determined by underlying disorder

ORGAN SYSTEMS

ORGAN SYSTEMS

Table 7 Differentiation of causes of vestibular syndrome by clinical signs

	Inner ear	Peripheral nerve	Cerebello-pontine angle	Brainstem	Cerebellum
Ear examination	May be abnormal – inflamed tympanic membrane	Normal	Normal	Normal	Normal
Other cranial nerves	Horner's syndrome Facial paralysis (VII)	Facial paralysis (VII)	Trigeminal (V) Abducens (VI) Facial (VII)	V, VI, VII Glossopharyngeal (IX) Vagus (X)	None or absent menace reflex
Balance	Abnormal	Abnormal	Abnormal	May be normal	May be normal
Ataxia	+	+	+	+	+
Pathological nystagmus	Constant Horizontal or rotatory	Constant Horizontal or rotatory	Constant Horizontal or rotatory	Positional Vertical or rotatory	Positional Vertical or rotatory
Paresis	–	–	+/–	+	–
Proprioceptive deficits	–	–	+/–	+	–
Tremor	–	–	+/–	–	+
Consciousness	Normal	Normal		Altered	
Reflexes	Normal	Normal		Exaggerated (UMN)	Normal
Gait (other than ataxia)					Dysmetria

INFLAMMATORY DISORDERS AFFECTING THE CNS

Aetiology
Infectious
- Viral, e.g. canine distemper, rabies, canine herpes, ICH, pseudorabies, postvaccinal (distemper, rabies)
- Protozoal, e.g. *Toxoplasma*, *Neospora*
- Bacterial – any, usually *Staphylococcus*, *Pasteurella*
- Mycotic, e.g. cryptococcosis
- Rickettsial, e.g. Rocky Mountain Spotted fever, ehrlichiosis
- Parasitic

Non-infectious
- Granulomatous meningoencephalitis (GME)
- Sterile steroid-responsive meningitis-arteritis (SRMA)
- Pug encephalitis (similar syndrome in Maltese terrier)
- White shaker dog syndrome

Major signs
- Anorexia
- Neurological deficits which can be focal, multifocal or diffuse
- Depression
- Lethargy
- Loss of condition
- Neck pain (owner may observe a reluctance to lower the head)
- Pyrexia (intermittent)
- Stiff/stilted gait

Minor signs
- Hyperaesthesia
- Other signs referable to the site of CNS inflammation

Predisposition
- Bacterial meningitis usually secondary to septicaemia/bacteraemia, e.g. bacterial endocarditis, bite wound, contaminated surgical instruments
- Pug encephalitis is seen in young pugs
- Specific inflammatory syndromes in Beagle and Bernese Mountain dog
- SRMA seen in young large-breed dogs
- White shaker dog syndrome is seen more commonly in dogs with white coats, e.g. Maltese terrier, WHWT

Sequelae
- Recovery

Historical clues
- None

Physical examination
- Hyperaesthesia
- Neck pain
- Photophobia
- Pyrexia
- Resistance to neck manipulation

Ophthalmological examination, including retinal examination
- Lesions of active chorioretinitis with some infectious disease
- Papilloedema suggesting raised intracranial pressure
- Optic neuritis – can be a component of GME

Neurological examination
- May detect abnormalities not observed by the owner or clinician, changing the assessment from a focal to multifocal or diffuse disease process
- Usually mild abnormalities, e.g. mild ataxia to paresis in all limbs

Laboratory findings
- Usually normal with immune-mediated meningitis
- Leukocytosis with neutrophilia may be present with immune-mediated meningitis
- Leukopenia may be seen with viral diseases

- Anaemia of chronic disease may be present (normocytic, normochromic and mild)

Imaging
- Thoracic and abdominal radiographs to check for underlying disease
- Spinal radiographs (plain ± myelogram) if signs not referable to central disease or are secondary to bone infection

Special investigations
- *Toxoplasma* and *Neospora* serology
  - Paired samples showing rising titre increases suspicions
- CSF tap and fluid analysis
  - Normal to increased pressure
  - Usually increased protein
  - Cytology
- Usually increased numbers; type depends on cause
  - Organisms may be seen on CSF examination, e.g. mycotic disease
  - Sterile, suppurative meningitis of young dogs: predominant cell is healthy, mature neutrophil, without organisms
  - Bacterial meningitis: neutrophils usually appear toxic and micro-organisms can be seen. Culture may yield the agent
  - GME – mixture of cells present
  - Lymphoma can be found

Treatment
Bacterial meningitis
- Treat for 4–6 weeks appropriate antibiotic (based on culture and sensitivity).
- Steroid therapy in first 24 hours may be beneficial at anti-inflammatory doses.

SRMA
- Immunosuppressive doses (2 mg/kg/day) of corticosteroids. If poor response, other immunosuppressive agents can be added, e.g. azathioprine

Viral meningitis
- Supportive therapy ± corticosteroids

Other infectious causes
- Identify appropriate therapy for the disease diagnosed and general supportive therapy

Monitor
- Clinical signs

Prognosis
- Prognosis is generally fair to good for sterile, suppurative meningitis of young dogs
- GME cases tend to have recurrence within 6 months to 1 year if they respond to initial therapy
- Bacterial meningitis – prognosis is more favourable with early diagnosis and aggressive therapy, e.g. intravenous antibiotics and on management of the underlying cause

MYASTHENIA GRAVIS (MG)

Aetiology
- MG may be congenital or acquired
- Acquired MG is an autoimmune disease with antibody directed at acetylcholine receptors
- MG may be associated with the presence of a thymoma
- Blockade of receptors at neuromuscular junction causes muscle weakness
- Repeated nerve stimulation provokes progressively worsening weakness
- MG may be generalised, affecting all striated muscle
- MG may be focal affecting the pharynx and/or oesophagus – see Megaoesophagus, pp. 161–4

Major signs
- Exercise intolerance

Minor signs
- Drooping of eyelids (ptosis)
- Dyspnoea
- Regurgitation

Potential sequelae
- Inhalation pneumonia if MO present
- Fulminating disease leading to respiratory failure

Predisposition
- Golden retriever seems to be over-represented

Historical clues
- Initially weakness at exercise
  - Dog is willing to walk, but tires/collapses rapidly
- Gradual worsening until complete collapse

Physical examination
- Normal spinal reflexes
- Muscle weakness, especially during exercise

Laboratory findings
- Usually unremarkable

Imaging
Plain radiographs
- MO and aspiration may be seen

Special investigations
- Edrophonium (*Tensilon*) response test
  - Dosage 0.1–0.2 mg/kg i/v to a maximum of 5 mg, after atropinisation
  - Temporary improvement after administration of very short-acting anticholinesterase
  - Response is transient, and may be subtle and difficult to detect if dog is not in a position to start exercising immediately
  - Neostigmine is longer acting, but causes adverse reaction if not MG
  - Response of MO cannot be assessed even by fluoroscopy
- Acetylcholine receptor antibody titre
  - Sensitive and specific test, but only available in USA, so delayed diagnosis
  - Negative in congenital MG

Treatment
- Anticholinesterase inhibition
  - Pyridostigmine @ 0.2–0.5 mg/kg PO BID-TID
- Immunosuppression
  - Prednisolone at 2–4 mg/kg/day
    - Starting slowly and increasing the dose to avoid initial added muscle weakness
    - Danger if inhalation present
  - Mycophenolate mofetil

Monitoring
- Clinical signs
- Acetylcholine receptor antibody titre

Prognosis
- Grave with fulminant form
- Guarded if MO present
- Guarded to good if medication can be optimised

RESPIRATORY SYSTEM

Problems
Clinical presentations (see Section 1)
- Cough
- Dyspnoea
- Haemoptysis
- Halitosis
- Nasal discharge
- Sneezing
- Weight loss

Physical abnormalities (see Section 2)
- Abnormal respiratory sounds (see below)
- Cyanosis
- Pleural effusion
- Pulmonary alveolar pattern
- Stridor

Laboratory abnormalities (see Section 3)
- Leukocytosis

Diagnostic approach
- Identify upper- or lower-airway problem by history and physical examination, e.g.
  - Upper-airway disease
    - Inspiratory respiratory effort/ dyspnoea
    - Non-productive cough
    - Positive tracheal pinch
  - Lower-airway disease
    - Expiratory respiratory effort/ dyspnoea
    - Productive cough
    - Cough in response to thoracic percussion

Upper-airway disease
- Radiographs
- Examination of larynx, pharynx and nose under GA

Lower-airway disease
- Thoracic radiographs
- Bronchoscopy and bronchoalveolar lavage (BAL)

Diagnostic methods
History
Age
- Young: congenital or infectious disease likely
- Older: bronchitis, cardiac failure, neoplasia more likely

Breed-associated disease
- WHWT: pulmonary fibrosis

- Toy breeds (e.g. Yorkshire terrier): tracheal collapse
- Irish setter: megaoesophagus (MO) and aspiration pneumonia

Environment
- Toxic access (e.g. paraquat, warfarin), parasite access

General details
- Vaccination status
- Respiratory signs: note previous signs, current signs: nature, timing, duration, etc.
- Exercise tolerance, weight loss, regurgitation, anorexia, etc.

Onset of signs
- Acute: trauma, foreign body, respiratory infection
- Chronic: chronic bronchitis, neoplasia

Clinical signs
- Coughing
- Dysphonia
- Dyspnoea
- Exercise intolerance (weakness or collapse uncommon)
- Oculo-nasal discharge
- Orthopnoea
- Respiratory noise
- Sneezing
- Tachypnoea
- Weight loss

Physical examination
- Observe general body condition, symmetry of nose, neck, chest
- Evaluate respiratory signs
  - Cough: frequency, nature (dry or moist)
  - Any swallowing after cough: suggests productive
  - Evidence of haemoptysis (neoplasia/ trauma/foreign body/coagulopathy)
- Examine mucous membranes for cyanosis

- Airway obstruction
- Severe pulmonary disease
- Reduced thoracic capacity, e.g. pleural effusion, ruptured diaphragm
- Right-to-left cardiac shunt
- Examine fundus for evidence of retinal lesions, e.g. fungal diseases
- Examine oral cavity: note halitosis, tonsils, etc.
- Examine nasal region: facial bone symmetry, pain, bilateral air flow through nares, nasal discharge
- Examine neck for laryngeal muscle wasting, check trachea is in midline at thoracic inlet
- Observe respiratory pattern: depth, effort, rhythm, rate (normal 10–30 per minute)
- Listen (without stethoscope) for respiratory noise (inspiratory or expiratory)
  - Inspiratory dyspnoea suggests upper-airway obstruction, restrictive disease, pulmonary fibrosis or pleural effusion
  - Expiratory dyspnoea suggests lower-airway disease
  - Mixed inspiratory/expiratory dyspnoea suggests CHF (pulmonary oedema), masses or obstruction at the carina (e.g. foreign body) and chronic bronchitis
- Dog's stance: does it suggest dyspnoea?
  - Standing, neck extended, lips drawn back: severe dyspnoea
  - Barrel chest: severe dyspnoea
  - Sternal recumbency/elbows abducted: orthopnoea
  - Lameness: consider hypertrophic pulmonary osteopathy (HPO)
  - Horner's syndrome: consider cervical/thoracic lesion

Thoracic auscultation
- Cardiac sounds
  - Cardiac abnormalities, e.g. murmur, tachycardia, gallop sounds, dysrhythmia

- Heart audibility
  - Increased by cardiomegaly, air, anaemia, thin dogs
  - Decreased/muffled by fluid, masses
- Location of heart sounds
  - Displaced by masses
  - Increased area if cardiomegaly
- Respiratory sounds
  - Normal
    - Can be displaced by fluid/mass
    - Airway: harsh/coarse/blowing to and fro sounds
    - Airway sounds audible at shoulder level, behind triceps
    - Pulmonary/alveolar/small bronchi: vesicular sounds: quiet, soft to and fro rustling sounds
    - Vesicular are difficult to hear in dogs
  - Abnormal
    - Crackles (bubbling) suggest small airway disease: obstruction with exudative material, e.g. bronchitis, pulmonary fibrosis or oedema
    - Wheezes (dry, squeaky and continuous) suggest small airway obstruction, e.g. bronchitis, secretions, neoplasia
    - Referred obstructive sounds: try to localise to upper respiratory tract with careful auscultation over larynx and trachea

Palpation
- Lymph nodes: local or generalised enlargement
- Airway
  - Larynx: deformity/obstruction/vibration
  - Trachea: collapse/foreign body/deviation/mass
- Cervical region for evidence of a dilated oesophagus or displacement of trachea by intrathoracic mass
- Thorax for evidence of swellings/pain/rib fractures/subcutaneous emphysema

- Abdomen for abdominal enlargement which may be compromising respiration
- Thickened distal limbs: consider HPO

Percussion
- Detect dull areas, e.g. pleural effusion, mass lesions, atelectasias, pneumonia, ruptured diaphragm
- Horizontal line of dullness = fluid line = effusion
- Hyper-resonance with pneumothorax or emphysema

Imaging
- Nasal radiographs under general anaesthesia if nasopharyngeal disease is suspected – see Nasal Discharge/Sneezing for investigation

Thoracic radiographs
- CARE IF DYSPNOEIC (DV is acceptable)
- Technique
  - Minimum of two views, e.g. right lateral and VD
  - Right and left laterals enhance ability to see metastatic lesions
  - Inflated films under anaesthesia may be necessary for best pulmonary images
  - Position well, with forelegs extended
  - Maximum contrast at maximum inspiration
  - Short exposure times reduce respiratory blur/movement
  - High kV increases penetration and reduces exposure time
  - Grids will help to reduce scatter in large/deep-chested dogs
- Assessment
  - Assess film for position/exposure/stage of respiration
  - Assess all on radiograph, i.e. bones and soft tissues as well as the contents of the thorax

- Evaluate cardiac silhouette, vasculature: see Section 4, Cardiovascular system
- Moderate cardiomegaly is often seen with chronic respiratory disease = cor pulmonale
- Evaluate lungs, mediastinum, lymph nodes and pleural space, diaphragm (intact?)
- Lung field abnormalities
  - Consolidation: localised, homogeneous increase in radiodensity – primary lung tumour, abscess, lobar collapse/torsion/haemorrhage
  - Alveolar disease
    - Ill-defined patchy/fluffy densities which coalesce
    - Air bronchograms: linear/spotty lucent (black) markings within the fluffy alveolar filling
    - Disseminated/diffuse pattern
    - Perihilar in left-sided CHF
    - Cranial and ventral in inhalation or bronchopneumonia
    - Local to individual lobes with haemorrhage
  - Interstitial disease
    - Diffuse, unstructured hazy densities: interstitial pneumonia/haemorrhage
    - Reticular, honeycombed appearance: bronchiectasis, focal fibrosis
    - Nodular, well-defined densities, visible if > 4 mm: metastatic neoplasia, granulomatous disease, calcification, fibrosis, abscesses
  - Bronchial pattern
    - Branching parallel lines and end-on rings ('doughnuts') due to bronchial wall thickening, e.g. infiltration, bronchitis
    - Uneven diameter of bronchi, e.g. sacculation with bronchiectasis ('bunch of grapes' appearance)
    - Luminal occlusion with exudates, foreign bodies, neoplasia (difficult to discern)

- Vascularity
  - Hypovascularity
  - Artefact of over-inflation or over-penetrated X-rays
  - General (increased lucency), e.g. right-to-left shunt, hypovolaemia, hypoadrenocorticism
  - Local: emphysema, bullae, cysts
  - PTE: often radiographically unremarkable
  - Hypervascular
  - Left-to-right shunts
  - Left-sided cardiac failure
  - Large distorted blood vessels
  - *Angiostrongylus* or *Dirofilaria* (distension and/or 'pruning' of artery)

Ultrasound
- Laryngeal: can be performed to assess laryngeal motor function and for the presence of laryngeal lesions, e.g. cysts, masses
- Ultrasound of mass/consolidated tissue ± ultrasound-guided FNA/biopsy

Laboratory findings
- Haematology for evidence of leukocytosis, e.g. with inflammation/infection
- Eosinophilia may be present in parasitic or immune-mediated disease (e.g. PIE)
- Serum biochemistry to assess other body systems
- Faecal examination to identify lungworm (not very reliable)
- Serology for specific diseases, e.g. *Dirofilaria immitis*, systemic mycoses

Special investigations
- Under GA
  - Examine laryngeal function (light plane of anaesthesia)
  - Examine nasopharynx/internal nares (choanae)
  - Rhinoscopy/nasopharyngoscopy (see Nasal discharge p. 51)
  - Bronchoscopy

- Bronchoscopy technique
  - Can use rigid bronchoscope to examine upper tracheobronchial tree
  - Ideally, flexible endoscope, allows examination of the smaller airways and for BAL to be performed
  - 'Top-up' i/v anaesthesia with propofol may be required during the procedure
  - Assess
    - Tracheal/bronchial mucosa: normally pink and glistening
    - Tracheal rings/conformation for distortion
    - Tracheal bifurcation for exudates, oedema, parasites
    - Mainstem bronchi (smaller airways dependent on scope available)
  - BAL fluid should be submitted for cytology and culture
  - Parasitic larvae may be found on bronchial washing
- Thoracocentesis
  - Performed to identify the nature of the effusion and to perform cytology and culture
  - Needle/catheter inserted in ventral chest cranial to rib at 7th or 8th intercostal space, or guided by ultrasound to wherever fluid is pocketing

Other procedures
- Angiography: rarely indicated
- Arterial blood gas analysis
  - To assess ventilation/perfusion, e.g. useful in the diagnosis of severe impairment, as with PTE
- Bronchography
  - Rarely indicated: used to outline defects in tracheal/bronchial walls
- Fluoroscopy
  - Useful for diagnosis of dynamic airway collapse airway obstruction
- Lung biopsy
  - Ultrasound-guided/bronchoscopic/thoracoscopic/at thoracotomy
- Perfusion scan (scintigraphy)
  - To identify PTE

- Thoracoscopy
  - To examine for lesions and obtain samples of tissue for diagnosis
- Tomography: for solitary densities to identify depth and density

UPPER AIRWAY

FUNGAL RHINITIS (NASAL ASPERGILLOSIS)
Aetiology
- *Aspergillus fumigatus* is an environmental contaminant, and its isolation from the nasal chamber is not necessarily significant
- In individual dogs it is an opportunistic invader, perhaps because of immunodeficiency, primary infections, anatomical defects in the nose or facial trauma

Major signs
- Sneezing/snorting
- Unilateral/bilateral profuse mucopurulent nasal discharge
- Epistaxis
- Nasal facial pain

Minor signs
- Anorexia/depression/dullness
- Nasal planum depigmentation

Potential sequelae
- Disease progression
- Systemic aspergillosis is seen, but is not usually a direct consequence of nasal infection

Predisposition
- Young adult dogs (aged 1–7 years)
- Dolicocephalic (and mesocephalic) breeds
- Increased incidence in Golden retriever and Collie

Historical clues
- Gradual onset of nasal discharge

Physical examination
- Normal air flow
- Nasal discharge
- Facial pain

Laboratory findings
- Inflammatory leukogram may be seen
- Usually normal

Imaging
- Loss of turbinate pattern
- No or minimal associated increase in soft tissue density
- May be a streaky appearance

Special investigations
- *Aspergillus* serology: false negatives can occur if early in disease process or on immunosuppressive therapy
- Nasal flush
- Rhinoscopy
- Biopsy

Treatment
- Oral: azole derivatives
  - Ketoconazole 5 mg/kg BID: 50% clinically normal
  - Itraconazole 5 mg/kg BID: 60–70% effective for treatment
- Topical
  - Topical application of povidone-iodine into frontal sinuses
  - Enilconazole flushing via tubes implanted in the frontal sinuses
    - Flush BID with 50% enilconazole suspension @ 10mg/kg BID in total volume 5–10 ml per side for 7–14 days or until discharge clears/ stops
    - Recurrence can occur
    - Not well tolerated by dog
  - Clotrimazole trephination protocol (Canesten)
    - Clotrimazole infused via sinus trephination under GA until solution fills nasal passages
    - Left in situ for 1 hour

- 90% cure rate
- Local irritation and tissue oedema reported causing upper-airway obstruction
- Non-invasive clotrimazole technique
  - Endoscopic placement of catheters and enilconazole administration
- Terbinafine: results not yet clear

Monitor
- Clinical signs
- Repeat radiographs and rhinoscopy

Prognosis
- Response in some cases is rapid and complete
- Some cases have recurrent disease or do not respond to therapy

HYPERPLASTIC RHINITIS
Aetiology
- Chronic inflammatory condition of the nasal chamber of unknown cause
- Once mucosal hyperplasia has occurred, inflammation may be self-perpetuating

Major signs
- Bilateral mucopurulent nasal discharge
- Normal air flow

Minor signs
- Epistaxis is uncommon
- Occasionally air flow blocked by mucus

Predisposition
- Possibly Whippet and Dachshund over-represented

Potential sequelae
- Poor response to treatment
- Disease will wax and wane

Historical clues
- Chronic nasal discharge, but no real disease progression

Physical examination
- Nasal discharge

Laboratory findings
- Usually unremarkable

Imaging
- Nasal radiographs: no turbinate destruction, mild hazy increase in soft tissue density

Special investigations
- Nasal biopsy
- Rule out other disease, e.g. aspergillosis

Treatment
- Symptomatic/tactical
  - Antibiotics: repeated long courses
  - Corticosteroids: questionable benefit, can be tried topically
  - Decongestants
  - Food trial
  - Mucolytics
- No proven benefit of any therapies long term

Monitor
- Clinical signs

Prognosis
- Guarded: often remains a chronic problem

LARYNGEAL PARALYSIS (LP)
Aetiology
- Disease/damage to the innervation of the intrinsic muscle of the larynx leading to paralysis of the vocal folds via arytenoid function failure
- A failure of arytenoid cartilage movement during the respiratory cycle

ORGAN SYSTEMS

causes a narrowing of the rima glottidis leading to airway obstruction

Major signs

- Inspiratory stridor
- Exercise intolerance
- Collapse/weakness/distress with cyanosis: usually on hot days or after extreme excitement
- Often cough (retch) when eating/drinking

Minor signs

- Dysphonia (change in character of the bark) but in only 50% of cases
- Dysphagia
- Signs resulting from aspiration pneumonia

Potential sequelae

- Aspiration pneumonia is a risk as dogs are unable to protect their airway via closure of the rima glottidis; this is a greater risk after tie-back surgery
- Death can occur in extreme situations
  - In hot weather, animals are unable to exchange heat adequately and become hyperthermic and hypoxic
  - Laryngeal oedema can occur and lead to respiratory obstruction
- Surgical correction improves the majority of cases. Many will still cough occasionally and still have the risk of aspiration pneumonia
- Surgical failure/breakdown of the tie-back can occur

Predisposition

Congenital
- Reported in Bouvier des Flandres and Siberian Husky
- Males more frequently affected

Idiopathic
- Medium to large breeds, e.g. Labrador retriever, Afghan hound, Irish setter, etc.

- Male > female (two to three times more likely)
- Usually aged > 10 years

Historical clues

- Gradual development of noisy breathing
- Change in bark
- Worsening signs in hot weather

Physical examination

- Auscultate over larynx: high-pitched whistling respiratory noise
- Complete physical examination for other disease, e.g. respiratory disease
- Neurological examination to ensure not part of a polyneuropathy

Laboratory findings

- Likely to be normal
- LP can be associated with hypothyroidism so assess cholesterol, triglycerides, haematology, and if indicated, thyroid status

Imaging

- Thoracic radiographs to assess for intrathoracic mass which may be affecting laryngeal nerve function (uncommon)
- Ultrasonography: identify movement of the arytenoids and vocal folds during the respiratory cycle. Preferably in non-sedated patient

Special investigations

- Electromyography/nerve conduction velocity/nerve and muscle biopsy can be performed to demonstrate abnormalities in the laryngeal nerves and intrinsic muscles. Not of clinical benefit
- Arterial blood gas analysis to quantify hypoxia: not of clinical benefit
- Thyroid status

Examination under GA

- Definitive diagnosis is made by examining the larynx under light plane of anaesthesia

- Examine at induction or on recovery
- Assessment of function must be made during *inspiration*
- During expiration, passive/paradoxical motion of the vocal folds can be seen due to expiratory air flow – do not confuse for active movement
- Assess if unilateral or bilateral

Treatment
If in acute crisis
- Oxygenation
  - Oxygen cage (can become too hot, which will further exacerbate signs)
  - Mask – can be stressful
  - Nasal catheter/nasal oxygen prongs – best tolerated
  - Humidification of the oxygen is beneficial
- Sedation: low-dose acepromazine
- Supportive therapy
  - Maintain normothermia
  - Maintain fluid intake
  - Antibiotics if any suspicion of aspiration pneumonia
- Emergency tracheostomy
- GA and intubation to be followed by surgery
- Laryngeal tie-back surgery (normally left-sided unilateral tie back) is effective in most cases

Monitoring
- If in acute crisis

Prognosis
- Guarded, but can be excellent response following successful surgery

NASAL TUMOURS
Aetiology
- Spontaneous neoplasm of nasal cavity
- Adenocarcinoma is most common type
- Nasal lymphosarcoma is rare in dogs, cf. cats

Major signs
- Epistaxis
- Nasal discharge
- Sneezing

Minor signs
- Facial/oral deformity
- Stertor
- Exophthalmus
- Epiphora

Potential sequelae
- Often present late in disease with extensive bony involvement
- Locally invasive as opposed to distant metastasis
- Usually malignant

Predisposition
- Middle- to old-aged dog
- No sex or breed predisposition

Historical clues
- Nasal discharge may initially be mucoid and unilateral
- As the tumour grows it is often bilateral and haemorrhagic

Physical examination
- Facial deformity
- Facial pain on palpation
- Nasal discharge (unilateral/bilateral)
- Airflow from nares often obstructed
- Epiphora (ipsilateral eye if unilateral disease due to pressure on nasolacrimal duct)

Laboratory findings
- Usually unremarkable

Imaging
- See Section 1, Nasal discharge (p. 51) for views
- Increased soft tissue density with loss of turbinate pattern
- Associated turbinate, vomer bone, hard palate and facial bone destruction

- Punctate areas of decreased opacity from bone destruction

Special investigations
- Rhinoscopy and biopsy
  - Pinch biopsy, catheter biopsy or nasal flush

NB – Do not insert biopsy instrument beyond a point level with medial canthus to avoid entering ethmoturbinates and brain.

  - Cytology and histopathology can be performed on tissue obtained
- CT/MRI to assess extent of tumour invasion

Treatment
- Radiotherapy: only therapy that significantly improves quality and duration of survival
- Tumour debulking: rhinotomy and radical turbinectomy produce no significant increase in survival time
- Chemotherapy: not been shown to improve outcome

Monitor
- Clinical signs
- Repeat imaging and rhinoscopy

Prognosis
- Poor without treatment (4 months)
- Combination of surgery and radiotherapy (median survival time 12 months) is best option

LARGE AIRWAYS

CHRONIC BRONCHITIS
Aetiology
- Chronic inflammatory condition of medium-sized airways, causing chronic cough

- The exact cause is unknown, but infection or inhalant allergy may precipitate it
- Signs are significantly worsened by obesity, and dusty, smoky rooms

Major signs
- Cough: dry, hacking, non-productive
- Paroxysmal coughing can occur
- Worse with exercise, excitement or at night

Minor signs
- Lethargy
- Gag/retch at end of coughing

Potential sequelae
- Chronic, progressive disease: dog is likely to continue to cough (intermittently or continuously) despite therapy
- Bronchiectasis and bronchopneumonia can develop as secondary complications
- Rarely emphysema/pneumothorax/pneumomediastinum can develop due to coughing

Predisposition
- Older dogs
- Often overweight
- Possible increased risk in Poodles, Terriers, Shetland Sheepdog

Historical clues
- See Signs and Predisposition

Physical examination
- Harsh bronchial sounds: inspiratory and expiratory crackles, wheezes
- Prolonged expiratory phase of respiration
- Heart rate should be normal
- Sinus arrhythmia is usually present
- Overweight (frequent finding)

Laboratory findings
- Usually unremarkable

Imaging

- Diffuse bronchial pattern with increased peribronchial markings ('doughnuts')
- May be interstitial pulmonary infiltrate
- Bronchiectasis in severe cases
- Right-sided cardiomegaly due to increased vascular resistance (cor pulmonale)

Special investigations

- Bronchoscopy
  - Exclude other diseases
  - Chronic bronchitis: roughening of airway mucosa, excessive mucus, inflammation
- BAL cytology
  - Mucus
  - Inflammatory cells: predominantly neutrophils (± eosinophils)
  - Bacteria may be present
- BAL culture

Treatment

- Maintain 'clean' atmosphere: minimise cigarette smoke, excessive dust
- Humidification and coupage: steamy bathroom can encourage mucus movement
- Diet: obesity increases the demands on the respiratory tract. Weight loss alone can improve many cases
- Exercise: limited exercise encourages loosening of the respiratory secretions and prevents pooling of secretions in dependent areas
- Use harness or 'Halti' restraint rather than a collar or choke chain
- Corticosteroids used at lowest effective dose
  - Anti-inflammatory doses
    - 1 mg/kg PO BID for 5 days, then reducing gradually to minimum effective dose, e.g. 0.1–0.25 mg/kg PO EOD or ETD

- Bronchodilators: methylxanthines, beta-2 agonists, anticholinergic drugs
  - Aids efficient ventilation
  - Encourage clearance of mucus, etc.
  - Theophylline sustained release 20 mg/kg q12–24 hours
- Antibiotics if complicated by bronchopneumonia or severe bronchiectasis
  - Base on culture and sensitivity
  - Prolonged courses may be necessary

Monitor

- Clinical signs
- Repeat radiography, BAL and culture if signs worsen

Prognosis

- Guarded: good control can be best achieved with significant weight reduction

INFECTIOUS TRACHEOBRONCHITIS (KENNEL COUGH)

Aetiology

- Acute infectious respiratory infection usually caused by a mixture of organisms
  - Parainfluenza virus
  - *Bordetella bronchiseptica*
  - Opportunistic invaders

Major signs

- Acute-onset cough – dry
  - Cough exacerbated by exercise/excitement

Minor signs

- Usually healthy otherwise, but occasionally
  - Anorexia
  - Dull/depressed
  - Serous oculonasal discharge and pyrexia

ORGAN SYSTEMS

Potential sequelae
- Self-limiting usually within 10 days to 3 weeks
- Occasionally disease is prolonged
- Can develop bronchopneumonia

Predisposition
- Younger dogs more susceptible
- Lack of vaccination

Historical clues
- Recent kennelling, dog training classes, etc. increase risk due to exposure to other dogs

Physical examination
- Coughing easily stimulated by tracheal palpation
- Mild/transient pyrexia

Laboratory findings
- Usually unremarkable

Imaging
- Usually unremarkable

Special investigations
- Virus isolation may allow identification of the specific cause in a major outbreak
- Tracheal washes may have increased numbers of neutrophils
- Culture and sensitivity may be useful

Prevention
- Regular vaccination including parainfluenza and *Bordetella* in high-risk dogs
- Isolation of coughing dogs from others (especially in kennels)
- Kennels must have strict attention to hygiene, ventilation and mixing of dogs

Treatment
- Restrict exercise
- If systemically ill or prolonged course of disease, treat with antibiotics

- Empirical or based on culture and sensitivity
- Amoxycillin, potentiated sulphonamides, tetracycline or enrofloxacin
- Expectorants may be useful if cough is productive
- Antitussives may be useful if non-productive cough

Monitoring
- Clinical signs, although cough may persist for weeks

Prognosis
- Excellent for recovery in the long term

TRACHEO-BRONCHIAL FOREIGN BODY
Aetiology
- Inhalation of foreign material
  - Radiolucent: grass awns
  - Radiodense: stones, toys, etc.

Major signs
- Acute-onset coughing (bronchial) or dyspnoea (tracheal)
- Haemoptysis

Minor signs
- Anorexia
- Halitosis

Potential sequelae
- Migration of grass awn causing:
  - Lung abscess
  - Pneumothorax
  - Infection elsewhere, e.g. pyothorax, retroperitoneal abscess
- Death from asphyxia because of airway obstruction

Predisposition
- Common in working dogs and gun-dogs
- Dogs exercising in overgrown fields, thickets, etc.

Historical clues
- Sudden onset of coughing after being in a field of ripe cereal grasses

Physical examination
- Halitosis (if foreign body has started to decompose)
- Abnormally dull percussion if local consolidation/abscess at foreign body site
- If focal consolidation: lack of normal respiratory sounds

Laboratory findings
- Often normal
- Haematology may show leukocytosis with inflammatory leukogram
- If severe inflammatory response, globulins may be increased

Imaging
- Radio-opaque foreign bodies will be evident on plain X-ray
- Radiolucent foreign bodies
  - May appear relatively normal
  - May have focal bronchopneumonia: usually right mainstem/diaphragmatic lobe bronchus (route straight down from trachea)
  - Ill-defined pulmonary infiltrate caudo-dorsal to heart base (right mainstem bronchus area)

Special investigations
- Bronchoscopy
  - Usually can identify the foreign body, although purulent material and haemorrhage around the area can obscure identification

Treatment
- i/v antibiotics before removal is attempted to achieve therapeutic concentrations at the site, e.g. cephalosporin, potentiated penicillin
- Bronchoscopy for removal

- Tracheal foreign bodies – rigid scope may be easier to use – allows airway maintenance and the use of large grabbing forceps
- Flexible bronchoscope is better for bronchial foreign body
- Plant material is often difficult to remove: friable nature and the effect of grass awn spikes embedding in airway
- Multiple attempts may be necessary, i.e. if marked inflammation and dog is stable treat with antibiotics ± anti-inflammatory dose prednisolone and attempt removal again after several days
- Surgical lobectomy is a last resort but necessary in cases where:
  - Foreign body is too firmly lodged for removal
  - Abscess formation

Monitor
- Clinical signs

Prognosis
- Prognosis excellent to good if removal of the foreign body is successful
- Surgery carries higher risks of respiratory obstruction from purulent material during surgery, and usual risks of thoracotomy

TRACHEAL COLLAPSE
Aetiology
- Probably an inherent weakness in tracheal cartilage or in the shape of the rings
- Bernoulli principle causes reduced intra-tracheal pressure when air velocity increases, e.g. during coughing, causing the tracheal walls to collapse inwards
- Air pressure changes cause
  - Cervical trachea to collapse on inspiration
  - Thoracic trachea to collapse on expiration

ORGAN SYSTEMS

Major signs
- Initially, a mild productive cough and mild exercise intolerance
- Progression to honking or wheezing cough and increased exercise intolerance
- Exacerbated by excitement/tracheal pressure
- Dyspnoea with respiratory noise
  - Inspiratory (cervical trachea)
  - Expiratory (thoracic trachea)
  - Both

Minor signs
- Cyanosis
- Often obese: exacerbates problem

Potential sequelae
- Many cases are adequately managed medically
- Surgery carries high risk of failure and should only be performed by experienced surgeons with ICU facilities for post-operative care

Predisposition
- Miniature/toy breeds, especially Yorkshire terrier
- Mid to old age
- Congenital disease has been reported

Historical clues
- Honking nature of cough

Physical examination
- If cervical trachea is affected – may be able to palpate collapsing segment – especially when neck is hyper-extended (beware in case of concurrent atlanto-axial subluxation!)
- Palpate lateral borders of collapsed segment as sharp edges
- Coincidental mitral valve disease is common in the same breeds: auscultate for murmur

Laboratory findings
- Usually normal
- HAC could be a precipitating factor: check for indicators on laboratory tests (see p. 234)

Imaging
- Inspiratory and expiratory radiographs of cervical and thoracic regions
  - Assess for collapse or widening of the cervical or thoracic trachea
  - Trachea may appear wide or irregular: due to billowing of the dorsal tracheal membrane

Special investigations
- Fluoroscopy: demonstrate dynamic collapse and extent of affected area
- Bronchoscopy: to diagnose the extent and grade the disease (I–IV)

Treatment
Medical
- Control exacerbating factors
  - Weight loss
  - Harness versus collar to avoid tracheal pressure
  - Cough suppression
- Antitussives, e.g. butorphanol @ 0.55–1.1 mg/kg PO BID-QID
  - Tactical corticosteroids @ anti-inflammatory doses/sedation in acute episodes
  - Bronchodilators, e.g. theophylline @ 20 mg/kg PO SID-TID
- Manage any underlying disease and treat any underlying chronic bronchitis
- Oxygen if severe distress

Surgical
- Only if medical management has failed due to inherent risks
- Intensive care is required post-operatively

Monitor
• Clinical signs

Prognosis
• Satisfactory control in milder cases is achievable
• Very guarded if severe, especially if requiring surgery

LUNGS

BACTERIAL BRONCHOPNEUMONIA
Aetiology
• Rarely due to primary respiratory infection except after kennel cough or distemper
• Most typically caused by inhalation
  • Aspiration of food or saliva (e.g. oesophageal disease)
  • Inhalation of foreign bodies

Major signs
• Dyspnoea
• Pyrexia
• Soft productive cough
• Tachypnoea

Minor signs
• Anorexia
• Cyanosis on excitement
• Dull/depressed
• Oculonasal discharge: mucopurulent

Predisposition
• Conditions associated with impaired airway mucus clearance
  • Chronic bronchitis
  • Ciliary dykinesia
  • Smoky environment.
• Immunosuppression
• Recumbent, severely ill large/giant breed dogs

Potential sequelae
• Death

Historical clues
• Dysphagia or regurgitation

Physical examination
• Thoracic auscultation
  • Crackles/wheezes
  • Areas of consolidation (no respiratory sounds)
• Dull areas on percussion
• Mucopurulent oculonasal discharge
• Dyspnoea/tachypnoea
• Pyrexia

Laboratory findings
• Neutrophilia with left shift
• Neutropenia in immunosuppressed patients/severe fulminant disease
• Chronic cases may have mild non-regenerative anaemia

Imaging
• Alveolar pattern: fluffy, indistinct, air bronchograms, local/diffuse often ventral lobes
• Bronchial and interstitial patterns may also be seen
• Hilar lymphadenopathy

Special investigations
• Arterial blood gas analysis
• Bronchoscopy
• BAL
  • Culture: aerobic and anaerobic and sensitivity
  • Cytology: numerous neutrophils which may contain intracellular bacteria

Treatment
• Identify and manage underlying disease
• Rest and symptomatic therapy
• Antibiotics

- Empirical (awaiting culture) based on Gram stain of mucopurulent discharge
- Definitive based on culture and sensitivity and antibiotic penetration to this site
  - i/v initially
- Humidification (nebulisation) and coupage to loosen secretions
- Fluid therapy to maintain systemic and airway hydration
- Oxygen supplementation (nasal, cage, mask, etc.)
- Bronchodilation, e.g. theophylline
- Mucolytics, e.g. bromhexine hydrochloride

Monitor
- Clinical signs
- Arterial blood gas analysis
- Radiographs

Prognosis
- Guarded unless underlying condition can be treated

EOSINOPHILIC RESPIRATORY DISEASE
Aetiology
- Inflammatory condition of the airways, characterised by eosinophilic infiltration
- It may be the result of parasitic disease, but when there is no infection it represents either an allergic reaction to aeroallergens, or is an immune dysregulation
- A variety of terms have been used depending on the anatomical site of the inflammation
  - Eosinophilic bronchopneumopathy
  - Pulmonary infiltrate with eosinophils
  - Eosinophilic pneumonia

Major signs
- Cough
- Dyspnoea
- Inappetence
- Weight loss

Minor signs
- Exercise intolerance

Potential sequelae
- Variable response
- Recurrent episodes
- Aggressive immunosuppression early yields more favourable results

Predisposition
- Seasonal
- Siberian Husky and perhaps Rottweiler and Dobermann

Historical clues
- See Clinical signs

Physical examination
- Thoracic auscultation: harsh crackles and wheezes

Laboratory findings
- Peripheral circulating eosinophilia: can be very marked ($> 5 \times 10^9$/L)
- Concurrent basophilia is seen more typically with parasitism

Imaging
Thoracic radiographs
- Areas of consolidation/infiltration (nodular): contain air bronchograms and poorly defined (differentiate from neoplasia)
- Increased interstitial markings
- Hilar lymphadenopathy

Special investigations
- Bronchoscopy: excessive greenish mucus production
- BAL: high proportion of eosinophils on cytology; usually sterile

Treatment
- Identify/remove underlying causes for inflammatory lesions:
  - Drug-related
  - Infectious
  - Neoplastic
  - Parasitic
  - Vaccine-related
- Most cases require prednisolone (no cause identified)
  - 2 mg/kg prednisolone SID-BID for 2–3 weeks, and then reduce by 25–33% every 2–3 weeks until on every other day therapy. Maintain treatment for minimum 2–3 months
- Antibiotics if secondary infection

Monitor
- Clinical signs
- Radiographic appearance

Prognosis
- Guarded: some do well, but others either need recurrent or continuous steroids or are refractory

HEARTWORM (ANGIOSTRONGYLUS VASORUM)
Aetiology
- Infection of pulmonary circulation by nematode
- Intermediate hosts are slugs and snails
- Infection acquired by eating mollusc deliberately or accidentally if ingesting grass
- Parasite migrates to right side of heart
- Signs caused by thrombosis of pulmonary vessels and pulmonary inflammation
- Larvae are coughed up, swallowed and excreted in faeces

NB – *Dirofilaria immitis* is a major cause of heartworm in the world but is restricted geographically by its mosquito vector. It is not currently present in the UK, although it should be considered in imported dogs. Readers are directed to specialist texts for further advice.

Major signs
- Cough/dyspnoea/tachypnoea
- Malaise
- Weight loss/stunting

Minor signs
- Anaemia/coagulopathy
- Subcutaneous swellings (haematoma)
- Cardiac failure (right-sided)
- Thromboembolism

Potential sequelae
- Recovery with treatment
- DIC and death

Predisposition
- Geographical location, e.g. south-west England, south Wales, Ireland, France
- Cases now being seen from wider geographical area in UK, including Midlands
- Particularly seen in Irish greyhounds
- Intermediate host slug/snail: dogs that eat a lot of grass are at increased risk in infected areas
- More commonly reported in young dogs

Historical clues
- Dog lives in or has visited endemic area
- Known ingestion of molluscs
- Known to eat grass, e.g. because of inflammatory bowel disease (inadvertently eat mollusc)

Physical examination
- Thoracic auscultation: abnormal respiratory noise, e.g. crackles
- Bleeding secondary to coagulopathy – check for evidence or mucosal bleeds or petechiation/ecchymoses

ORGAN SYSTEMS

- Ocular/retinal examination: active chorioretinitis lesions can be seen in *Angiostrongylus*, also changes secondary to hyperglobulinaemia

Laboratory findings
- Circulating eosinophilia can be marked
- Hyperglobulinaemia can be seen (polyclonal)
- Anaemia has been reported: probably secondary to haemorrhage into pulmonary tissue
- Thrombocytopenia reported: consumptive coagulopathy (DIC)
- Faecal examination may demonstrate parasitic larvae

Imaging
Thoracic radiographs
- Mixed pattern is often seen
  - Patchy alveolar infiltrate
  - Diffuse interstitial pattern
- Large pulmonary vessels
- Right-sided cardiomegaly
- Sometimes nodules can be seen: need to differentiate from metastatic neoplasia

Echocardiography
- May demonstrate adult worms in right ventricle/pulmonary artery
- Right-sided cardiomegaly
- Enlarged pulmonary outflow

Special investigations
- Bronchoscopy
  - BAL may demonstrate larvae
  - Eosinophils predominate on cytology
- Coagulation tests/D-dimer/FDPs to assess for DIC
- Arterial blood gas analysis to assess oxygenation

Treatment
- Fenbendazole (as *Oslerus* – same group of worms)

- Prednisolone: anti-inflammatory doses to reduce immune reaction to dying worms and reduce long-term pulmonary damage
- Management of any coagulopathy
- Antibiotics: pulmonary haemorrhage provides a good environment for microbial proliferation

Monitor
- Clinical signs
- Radiographic appearance

Prognosis
- Can be successfully treated if recognised before complications develop

LUNGWORM (*OSLERUS OSLERI*)
Aetiology
- *Oslerus* (formerly *Filaroides*) is a nematode which forms granulomas in trachea and main bronchi
- Life cycle may or may not involve intermediate host
- Larvae coughed up, swallowed and excreted in faeces
- Clinical signs are related to airway irritation and obstruction
- Other lungworms are uncommon in dogs in UK
  - *Filaroides hirthii*
  - *Crenosmoma vulpii*

Major signs
- Cough: dry, paroxysmal, non-productive with retch
- Wheezing
- Exacerbated with excitement/exercise

Minor signs
- Cyanosis if nodules are very large

Predisposition
- Young dogs aged < 5 years
- Kennelled dogs

- Infected bitch easily transmits infective larvae to pups
- No intermediate host needed so easily spread dog-to-dog

Potential sequelae
- Airway obstruction
  - Dyspnoea
  - Exercise intolerance
- Persistent infection

Historical clues
- Contact with infected dog

Physical examination
- Possibly harsh respiratory sounds over trachea if large nodules
- Usually unremarkable

Laboratory findings
- Circulating eosinophilia may be present
- Faecal parasitology (Baermann technique) may demonstrate larvae, but false negatives are common

Imaging
- Thoracic radiographs may demonstrate nodules in trachea if large

Special investigations
- Bronchoscopy: 1–1.5 cm nodules in distal trachea/bronchi
- Larvae in BAL

Treatment
- Fenbendazole @ 50 mg/kg PO SID for 7 days
- Praziquantel/febantel/pyrantel embonate combination, benzimidazoles and levamisole also have been used
- Remove faeces from environment
- Check in-contact animals

Monitor
Clinical signs

Prognosis
- Can be difficult to treat: nodules remain and may calcify, then cough can persist

PULMONARY NEOPLASIA – PRIMARY OR SECONDARY
Aetiology
- Primary lung tumour arises *de novo* in bronchus or small airway
- Adenocarcinoma is most common type
- Lungs are a common site for secondary, metastatic tumours, e.g. all carcinomas, haemangiosarcoma
- Clinical signs are related to airway obstruction by tumour, haemorrhage or fluid

Predisposition
- Mid- to old-aged dogs

Major signs
- Dry cough
- Dyspnoea more common with metastasis (cough less frequently)
- Exercise intolerance or lethargy or depression
- Increasing tachypnoea/orthopnoea
- Weight loss

Minor signs
- Lameness (HPO or metastasis to bone)
- Haemoptysis – more common with primary tumour

Potential sequelae
- Death

Historical clues
- Presence of a primary tumour elsewhere, that may have already been excised

Physical examination
- Thoracic auscultation
  - Areas of increased/decreased or abnormal sounds

ORGAN SYSTEMS

- Heart sounds may be muffled or in abnormal position due to displacement by mass
- Tachypnoea/dyspnoea/orthopnoea

Laboratory findings
- Usually unremarkable
- Inflammatory leukogram may be seen with necrotic centres of tumours
- Anaemia if significant haemorrhage
- Abnormal circulating lymphocytes may be seen in lymphoma

Imaging
- Left and right lateral recumbent radiographs
- Primary lung tumour
  - Lobar consolidation: no air bronchograms
  - Increase pulmonary interstitial markings
  - One or more discrete soft tissue masses
  - Right caudal lobe more commonly affected than other lobes
  - Pleural effusion
  - Hilar/sternal lymphadenopathy
- Metastatic neoplasia
  - Multiple, discrete, round soft tissue masses 'cannonballs' or more miliary nodular pattern in interstitium: best seen over other soft tissue structures, e.g. diaphragm and heart (DDx pleural nodules, end-on blood vessels)
  - Pleural effusion

Special investigations
- Bronchoscopy and BAL cytology and culture: some neoplastic cells may be seen in the wash

- FNA/biopsy: with ultrasound guidance for cytology/histopathology
- Thoracoscopic biopsy
- Thoracotomy and biopsy/resection

Treatment
- Primary lung tumour
  - Surgical lobectomy of the affected lobe(s) and removal of associated LNs
  - Adjuvant chemotherapy for patients with non-resectable masses or evidence of lymph node metastasis, e.g. cisplatin, vinblastine
- Secondary/metastatic
  - One or two metastatic masses – excision can be considered – rarely appropriate as micrometastasis is often already present elsewhere
  - Attempt excision or pleurodesis if metastasis has eroded visceral pleura and is causing pneumothorax
  - Systemic chemotherapy: generally disappointing

Monitor
- Check for recurrence of tumour by radiographs

Prognosis
- Primary lung tumours tend to have slow growth, so even incomplete resection can provide a prolonged period of good quality of life
- Surgical/anaesthetic complications should be considered
- Survival times after surgery
  - Lobe and LN affected – 4 months
  - Lobe only – 12 months
- For metastatic neoplasia, the prognosis is guarded/poor

UROGENITAL TRACT

- Diseases of the urinary tract typically affect either the:
  - kidneys, or
  - lower urinary tract comprising ureters, bladder, urethra (and prostate)
- Urinary tract infection (UTI) can affect the whole tract
- Urolithiasis may be solitary or multiple and can occur anywhere from the renal pelvis to the urethra

RENAL SYSTEM

- Azotaemia is the increase in the plasma concentration of nitrogenous substances (see pp. 135–6)
- Uraemia is the clinical syndrome associated with azotaemia
- The kidneys have significant reserve capacity, and azotaemia only occurs when glomerular filtration is < 25% of normal

Problems
Clinical presentations (see Section 1)
- Abdominal discomfort/pain
- Anorexia
- Constipation
- Diarrhoea
- Dysuria
- Haematemesis
- Haematuria and discoloured urine
- Halitosis
- Polyuria/polydipsia
- Seizures
- Urinary incontinence
- Vomiting
- Weakness-lethargy-(collapse)
- Weight loss

Physical abnormalities (see Section 2)
- Abdominal enlargement
- Anaemia
- Ascites
- Hyperthermia and pyrexia
- Peripheral oedema
- Pleural effusion
- Stomatitis
- Systemic hypertension

Laboratory abnormalities (see Section 3)
- Anaemia (see above)
- Azotaemia (urea and creatinine)
- Hypercalcaemia
- Hyperlipidaemia/hypercholesterolaemia
- Hyperkalaemia
- Hypernatraemia
- Hypoproteinaemia (hypoalbuminaemia)
- Proteinuria
- Leukocytosis

Diagnostic approach
- Identify renal insufficiency and renal failure from clinical signs and azotaemia
- Identify significant proteinuria caused by protein-losing nephropathy
- Distinguish:
  - Acute renal failure (ARF) versus chronic renal failure (CRF)
  - Progressive versus non-progressive
  - Reversible versus irreversible

Diagnostic methods
History
- Clinical presentation – signs of uraemia

Endocrine and metabolic disturbances
- Muscle atrophy
- Osteodystrophy
- Weight loss

Fluid, electrolyte disturbances
- Dehydration
- Nocturia – urination at night due to PU/PD (distinguish from incontinence)
- PU/PD

Gastrointestinal disturbances
- Anorexia

ORGAN SYSTEMS

- Gastritis/gastric ulceration
- Gastrointestinal bleeding
- Halitosis
- Oral ulceration/stomatitis
- Vomiting

Haematological disturbances
- Pallor (chronic renal disease)

Hypertensive complications
- Blindness
- Hyphaema

Neuromuscular disturbances
- Depression
- Lethargy
- Weakness

Physical examination
General
- Dehydrated – poor skin turgor, sunken eyes, pale/tacky mucous membranes, tachycardia
- Halitosis
- Loss of muscle mass
- Oral ulceration in uraemic patients: buccal mucosa around molars and premolars and tongue ulceration and necrosis
- Osteodystrophy – thickened bones with abnormal flexibility 'rubber jaw' – young, growing, uraemic puppies
- Pale mucous membranes can be due to dehydration and/or anaemia
- Poor hair coat
- Pyrexia – pyelonephritis, neoplasia, inflammatory disease (± related to azotaemia)

Bladder palpation
- Dehydrated, uraemic patients with CRF often have large, normal-shaped bladder full of dilute urine

Rectal examination
- Anal sac adenocarcinoma associated with paraneoplastic hypercalcaemia

Renal palpation
- Abnormal renal size/shape
  - Small: suspect CRF
  - Large: neoplasia, hydronephrosis, peri-renal cysts, haemorrhage, poly-cystic disease, haematoma, acute renal inflammation, PSS
- Pain on palpation of kidneys or dorsal abdomen – pyelonephritis, acute hydronephrosis, large renal calculi, ureteral obstruction

Retinal examination
- Hypertensive retinal lesions associated with CRF
  - Initially:
    - Dilation and tortuosity of retinal vessels
  - Then:
    - Bullous retinal detachment through to complete detachment
    - Retinal haemorrhage
  - Finally:
    - Hyphaema

Laboratory findings
Haematology
- Moderately severe non-regenerative normocytic, normochromic anaemia with CRF due to failure of red cell production, i.e. takes weeks to months to develop.
- ARF and post-renal causes azotaemia are not associated with anaemia unless secondary GI blood loss or combined anticoagulant and cholecalciferol toxicity.
- Moderate to more than severe neutrophilia may indicate septic process or urinary tract infection.
- Mild lymphopenia and neutrophilia seen in some uraemic patients (non-specific).
- Due to dehydration, the PCV may be normal at presentation (haemoconcentration); assess PCV and total plasma protein to allow recognition of anaemia in dehydrated patient.

Serum biochemistry
- Calcium
  - Total may be high, low or normal in uraemic patients
  - Hypercalcaemia may cause intrinsic renal failure
  - More appropriate to assess ionised calcium
- Hyperkalaemia
  - Advanced post-renal azotaemia and oliguric or anuric acute renal failure ± end-stage CRF
- Hyperphosphataemia
  - Can be seen with all forms of azotaemia – least likely with pre-renal
- Hypokalaemia
  - Patients with CRF – weakness, inappetence and polymyopathy
  - Post-obstructional diuresis
- Urea and creatinine will not rise above normal until more than 75% of the glomeruli are not filtering. Creatinine is a more accurate reflection of GFR than urea (see pp. 135–6)

Urinalysis
- A full urinalysis = dipstick and sediment examination
- Dehydrated patient with azotaemia and concentrated urine should be investigated for causes of pre-renal azotaemia
- Dehydrated patient with azotaemia producing no urine suggests anuric renal failure or post-renal causes
- Dilute isosthenuric urine (SG 1.007–1.016) in dehydrated patient with azotaemia suggests renal failure
- Exceptions to the above rules are patients with normal GFR but deficient renal tubular concentrating ability that are deprived of water, i.e. azotaemic without appropriate hypersthenuric urine but not in renal failure (yet)
  - Pyometra
  - Hypoadrenocorticism
  - Diabetes insipidus
  - Hypercalcaemia

- Excess glucocorticoids
- Diuretic therapy (excessive)
- Intrinsic renal tubular disease
  - Fanconi
  - Renal glycosuria
  - Renal tubular acidosis
- Urine bacterial culture if sediment examination shows pyuria or bacteriuria on cystocentesis sample or if indicated for other reasons

The significance of findings on urine examination are detailed in Table 8.

- Proteinuria assessment by urine protein:creatinine ratio:
  - Normal   < 1.0
  - Uncertain   1.0–2.0
  - Abnormal   > 2.0

Imaging
Abdominal radiography
- Assess renal size ± shape
- Intact urinary bladder?
- Presence of radio-opaque calculi – azotaemia associated with bilateral renal or ureteral calculi or urethral calculi causing obstruction
- Renal and/or cystic calculi in young animals should raise the likelihood urate calculi secondary to PSS
- Urinary tract rupture –intrapelvic soft tissue swelling, caudal peritonitis, ascites – perform positive contrast studies to identify the site of leakage

Thoracic radiography
- If cardiorespiratory signs or checking for metastasis from urinary tract neoplasia
- Uraemic pneumonitis is very rare finding in advanced disease – patchy alveolar and diffuse interstitial pulmonary infiltrates

Contrast radiography
- i/v urography to assess renal excretion
- Lower-urinary tract contrast studies to assess for causes of urinary tract obstruction

Table 8   Interpretation of urinalysis findings

Urine	Significance
SG >1.030 Hypersthenuric	If azotaemic likely pre-renal, could be peracute renal
SG >1.016 < 1.030 Hypersthenuric	Could have renal disease – if azotaemic, first look for pre-renal cause or other cause of decreased concentrating ability
SG >1.007 <1.016 Isosthenuria	If azotaemic with uraemic signs and no other identifiable cause for failure to concentrate – likely to be renal failure
SG <1.007 Hyposthenuria	Active dilution of glomerular filtrate by renal tubules – if dehydrated then renal failure is possible but more likely due to other causes, e.g. diabetes insipidus
++++ Proteinuria (dipstick)	If no haemoglobinuria and not ++ white cells or debris on sediment, then may be protein-losing nephropathy – perform urine protein:creatinine ratio to assess
Glycosuria	If normoglycaemic, indicates proximal renal tubular dysfunction – can also be seen with amyloidosis + some familial nephropathies
	If hyperglycaemic, indicates diabetes mellitus
Bacteria and WBCs on sediment examination (not free catch urine sample)	Bacterial urinary tract infection could be cause of renal failure (pyelonephritis) or secondary complication. Culture and sensitivity indicated
Cylinduria (casts)	Toxic, infectious, ischaemic and traumatic renal disease can lead to cast formation secondary to tubular damage

Ultrasonography
- Check bladder for size, mural lesions or intravesical abnormalities, e.g. calculi
- Check prostate for enlargement and echoarchitecture
- Check renal size, shape and echoarchitecture
- Are sublumbar lymph nodes enlarged? ± biopsy?
- Check ureteral emptying into bladder neck to assess ectopic ureters

Special tests
- Systemic blood pressure: indicated in all azotaemic patients
- Fractional clearance of electrolytes
- GFR assessment
  - Endogenous creatinine clearance
  - Iohexol clearance
  - Radioisotopes
- Blood gas for acid–base status

- Renal biopsy (ultrasound guidance or surgical) for histology and culture
  - Most reliable method to distinguish ARF versus CRF for a specific diagnosis and prognosis, but may not be justifiable if markedly azotaemic because of risk of haemorrhage and post-biopsy deterioration
  - May have little impact on prognosis
    - Use in the following patients:
    - Suspected of having disease other than CRF
    - Owner requests accurate prognosis before deciding upon management
    - Marked proteinuria before azotaemia develops

Differentiation between ARF and CRF
(See Table 9)

ACUTE RENAL FAILURE (ARF)
Aetiology
- An acute reduction in GFR in previously healthy kidneys due to renal causes, and that results in azotaemia

Causes
- Hypercalcaemia
- Hyperthermia
- Hypothermia
- Hypovolaemia/ischaemia
  - Cardiac arrest/acute cardiac failure
  - Shock

- Profound anaesthesia and prolonged surgery
- Trauma
- Infection
  - Pyelonephritis
  - Leptospirosis
- Toxins
  - Aminoglycosides (gentamicin, amikacin)
  - Cisplatin
  - Cyclosporin
  - Ethylene glycol
  - Haemoglobin (haemolysis)
  - Heavy metals (mercury, arsenic, cadmium)
  - I/v iodinated contrast agents
  - Myoglobin
  - NSAIDs
  - Raisins

Major signs
Acute onset of:
- Lethargy
- Anorexia
- Vomiting
- Diarrhoea

Minor signs
- Weakness
- PU/PD, weight loss and anaemia usually absent

ORGAN SYSTEMS

Table 9

	ARF	CRF
Polydipsia	No	Yes
Urine volume	Variable	Increased, except terminally
Precipitating event	Yes	No, but may cause acute exacerbations
Kidney size	Normal	Small, irregular
Weight loss	No	Yes
Anaemia	No	Yes
Serum potassium	Normal/high	Normal/low
Metabolic acidosis	Moderate/severe	Mild/moderate
Cylinduria (casts)	Yes	No

Potential sequelae
- Slow recovery
- Death

Predisposition
- Acute insult in previously healthy dog in the absence of pre- and post-renal causes

Historical clues
- Duration of illness: ARF more likely to have acute onset
- PU/PD and nocturia often with CRF
- ARF also present with anorexia, lethargy and vomiting
- Acute onset of signs: check for toxic access, e.g. antifreeze/ethylene glycol
- Some medication can be nephrotoxic, e.g. NSAIDs, aminoglycosides
- Recent GA: hypovolaemia may have initiated ARF
- ? Back pain can be seen with renal, perirenal or ureteral inflammation/obstruction

Physical examination
- Dehydration
- Renal pain
- Renomegaly
- Urine volume decreased in proportion to degree of damage (normal >1 ml/kg/hour)
- Weakness

Laboratory findings
Haematology
- Leukocytosis may accompany pyelonephritis
- Anaemia usually absent

Biochemistry
- Azotaemia
- Variable elevations in phosphorus and potassium

Urinalysis
- SG < 1.030, despite dehydration

- Mild proteinuria and glycosuria sometimes
- Epithelial and granular casts
- Calcium oxalate crystals in ethylene glycol intoxication

Imaging
Radiographs
- Renomegaly

Ultrasound
- Renomegaly
- Increased echogenicity of cortex
- Calcification of cortico-medullary junction in hypercalcaemia

Special tests
- Blood gas analysis for acid–base evaluation
- Urine culture

Treatment
- i/v fluid therapy to correct extracellular fluid volume and restore urine output
  - Dehydration
  - Hypo- or hyperkalaemia
  - Acidosis
- Forced diuresis
  - i/v fluids
  - Mannitol
  - Furosemide
  - Dopamine infusion
- Anti-emetics
- Dialysis
  - Peritoneal
  - Haemodialysis
- Enteral tube feeding
- Treat underlying toxins
  - Induction of emesis
  - Activated charcoal
  - Forced diuresis
  - Ethanol or 4-methypyrazole for ethylene glycol

Monitor
- Azotaemia

Prognosis

- ARF carries a better prognosis than CRF for recovery of renal function from tubular regeneration
- Prognosis for ARF depends on severity and nature of damage – response to therapy is the best indicator
- Failure to produce urine after appropriate fluid therapy is a negative prognostic indicator
- Overall prognosis with ARF is guarded to poor

CHRONIC RENAL FAILURE (CRF)
Aetiology

- Long-standing primary renal failure associated with irreversible structural lesions
- Has a tendency to deteriorate with time, and so is usually progressive and irreversible
- Renal function may remain relatively stable for a long time, but may become decompensated by non-renal disease causing additional fluid loss
- The kidneys have significant reserve capacity, and azotaemia only occurs when glomerular filtration is < 25% of normal

Causes

- Chronic interstitial nephritis
- Chronic glomerulonephritis
- Chronic pyelonephritis
- Congenital renal aplasia/dysplasia
- Hypercalcaemia and nephrocalcinosis
- Hydronephrosis from chronic obstruction

Major signs

- Halitosis
- Inappetence
- Lethargy
- Nocturia
- PU/PD
- Vomiting

Minor signs

- Diarrhoea
- Vision loss secondary to hypertension
- Weight loss

Potential sequelae

- Osteopenia
- Death

Predisposition

- Acquired bacterial infection (severe) can cause azotaemia – female dogs predisposed
- Acquired degenerative/neoplastic renal disease tends to be seen in older animals
- Familial nephropathies – first months to years of life associated with many breeds:
  - Alaskan Malamute, Basenji, Bernese Mountain dog, Bull terrier, Chow Chow, Cocker spaniel, Doberman, Golden retriever, Lhasa Apso, Newfoundland, Norwegian Elkhound, Rottweiler, Samoyed, Schnauzers, Shar pei, Shih tzu, Standard poodle, Soft-coated Wheaten terrier, etc.
- Middle age to older for chronic interstitial nephritis

Historical clues

- CRF patients have a pre-existing history of clinical signs, e.g. weight loss, lethargy, inappetence, halitosis and vomiting, but often acute onset of signs being noticed by owner
- ? Back pain can be seen with renal, perirenal or ureteral inflammation/obstruction
- Inherited/familial nephropathies can cause uraemia or proteinuria or both
  - Kidneys are normal at birth but deteriorate in structure and function over the first months to years of life
- PU/PD and nocturia often with CRF
- Vision loss secondary to hypertension

Physical examination
- Bladder palpation
  - Dehydrated, uraemic patients often have large, normal-shaped bladder on palpation full of dilute urine in PU/PD animals with CRF
    - Combine with abdominal palpation to try and palpate calculi
- Dehydration
- Halitosis
- Loss of muscle mass
- Oral ulceration
- Osteodystrophy
- Pale mucous membranes
- Poor hair coat
- Pyrexia – pyelonephritis, neoplasia, inflammatory disease (± related to azotaemia)
- Small kidneys

Laboratory findings
Haematology
- Mild lymphopenia and neutrophilia seen in some uraemic patients (non-specific)
- Moderate to severe neutrophilia may indicate septic process or urinary tract infection
- Normocytic, normochromic non-regenerative anaemia

Serum biochemistry
- Acidosis
- Azotaemia
- Hyperphosphataemia
- Hyperkalaemia (end-stage)
- Hypokalaemia
- Hyper- or hypocalcaemia

Urinalysis
- Isosthenuria, i.e. fixed urine SG of 1.007–1.015 in the face of dehydration
- Variable degrees of proteinuria, depending on the cause

Imaging
Radiographs
- Small, irregular kidneys usually
- Normal or increased size with neoplasia, amyloidosis

Ultrasound
- Reduced renal size
- Increased echogenicity
- Loss of cortico-medullary definition

Special tests
- Acid–base status
- Fractional clearance of electrolytes
- GFR assessment
- Renal biopsy rarely indicated
- Retinal examination
- Systemic blood pressure

Treatment
i/v fluid therapy
- In decompensated chronic renal failure to correct
  - Dehydration
  - Hypo- or hyperkalaemia
  - Acidosis

Diet
- Low-phosphate diet
  - Phosphate restriction reduces rate of progression of chronic renal failure
- Moderate protein restriction if uraemic, to reduce signs of uraemia, but has no clear benefit for halting disease progression
- If diet does not control hyperphosphataemia and secondary renal hyperparathyroidism persists:
  - Oral phosphate binders (aluminium hydroxide)
  - Calcitriol

ACE inhibitors
- Use if proteinuric
- Use cautiously if proteinuric and azotaemic

- Do not oversupplement protein
- Used to reduce blood pressure if hypertensive

Antibiotics
- If UTI present, choice depends on:
  - Culture and sensitivity
  - Renal excretion
  - Potential for nephrotoxicity

Dialysis
- Peritoneal dialysis difficult to perform chronically
- Haemodialysis rarely available

Transplantation
- Not yet successful in dogs

Miscellaneous
- Antibiotics if UTI
- Recombinant erythropoietin if anaemic
- Water-soluble vitamin supplementation

Monitor
- Anaemia
- Azotaemia
- Body weight

Prognosis
- Medical management of CRF can decrease severity of uraemia and improve duration and quality of life – rehydration decreases the pre-renal component of azotaemia which exists in most of these patients
- CRF is associated with chronic, irreversible, progressive renal damage – prognosis is poor
- Treatment of concurrent disease/complicating factors, e.g. UTI, systemic hypertension, will improve the long-term prognosis

PROTEIN-LOSING NEPHROPATHY/NEPHROTIC SYNDROME
Aetiology
Glomerular disease causing significant proteinuria can result in nephrotic syndrome:
- Proteinuria
- Hypoalbuminaemia
- Hypercholesterolaemia
- Oedema and effusions
- Risk of thromboembolism

Causes
- Glomerulonephritis
  - Primary idiopathic
  - Familial
  - SLE
  - Immune complex deposition from primary inflammatory/immune-mediated disease elsewhere
- Amyloidosis

Major signs
- Ascites
- Dyspnoea from pleural effusion or PTE
- Subcutaneous oedema
- Uraemia-related signs when CRF develops
- Weight loss

Minor signs
- Blindness from hypertensive ocular disease
- Lameness or paresis from thromboembolism

Potential sequelae
- Progressive deterioration resulting in CRF
- Risk of thromboembolism

Predisposition
Glomerulonephritis
- Middle-aged dogs
- No sex or breed predisposition

ORGAN SYSTEMS

Amyloidosis
- Familial disease in dogs aged < 6 years, but otherwise older dogs
- Shar pei, and possibly Beagles, Collies

Historical clues
- May be clinically silent or PU/PD
- Eventual development of ascites, etc.

Laboratory findings
Haematology
- Non-regenerative anaemia when CRF develops

Serum biochemistry
- Azotaemia and hyperphosphataemia when CRF develops
- Hypercholesterolaemia
- Hypoalbuminaemia (see p. 144)
- Normoglobulinaemia
- Raised liver enzymes, etc. if concurrent hepatic amyloidosis

Urinalysis
- Hyaline casts
- Isosthenuria when CRF develops
- Proteinuria in absence of active sediment

Imaging
Radiographs
- May be normal size or enlarged

Ultrasound
- Occasionally increased cortical echogenicity

Special tests
- Renal biopsy: not readily justifiable if already azotaemic

Treatment
Supportive
- Sodium restriction
- Moderate protein restriction, but sufficient to avoid malnutrition
- High protein may worsen glomerular injury

- Antihypertensive drugs
- Plasma transfusion
- Diuretics
- Thoraco- and abdominocentesis if fluid accumulation is causing respiratory distress

Specific
Glomerulonephritis
- Treat any underlying disease
- ACE inhibitors have been shown to be beneficial
- Immunosuppressive drugs have not been shown to be effective
- Low-dose aspirin
- Omega-3 fatty acids

Amyloidosis
- Treat underlying condition
- Dimethyl sulphoxide (DMSO) – effectiveness controversial
- Colchicine – may slow progression, but does not reverse changes

Monitor
- Serum albumin
- Azotaemia

Prognosis
- Ultimately grave
- Survival in glomerulonephritis is significantly prolonged by ACE inhibitors
- Survival times in amyloidosis are short

RENAL TUBULAR DISORDERS
Aetiology
- Abnormal renal tubular function results in diminished reabsorption of water and various constituents with clinical signs related to their loss or the formation of calculi
- Tubular defects are often genetic, or secondary to infection

Specific disorders
- Cystinuria

- Distal renal tubular acidosis – idiopathic rarely, pyelonephritis
- Fanconi's syndrome – variable reabsorption defects
  - Water, sodium, potassium, glucose, phosphorus, bicarbonate and amino acids
- Primary renal glycosuria
- Proximal renal tubular acidosis – usually part of Fanconi's syndrome
- Urate excretion

Major signs
- PU/PD
- Muscle weakness if hypokalaemic
- Uraemic signs if CRF develops
- Weight loss

Predisposition
- Usually congenital, and often inherited
- Signs only develop when metabolic abnormalities become profound or when calculi are formed
- 75% of Fanconi's cases are Basenjis
- Renal glycosuria in Scottish terrier, Norwegian Elkhound

Potential sequelae
- Recurrent UTI from glycosuria
- CRF

Historical clues
- Breed association
- Glycosuria in face of normoglycaemia

Laboratory findings
Haematology
- Unremarkable unless CRF develops

Serum biochemistry
- Hypokalaemia
- Euglycaemia
- Azotaemia if CRF develops

Urinalysis
- Low urine SG

- Glycosuria in the absence of hyperglycaemia is common defect: Fanconi's and renal glycosuria
- Glycosuria can also be seen with ARF and amyloidosis

Imaging
- Usually unremarkable

Special tests
- Blood gas

Treatment
- Address
  - Hypokalaemia
  - Metabolic acidosis – give bicarbonate
    - CRF – see above

Monitor
- Blood gas
- Azotaemia

Prognosis
- Ultimately grave, but may only be slowly progressive towards CRF, especially with treatment

LOWER-URINARY TRACT DISEASES

Problems
Clinical presentations (see Section 1)
- Abdominal discomfort/pain
- Anorexia
- Bleeding
- Constipation
- Dysuria
- Haematuria and discoloured urine
- Urinary incontinence
- Vomiting
- Weakness-lethargy-collapse/syncope

Physical abnormalities (see Section 2)
- Abdominal enlargement

ORGAN SYSTEMS

- Bradycardia
- Prostatomegaly

Laboratory abnormalities (see Section 3)
- Azotaemia (urea and creatinine)
- Hyperkalaemia
- Hyperglobulinaemia
- Proteinuria
- Leukocytosis
- Leukopenia

Diagnostic approach
- Dysuria must be distinguished from urinary incontinence and from increased frequency because of PU/PD
- Distinguish inflammatory from obstructive disease by noting the dog's ability to pass urine and whether the bladder tends to be full or empty
- Urinalysis to detect inflammatory and neoplastic disease
- Identify UTI and treat. If relapses occur, look for underlying disease such as urolithiasis
- Radiographs and ultrasonography to image the lower urinary tract, and detect urolithiasis, neoplasia, structural abnormalities
- See Section 1: Dysuria, Haematuria, Urinary incontinence

Diagnostic methods
History
- Duration of current episode
- Number of past episodes and response to treatment
- Presence of gross haematuria
- Ability to pass urine
- Presence or absence of urination, tenesmus and haematuria
- Pollakiuria suggests inflammation of lower urinary tract

Clinical signs
- Dysuria = painful or difficult urination
- Stranguria = slow or painful urination characterised by straining

- Pollakiuria = increased frequency of urination
- Haematuria = blood in urine
- Incontinence

Physical examination
Observation
- Check whether dog strains to urinate, and whether it actually passes urine

Inspection
- Pyrexia – pyelonephritis, neoplasia, inflammatory disease
- Urine staining of perineum is more suggestive of incontinence than dysuria

Palpation
- Abdominal palpation for empty or distended bladder
  - Urinary tract inflammation – tight small bladder after urination, tense abdomen
  - Acute/complete urethral obstruction – bladder feels very round, firm and distended
  - Ruptured bladder – non-palpable or empty bladder
  - A full bladder despite attempts to urinate indicates either an obstruction or a hypotonic bladder
  - If not obstructed, the bladder can be expressed or catheterised
- Rectal palpation for prostate, intrapelvic urethra and bladder neck
  - Check prostate for size, symmetry, pain, and fluctuance by rectal examination
  - Normal prostate is smooth, softish, bilobed, bilaterally symmetrical and occupies less than one-third of the vertical height of the pelvic canal
  - Pelvic floor for urethral, prostatic or mass
  - Sublumbar area for lymphadenopathy
  - Combine with abdominal palpation to try and palpate calculi

- Pain on palpation of kidneys or dorsal abdomen
  - Pyelonephritis, acute hydronephrosis, large renal calculi, ureteral obstruction

Laboratory findings
Haematology
- Generally unremarkable

Serum biochemistry
- Azotaemia if urinary obstruction or polyuric renal failure
- Acquired bacterial infection (severe) can cause azotaemia – female dogs predisposed
- Dehydrated patient with azotaemia producing no urine suggests post-renal causes

Urinalysis
- Full urinalysis essential = dipstick and sediment examination
  - Catheterised
  - Cystocentesis
    - Presence of microscopic haematuria expected
  - Midstream free-catch
    - Some bacterial contamination likely; therefore not ideal for culture
    - $> 10^5$ organisms per ml considered significant
- Urine bacterial culture if sediment examination shows pyuria or bacteriuria on cystocentesis sample or if indicated for other reasons

Imaging
Plain radiographs
- Abdominal and pelvic radiographs
- Include extra-pelvic urethra in male if obstruction suspected
- Presence of radio-opaque calculi
  - Renal and/or cystic calculi in young animals raise the likelihood urate calculi secondary to PSS

- Urinary tract rupture – intrapelvic soft tissue swelling, caudal peritonitis, ascites – perform positive contrast studies to identify the site of leakage
- Thoracic radiographs if urinary tract neoplasia

Contrast radiographs (after enema)
- i/v urography
  - To demonstrate ectopic ureters
- Lower-urinary tract contrast studies
  - To assess causes of urinary tract obstruction and haematuria
- Pneumocystogram
- Positive contrast retrograde (vagino)-urethrogram
  - To assess bladder and urethra

Ultrasonography
- Renal size, shape and echoarchitecture
- Sublumbar lymph nodes
- Ultrasound examination of bladder and prostate
  - Bladder for size, mural lesions or intravesical abnormalities, e.g. calculi
  - Prostate – enlargement, echoarchitecture – masses, cysts, abscess
  - Ureteral emptying into bladder neck to assess ectopic ureters

Special investigations
- Acid–base status
- Biopsy – surgical, catheter suction
- Fractional clearance of electrolytes
- Myelogram
- Neurological examination
- Passage of urinary catheter
  - Check patency: strictures, urethral calculi
  - FNA/biopsy of prostate and sublumbar LN
  - Prostatic wash
- Urethrocystoscopy
- Urodynamic pressure profile

ORGAN SYSTEMS

Treatment
- Modification of urine composition (minerals, pH) if calculi
  - Diets
  - Urinary acidifiers
- Antibiotics if UTI
  - Choice depends on
    - Culture and sensitivity
    - Renal excretion
    - Potential for nephrotoxicity
    - Penetration of prostate
- Autonomic control if incontinent
  - Phenylpropanolamine
  - Bethanecol
  - Phenoxybenzamine
  - Diazepam
- Surgery if incontinent
- Urethral hydropulsion if small calculi

PROSTATIC DISEASE
Aetiology
- Benign and malignant causes of prostatic enlargement cause clinical signs through interference with normal urinary and faecal flow

Causes
- Benign prostatic hypertrophy (BPH)
- Cyst ± paraprostatic cyst
- Neoplasia
- Prostatitis/prostatic abscess
- Squamous metaplasia (Sertoli cell tumour, exogenous oestrogen)

Major signs
- Dysuria
- Tenesmus – urinary and/or faecal
- Haematuria
- Intermittent haemorrhage from penis, not associated with urination
- 'Ribbon' stool

Minor signs
- Fever
- Hindlimb lameness
- Hindlimb oedema

Predisposition/patient details
- Uncastrated male dog
- Increased incidence with age

Potential sequelae
- Recurrent infection if squamous metaplasia or cysts
- Neoplasia may still occur in neutered dogs

Historical clues
- Disease more likely if older intact male
- Dripping blood from penis outwith urination is characteristic

Physical examination
- Rectal examination
  - Abnormal prostate may be enlarged (may be intra-abdominal), asymmetric, firm, and have areas of fluctuance and pain
  - Sublumbar lymphadenopathy suggestive of neoplasia

Laboratory findings
- Rarely any abnormalities in haematology and serum biochemistry
- Inflammatory leukogram in prostatitis
- Azotaemia and hyperkalaemia if urinary obstruction

Urinalysis
- Haematuria sometimes in BPH, prostatic cyst
- Pyuria in prostatitis
- Abnormal cells in prostatic carcinoma

Imaging
Plain radiographs
- Prostatic enlargement
- Sublumbar lymph node enlargement with periosteal reaction on lumbar vertebral bodies
- Thoracic radiographs for metastatic disease

Contrast radiographs
- Irregular urethra
- Extravasation of contrast on retrograde urethrogram
- Asymmetric position of urethra if neoplasia or cyst

Ultrasound
- Prostate size and changes in echoarchitecture
- Cysts, abscess, neoplasia

Special tests
- Prostatic wash for culture and cytology
- (Ultrasound-guided) FNA and Tru-cut biopsy

Treatment
BPH
- Anti-androgens (delmadinone)
- Castration

Squamous metaplasia
- Castration
- Remove Sertoli cell tumour or discontinue oestrogen therapy

Prostatitis
- Antibacterials
- Surgical drainage ± omentalisation for abscess or large cyst

Prostatic cyst
- None unless infected or causing obstruction

Neoplasia
- None successful
- Palliative radiotherapy

Monitor
- Prostate size

Prognosis
- Good for BPH
- Guarded for prostatitis
- Poor for carcinoma

PYOMETRA
Aetiology
- Cystic endometrial hyperplasia is the accumulation of uterine fluid following hormone-related hypertrophy and hyperplasia of endometrial glands
- Pyometra is bacterial infection of the uterus predisposed by cystic endometrial hyperplasia

Major signs
- Polyuria/polydipsia
- Vomiting
- Vulval discharge

Minor signs
- Abdominal distension
- Anorexia
- Lethargy

Predisposition
- Entire, nulliparous bitches
- Recent oestrus (within past 2 months, i.e. metoestrus), or after administration of progestins ± oestrogens

Potential sequelae
- Septic peritonitis if ruptures
- Septicaemia, renal failure, shock and death

Historical clues
- Recent season followed by increased thirst

Physical examination
- Dehydration
- Tubular mass in caudo-ventral abdomen, extending cranially

Laboratory findings
Haematology
- Inflammatory leukogram
- Mild non-regenerative anaemia

Serum biochemistry
- Azotaemia
- Raised ALP

ORGAN SYSTEMS

Urinalysis
- Isosthenuria
- Pyuria

Imaging
Plain radiography
- Fluid-dense tubular structure in caudal abdomen, unless open pyometra

Ultrasound
- Distinguish pyometra from pregnancy
- Fluid-filled uterus lying between bladder and colon

Special tests
- FNA not recommended due to risk of uterine rupture
- Vaginal cytology

Treatment
- Correct dehydration
- Ovariohysterectomy (OHE)
- Medical therapy with prostaglandins and antibiosis only relatively safe for open pyometra, carries risk of recurrence if not bred from, and is not generally recommended

Monitor
- Renal function post-operatively

Prognosis
- Good if OHE performed successfully

SPHINCTER MECHANISM INCONTINENCE (SMI)
Aetiology
- Involuntary urinary incontinence due to dysfunction of the urethral sphincter mechanism

Major signs
- Involuntary incontinence
- Usually occurs at rest

Minor signs
- Bitch can also empty bladder normally

- Usually occurs without evidence of UTI
- May be 'unmasked' if there is a primary cause of PU/PD

Predisposition/patient details
- Middle-aged to older females
- Pelvic bladder (intra-pelvic position to bladder neck)
- Previous OHE

Potential sequelae
- Incontinence may get progressively worse unless treated

Historical clues
- History of spaying, often at an early age

Physical examination
- Generally unremarkable except for urine staining of perineum
- Bladder not over-distended

Laboratory findings
- Unremarkable unless concurrent UTI or underlying cause of PU/PD

Imaging
- Retrograde vagino-urethrogram
  - Pelvic bladder
  - Short urethra
  - No other abnormalities

Special tests
- Urethral profilometry

Treatment
- Phenypropanolamine
- Surgical colposuspension

Monitor
- Clinical signs

Prognosis
- Mild cases can be controlled medically

- Severe cases benefit from surgery: success rate is operator-dependent but is up to 80%

TESTICULAR TUMOURS
Aetiology
- Spontaneous neoplasms
- Sertoli cell
- Interstitial cell
- Seminoma

Major signs
- Testicular enlargement
- Atrophy of contralateral testis

Minor signs
- Associated with oestrogen production, especially by Sertoli cell tumour
  - Aplastic anaemia
  - Attractiveness to males
  - Bilaterally symmetrical hair loss
  - Feminisation
  - Gynaecomastia
  - Pendulous prepuce
- Prostatic enlargement

Predisposition
- Entire, aged dogs
- Cryptorchidism

Potential sequelae
- Metastasis uncommon (mainly Sertoli cell)
- Haemorrhage or infection secondary to aplastic anaemia

Historical signs
- No clinical signs initially
- Incidental finding
- Found as a result of hyperoestrogenism

Physical examination
- Non-painful enlargement of one testicle
- Palpable abdominal mass if intra-abdominal
- Contralateral testis small and soft

Laboratory findings
- Pancytopenia if oestrogen excess causes aplastic anaemia

Imaging
Radiography
- To show abdominal tumour
- Hepatomegaly or pulmonary metastases

Ultrasound
- To identify mass within testis

Special tests
- Plasma oestrogen and testosterone concentrations not very helpful
- FNA/biopsy

Treatment
- Neutering
- Aplastic anaemia
  - Blood transfusion
  - Recombinant erythropoietin, G-CSF
  - Lithium?

Monitor
- Haematology

Prognosis
- Good if neutering occurs before metastasis
- Very guarded if aplastic anaemia develops

URETHRAL OBSTRUCTION
Aetiology
- Partial or complete obstruction of the urethra by:
  - Benign prostatic hypertrophy
  - Displacement of bladder causing kinking of urethra
    - Retroflexion of bladder into perineal hernia
  - Intraluminal material
    - Cystic calculi passing into urethra
    - Foreign bodies (rare)

- Intramural tumour
- Penile tumours
- Prostatic carcinoma
- Transitional cell carcinoma at bladder neck
- Urethral stricture
  - Trauma from calculus, catheterisation or surgery
  - Vaginal tumours
- Clinical signs are related to difficulty urinating and metabolic effects of urine retention, especially hyperkalaemia

Major signs
- Dysuria
- Haematuria
- Pollakiuria
- Stranguria

Minor signs
- Metabolic effects of urine retention and hyperkalaemia
  - Coma
  - Vomiting
  - Weakness

Predisposition
- As for urolithiasis (see p. 330)
- Males
- Longer urethra more prone to blockage
- Perineal hernia in intact males
- Prostatic enlargement

Potential sequelae
- Post-renal azotaemia carries a good prognosis if the obstruction can be relieved and the patient nursed through the uraemic crisis
- Recurrence of urolithiasis
- Urethral stricture

Historical clues
- Dysuria or haematuria previously

Physical examination
- Bladder neck mass

- Cystic calculi
- Failure to pass urinary catheter
- Large, distended bladder
- Prostatic enlargement
- Rectal examination of prostate urethra, and pelvic cavity
  - Sublumbar lymphadenopathy
  - Tense swelling in perineal region if perineal hernia and retroflexed bladder
  - Urethral calculi

Laboratory findings
Haematology
- Usually unremarkable

Serum biochemistry
- Azotaemia and hyperkalaemia if complete obstruction

Imaging
Plain radiographs
- Distended bladder
- Cystic and urethral calculi
- Prostatic or bladder mass ± sublumbar lymphadenopathy
- Hind-leg drawn forward to visualise urethra and possible calculi

Contrast radiographs
- Retrograde urethrogram (males) or vaginourethrogram (females)

Ultrasound
- Radiolucent cystic calculi
- Mural cystic and prostatic lesions

Special tests
- Catheter biopsy

Treatment
If obstructed
- Treat acute post-renal azotaemia
  - i/v fluid therapy to correct dehydration
  - Post-obstructive diuresis
  - Correct hyperkalaemia
    - NaCl

- Soluble insulin plus dextrose
  - Bicarbonate
- Voiding urohydropulsion
- Catheterisation, retropulsion and bladder lavage or cystotomy
- Perineal or penile urethrostomy
- Surgical removal or medical dissolution of calculi
- Surgical repair of perineal hernia
- Palliative treatment with piroxicam for urethral neoplasia

Monitor
- Ability to urinate

Prognosis
- Good for complete recovery, but tendency to recur or urethral stricture

URINARY TRACT INFECTION (UTI)
Aetiology
- UTIs may affect any part of the urinary tract, and most frequently arise as ascending infections
- They may exist in isolation, or in combination with other causes of dysuria

Major signs
Upper UTI
- Asymptomatic
- Systemic illness
- Fever, lethargy, anorexia, lumbar pain, PU/PD

Lower UTI
- Stranguria
- Pollakiuria
- Haematuria

Minor signs
- Pain

Predisposition
- Chronically dilute urine (CRF)
- Diverticula
- Ectopic ureters
- Females have shorter urethra than males
- Glycosuria
  - DM
  - Fanconi's syndrome
  - Renal glycosuria
- Immunosuppressed, e.g. hyperadrenocorticism, exogenous steroids
- Incomplete emptying (neurogenic, post-obstructive atony)
- Neoplasia
- Pelvic bladder
- Previous urethral catheterisation
- Prostatic squamous metaplasia

Potential sequelae
- Relapses with same organism – re-evaluate antibiotic choice and treat for longer
- Re-infection with new organism – assess risk factors

Historical clues
- Clinical signs
- Discoloured urine

Physical examination
- Bladder often empty because of pollakiuria
- Crackling from emphysematous cystitis most commonly seen with glycosuria
- Pyrexia if pyelonephritis

Laboratory findings
Haematology
- Usually unremarkable
- Leukocytosis seen sometimes with pyelonephritis

Biochemistry
- Usually unremarkable

Urinalysis
- Bacteriuria
  - Increased pH in presence of urease-positive bacteria
  - Positive culture if off antibiotics

- Cellular casts suggest renal involvement
- Haematuria
- Proteinuria
- Pyuria

Imaging
Plain radiographs
- Urolithiasis

Contrast radiographs
- Anatomical abnormalities

Ultrasound
- Underlying urolithiasis, neoplasia, etc.
- Prostatic abscess

Special tests
- Prostatic wash

Treatment
Uncomplicated urethrocystitis
- 10–14 days antibiotics
- Encourage urination by increased fluid input

Complicated urethrocystitis (recurrent infection or underlying risk factor)
- Identify and correct risk factor
- Antibiotics for 3–4 weeks based on culture/sensitivity
- Repeat urine culture 7 days after stopping first course

Pyelonephritis
- 4–6 weeks of antibiotics based on culture/sensitivity
- Supportive care if renal impairment

Monitor
- Azotaemia
- Urinalysis and culture

Prognosis
- Good for simple infection
- Guarded for chronic or complicated (e.g. urolithiasis) infection

UROLITHIASIS
Aetiology
- Urolithiasis is the concretion of minerals within the urinary tract
  - Calcium oxalate
  - Calcium phosphate
  - Cystine
  - Mixed
  - Silica
  - Struvite – magnesium ammonium phosphate (triple phosphate)
  - Urate
- Nephroliths and ureteral calculi are uncommon: cystic calculi are quite common
- Cystic calculi may be passed via the urethra but may cause obstruction, more typically in males
- Urinary obstruction by uroliths causes acute post-renal azotaemia (see p. 327) and uraemia (see p. 311–12)

Major signs
Upper urinary tract
- Haematuria
- Lumbar pain
- Signs of renal dysfunction

Lower urinary tract
- Dysuria
- Haematuria
- Pollakiuria
- Stranguria

Potential sequelae
- Recurrence
- CRF

Predisposition
- Young – urate urolithiasis in congenital PSS
- Older – neoplasia, urolithiasis
- Breed associations: see below
- Struvite calculi associated with UTI by urease-positive bacteria

Historical clues
Typical clinical features of urolithiasis are detailed in Table 10.

Physical examination
Palpation
- Distended, turgid, painful bladder if obstructed
- Uroliths may be palpated in the bladder

Rectal palpation
- Failure to pass catheter if urethral calculi
- Uroliths in proximal urethra

Laboratory findings
Haematology
- Usually unremarkable unless extreme blood loss

Biochemistry
- May reveal evidence of metabolic cause of urolith, e.g. PSS

Urinalysis
- Haematuria
- Pyuria
- Bacteriuria
- Crystalluria
  - Does NOT prove presence of uroliths
  - May help identify confirmed uroliths
- Urine pH
  - Influences urolith formation and dissolution

Imaging
Plain radiographs
- Include extra-pelvic urethra in male if obstruction suspected
- Presence of radio-opaque calculi

NB – Urate and cystine calculi may be radiolucent.

Contrast radiographs (after enema)
- Lower-urinary tract contrast studies to assess causes of urinary tract obstruction and haematuria
- Pneumocystogram
- Positive contrast retrograde (vagino)-urethrogram

Ultrasonography
- Bladder and urethra for calculi

Special tests
- Mineral analysis
- Urine culture

Treatment
Medical dissolution
- Indications
  - Poor anaesthetic/surgical candidate
  - Repeated urolith recurrence
  - Urolith amenable to dissolution

Calcium oxalate
- Alkalinisation: potassium citrate?
- Correct hypercalcaemia
- Reduced protein, calcium and oxalate diet

Cystine
- Protein-restricted diet
- Alkalinisation
- N-2 mercaptopropionyl glycine
- D-penicillamine

Silicate
- None

Struvite
- Acidification
- Antibiotics for UTI
- High-sodium diet for diuresis
- Protein- and mineral (Pi, Mg)-restricted diet

Urate
- Alkalinisation (pH 7): sodium bicarbonate, potassium citrate

ORGAN SYSTEMS

ORGAN SYSTEMS

Table 10 Characteristic features of urinary calculi formation

Predisposition	Breed	Signs	Urine pH	Radiographic appearance	Probable composition
Female	Miniature Schnauzer, Dachshund, Poodle, Dalmatian	UTI with urease-positive bacteria	Alkaline	Radiodense	Struvite
			Acidic to neutral	Radiolucent	Urate
		PSS	Acidic to neutral	Radiolucent	Urate
Middle-aged male	Bulldog, Dachshund	Cystine crystalluria	Acidic to neutral	Radiolucent	Cystine
Middle-aged to older male	GSD, Retriever	High plant protein diet	Acidic to neutral	Radiodense jack-stone shape	Silicate
Middle-aged to older male	Miniature Schnauzer, Lhasa Apso, Yorkshire terrier	Hypercalcaemia, hyperadrenocorticism	Acidic to neutral	Radiodense	Calcium oxalate

- Allopurinol
- Correct PSS
- Protein restriction of diet

Surgical removal
- Indications
  - Acute urinary obstruction
  - Anatomic defect in urinary tract
  - High risk of obstruction (male)

- Urolith not amenable to medical dissolution, e.g. oxalate, silica

Monitor
- Recurrence by urinalysis and imaging

Prognosis
- Guarded: tendency for stones to recur

ORGAN SYSTEMS

INDEX